Nursing Care of the Aged

Edited by
Karen Kay Esberger, R.N., Ph.D.
Samuel T. Hughes, Jr., R.N., Ed.D.

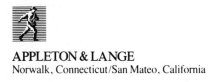

APPLETON & LANGE
Norwalk, Connecticut/San Mateo, California

ISBN: 0-8385-7010-0

Notice: Our knowledge in clinical sciences is constantly changing. As new
information becomes available, changes in treatment and in the use of drugs
become necessary. The authors and the publisher of this volume have taken
care to make certain that the doses of drugs and schedules of treatment are
correct and compatible with the standards generally accepted at the time of
publication. The reader is advised to consult carefully the instruction
and information material included in the package insert of each drug or
therapeutic agent before administration. This advice is especially
important when using new or infrequently used drugs.

Prentice-Hall International (UK) Limited, *London*
Prentice-Hall of Australia Pty, Limited, *Sydney*
Prentice-Hall Canada, Inc., *Toronto*
Prentice-Hall Hispanoamericana, S.A., *Mexico*
Prentice-Hall of India Private Limited, *New Delhi*
Prentice-Hall of Japan, Inc., *Tokyo*
Simon & Schuster Asia Pte. Ltd., *Singapore*
Editora Prentice-Hall do Brasil Ltda., *Rio de Janeiro*
Prentice-Hall, *Englewood Cliffs, New Jersey*

Library of Congress Cataloging-in-Publication Data

Nursing care of the aged.

   Includes index.
   1. Geriatric nursing. I. Esberger; Karen Kay.
II. Hughes, Samuel T. [DNLM: 1. Aging—physiology.
2. Aging—psychology. 3. Geriatric Nursing.
Wy 152 N9744]
RC954.N883   1989   610.73'65   88-19269
ISBN 0-8385-7010-0

Production Editor: Christine Langan
Designer: Steven M. Byrum

PRINTED IN THE UNITED STATES OF AMERICA

This book is lovingly dedicated to our parents:

Phama Duke Kay and the late James T. Kay, Jr.
and
Lula McCormack Hughes and Samuel Thomas Hughes, Sr.

CONTRIBUTORS

Dolores M. Alford
M.S.N., F.A.A.N., R.N.
Gerontic Nursing Consultant
Nursing Associates
Dallas, Texas

Helen A. Bush
Ph.D., R.N.
Professor & Assistant Dean, College of
Nursing
Texas Woman's University
Denton, Texas

Karen Kay Esberger
Ph.D., R.N.
School Nurse
Midlothian (Tx) ISD
formerly Associate
Professor of Nursing

Bert Hayslip, Jr.
Ph.D.
Associate Professor Psychology
University of North Texas
Denton, Texas

Samuel T. Hughes, Jr.
Ed.D., G.N.P., R.N.
Professor of Nursing

The University of Texas at Arlington
Arlington, Texas

Hazel M. Jay
M.Ed., M.S., R.N.
Professor Emeritus
The University of Texas at
Arlington School of Nursing
Arlington, Texas

Cora A. Martin
Ph.D.
Professor of Sociology and
Community Service
University of North Texas
Denton, Texas

Frances Martin
M.S.N., R.N.
Specialist
The University of Texas at Arlington
School of Nursing
Arlington, Texas

Janet A. Moll
M.S., G.N.P., R.N.
Geriatric Nurse Practitioner
Nursing Associates
Dallas, Texas

Jacquelin S. Neatherlin
M.S.N., C.N.R.N., R.N.
Neurological Clinical Specialist
Harris Methodist
Fort Worth, Texas

John C. Reed
Ed.D.
Associate Professor
The University of Texas at Arlington
School of Nursing
Arlington, Texas

Ann Robbins
M.S.N., R.N.
Director of Nursing and Health Services
American Red Cross
Dallas, Texas

Carol A. Stephenson
Ed.D., R.N.
Associate Professor
Harris College of Nursing
Texas Christian University
Fort Worth, Texas

Wanda J. Thompson
Ed.D., C.F.N.P., R.N.
Associate Professor of Nursing
The University of Texas at Arlington
Arlington, Texas

Mary Ellen Wyers
Ed.D., R.N.
Associate Dean & Professor
The University of Texas at Arlington
School of Nursing
Arlington, Texas

CONTENTS

PREFACE

The heterogeneity of older persons is most striking. Genetic inheritance, culture, environment, education, religious beliefs, and other experiences contribute to the uniqueness of each aged person. We believe that each person should be nursed in a holistic manner, with attention to social and spiritual needs, as well as the psychological and biological requisites.

It must be emphasized that aging is not necessarily a pathological process. Many older people adapt readily to aging and do not succumb to the problems presented in a gerontological nursing textbook. Nursing care must be individualized for each client, therefore, and the nurse chooses among the possible plans of care for each person.

Nursing Care of the Aged has been prepared to aid students, both undergraduate and graduate, gerontological nurse practitioners, and other nurses specializing in gerontological nursing to practice more effectively. These students and nurses may encounter the aged in many settings, both acute and long term care, and in the community.

The book provides comprehensive information on both the physical and psychological changes often associated with aging. This is one of the first books that discusses the physiological changes of aging from a nursing perspective. By including both physiological and psychosocial changes of aging, *Nursing Care of the Aged* provides the nurse with a comprehensive source of information on the aging process and suitable nursing care. The organization of physiological alterations on a body systems basis provides a familiar and convenient format in order to help the reader locate desired information more rapidly.

We perceive the A.N.A. Standards And Scope Of Gerontological Nursing Practice as a relevant document. The nursing process, which that statement encompasses, is an important basis of this book. Emphasis on data collection has been stressed in the assessment parameters, as is planning of care and intervention. The ongoing process of evaluation would lead to revised plans and intervention. Individualized care will maximize the functional abilities, both physiological and mental, of each person, minimizing their disabilities and maintaining their dignity.

Chapter One, an introductory chapter, focuses on sociological topics pertinent to aging including demography and social changes such as roles, abuse, retirement, economics, housing, safety, politics and ethnicity. The Standards And Scope Of Gerontological Nursing Practice are presented. Assessment of the aged person is discussed as a means to delineate pertinent points that should be considered in that process.

Chapter Two provides a current and comprehensive review on theories of aging.

Drug therapy, including use, abuse, and noncompliance, follows in Chapter Three. Abuse in the form of health care workers overmedicating elderly clients is discussed along with abuse of prescriptions and over-the-counter medications by the aged themselves. Bases of drug interactions are described as they interact with each other and with food or alcohol, and affect lab values. Specific classifications of drugs are summarized.

Chapters Four through Eleven deal with physiological topics, in each chapter the problem or disease process is discussed in terms of assessment parameters and appropriate nursing care.

Neurological/sensory changes are the subject of Chapter Four, the first chapter to deal with specific physiological changes of aging. Common nervous system changes and sleep alterations are discussed; then specific neurological problems are described. Age-related changes in each of the five senses follow. Both prescription and non-prescription medications commonly used for the nervous system are identified.

Age-related changes of the integument open Chapter Five which then deals with problems of the aging skin. Tumors, infections, and other problems such as decubiti are presented.

In Chapter Six gastro-intestinal changes progress from problems involving the mouth and esophagus to the lower GI tract with special attention to the management of constipation. Other problems of the lower GI tract, such as diverticulosis and cancer, are discussed, as are gall bladder, pancreatic, and liver disorders.

The genito-urinary tract receives extensive coverage in Chapter Seven, as the female and male reproductive tracts are separately discussed in terms of normal aging and physiological problems that may be found in older persons. The sexual response cycle is presented with physiological and psychological changes of both females and males that affect the cycle. Aging of the kidney and the lower urinary tract complete

the chapter along with a discussion of fluid and electrolyte disorders.

Chapter Eight presents aging and disorders of the musculoskeletal system, along with general health parameters of that system, such as exercise, rest, nutrition, and safety.

Chapter Nine begins with the aging of the endocrine system. Thyroid dysfunction, obesity, and diabetes are discussed. Attention to diabetes mellitus, including management and complications, is extensive.

Respiratory changes are the subject of Chapter Ten, which opens with a discussion of common age-associated changes. Many disease processes, such as pneumonias, chronic obstructive diseases, asthma, tuberculosis, and cancer are described. Smoking and drug therapy are the topics that conclude the chapter.

Cardio-vascular changes appear in Chapter Eleven. Aging of the heart and vessels is described as are specific disorders such as hypertension, ischemia, infarctions, peripheral and cerebral vascular disease, and congestive heart failure. Iron deficiency and megaloblastic anemias conclude the chapter.

Chapter Twelve discusses communicating with the aged based on possible changes in the cognitive processes. Assessment of learning needs and selection of teaching strategies is a particular feature of this chapter.

Variations in mental health is the topic of Chapter Thirteen. Maintenance of self-esteem is discussed along with the concepts of sensory deprivation, territoriality, and loss. Common disorders ranging from loneliness to anxiety to depression, and others, are covered.

Treatment modalities for mental health problems are found in Chapter Fourteen. Therapies such as life review, reality orientation, and remotivation are included, along with more traditional approaches.

Death is the topic of Chapter Fifteen. Bereavement, suicide, and the dying person are considered, and helpful approaches are emphasized.

The Appendix discusses normal nutritional

needs of the aged person and needs for specific nutrients. A chart on physical indicators of poor nutrition is especially helpful.

While this book is designed as a means of professional development, the nurse is urged to read current professional journals and participate in additional professional activities. Information sheets on drugs and other products that the nurse uses should be studied carefully along with pro-cedure manuals and lists of laboratory values considered ''normal'' in each setting.

We wish to thank the contributors for their time and energy in helping complete this text and the editors at Appleton & Lange for their guidance and expertise.

Karen Kay Esberger
Samuel T. Hughes, Jr.

Issues Associated with Nursing Care of the Aged

Stereotypes regarding the health, happiness, and housing of the aged continue to pursue this population. Changes such as a decline in energy, retirement, and health problems may be mitigated to various extents by such measures as periodic medical examinations for early detection of diseases, accident prevention, good nutrition, exercise, and rehabilitation. Some restriction on activities is inevitable, but most of the aged learn to conserve their energy and pace themselves by participating in only those activities that they particularly value. The aged have learned to focus their energy more effectively and are highly motivated to participate in their chosen activities. They can recognize the need for change and can utilize their experiences effectively. Even more than age, personality may be the main factor in determining one's behavior, in addition to the circumstances of one's life. "Time does not just take; it also gives— wisdom, skills, insight" (Dolan, 1987, p. 57).

DEMOGRAPHY

In the 1980 United States census, 11.3% of the population was found to be age 65 and over, an increase from 9.9% in 1970, and a substantial increase from the 1900 figure of 4.0 percent (U.S. Bureau of the Census, 1983, p. 3). The current growth rate of the older population is popularly assumed to be due to increased longevity. In fact, this is considered a secondary cause, with the primary cause being "a steady increase in the annual number of births in the years prior to 1920" (U.S. Bureau of the Census, 1983, p. 4).

Between 1970 and 1980, the median age of the population rose from 28 years to 30 years. The age composition in 1980 of various racial groups varied substantially. Among the white population, 12.2% were 65 years and older. Among Hispanics, this figure was 4.9% and among blacks it was 7.9% (Age, Sex, Race, 1980, p. 1).

In 1980, more than 15 million people in the United States were between 65 and 74 years of age; the older aged (those older than 75 years) numbered nearly 10 million. Females predominate in both these groups, numbering nearly 9 million aged 65–74 years, as compared to 6.5 million males. In the 75 years and older group, females number 6.5 million to 3.5 million males (Age, Sex, Race, 1980, p. 1). Of particular import in the United States is the steadily climbing ratio of aged females to aged males. This trend continues in spite of the growing convergence of life-styles between the sexes. Although genetic and environmental factors influencing this trend are being studied, there remain the resultant problems of widowhood, economic losses, and lessened psychological support for aged women. It has been suggested that women live longer because they are better able to deal with environmental stress and have more alternative coping methods open to them (Haynes & Feinleib, 1980).

The life expectancy at birth in 1980 was 73.6 years, an increase from the life expectancy of 70.8 years in 1970, and a substantial increase from 49 years in 1900. The 1980 figure can be broken down in this manner: "white females 78.1 years; all other females 74.0 years; white males 70.5 years; all other males 65.3 years" (Annual Summary of Births, 1982, p. 3). The difference in life expectancy at birth between whites and blacks is rapidly closing: in 1940 it was 11 years and in 1978 it was 5 years (U. S. Bureau of the Census, 1983, p. 5).

The geographical area with the greatest number of aged is the South, where $8\frac{1}{2}$ million people are age 65 and over. Nevertheless, the median age in the South is only 29.7 years whereas in the Northeast it is 31.8 years. The total number of aged persons in the Northeast is about 6 million. The other two geographical categories established by the Bureau of the Census are the North Central, where there are more than $6\frac{1}{2}$ million aged persons and the median age is 29.6 years, and the West, where there are slightly more than 4 million aged persons and the median age is 29.8 years (Age, Sex, Race, 1980). Specific states having more than 1 million persons aged 65 and over in 1980 included California (2.4 million), New York (2.2 million), Florida (1.7 million), Pennsylvania (1.5 million), Texas (1.4 million), Illinois (1.3 million), and Ohio (1.2 million) (United States Bureau of the Census, 1983, p. 19).

It is projected that the number of people above 65 years of age will be 36 million in the year 2000 and 68 million in 2040. Further, the number of Americans above the age of 85 is expected to be 5 million in 2000 and 13 million in 2040 (Ubell, 1984). These figures have grave

implications for the health care system in the United States because the aged use the largest share of health resources. Expected increases in their utilization of these resources may occur because of broader insurance coverage and increased educational levels among the aged. The present imbalance in availability of health care in rural as opposed to urban areas holds particular importance for the aged.

With the proportion of aged persons increasing in this country, persons in the usual working ages (18–64) are comprising smaller and smaller percentages of the total population. Thus, fewer persons will be contributing to the national economy and fewer of the aged will have family members available for support during times of crisis—health, financial, or otherwise. The government may have to assume a greater role in providing services to these citizens.

The United States shares this concern regarding aged populations with other advanced industrialized nations, primarily those of northern and western Europe. The growth in aged populations is a relatively recent phenomenon due to the technological development of these societies. Because the majority of people in the world live in nonindustrialized nations, in which life expectancy is considerably lower than it is in the industrialized nations, the aged comprise only a very small percentage of the total world population (Hendricks & Hendricks, 1981).

TERMS OF INTEREST

Senescence can be defined as "a period characterized by cell death exceeding cell birth" (Levenson & Porter, 1984, p. 6). This term must be carefully distinguished from *senility,* an archaic word usually applied in a general manner to any older person who appears the least bit confused. The continued use of "senility" or "senile" is inappropriate and often indicates a prejudice against the aged.

Behavior of an aged person that is labeled confused by observers is often the result of inadequate communication. The family, nurse, or other may not have taken time to look behind the communication barrier for such possible problems as sensory defects, slowed comprehension, articulation difficulties, depression, or general lack of daily environmental stimulation. Many of the psychological changes of the aged, commonly labeled senility, are blamed solely on old age, whereas chronic diseases may be the actual culprits. Expecting that mental deterioration will accompany aging becomes a self-fulfilling prophecy as prevention and treatment are neglected.

The balance between interaction and isolation is of significance in its relation to confusion and other mental changes associated with aging. Isolation, whether its origin is emotional, social, or physiological, tends to exacerbate neurotic traits, as well as depressed or paranoid reactions. This interaction/isolation balance also has somatic implications for the aged.

Sensory loss in isolation states associated with "a changed social environment, a loss of past sources of emotional satisfaction and pride of accomplishment, a constriction of the circle of family and friends" (Ernst, Beran, Safford, & Kleinhauz, 1978, p. 472) may ultimately lead to psychosis. Thus, the problem may not be physical in origin, but a result of the changed world in which the aged find themselves.

Organic brain syndrome (OBS) (American Psychiatric Association, 1980) is another frequently misused term. It is associated with the following symptoms: shallow and labile affect, disorientation, and impairment of judgment, memory, and intellectual function. Types of OBS are delirium, of sudden onset and reversible, and dementia, of insidious onset and progressive, static, or remitting. Any individual may have more than one form of OBS simultaneously, or one type may be followed by another. Manifestations of brain syndromes include disintegration of social manners, deterioration of physical appearance, wandering, frequent spilling of food, alteration of sleep patterns, and incorrect schedule of taking medications.

Specific disease processes that may lead to neuronal degeneration include Alzheimer's disease, Pick's disease, Huntington's chorea, and senile dementia. These diseases lead to the state of chronic confusion often referred to as OBS.

Confusion can be caused by many metabolic problems such as medication toxicity, febrile conditions, and vitamin deficiencies. Other causes include diabetes, or thyroid, liver, or kidney dysfunctions. Any state resulting in decreased oxygen to the brain, e.g., pulmonary disease, decreased cardiac output, and cerebrovascular insufficiency, causes impairment.

In summary, before such terms as OBS are applied to confused or disoriented states it is necessary to rule out underlying physical or psychological changes that might be causing the problem. The client exhibiting confusion or disorientation needs a complete assessment and such treatment modalities as increased sensory stimulation and adequate diet and fluids.

SOCIAL CHANGES

Role

Numerous role realignments, both ascribed and acquired, become necessary as one ages. In addition to differences resulting from one's personality and life-style, there are cultural, economic, and rural/urban variations that affect the evolvement of individual roles. It must be emphasized that there is no single ideal, optimal role for all aged persons. Individual capacities and values greatly influence the alterations.

Each aged person has a distinctive variety of roles, e.g., spouse, son/daughter, parent, grandparent, sibling, friend, employer or employee, homeowner, neighbor, citizen, and member of church or other organization. A person's number of social roles generally decreases with increasing age. Unfortunately, the aged have few sources of information to help them make the transition, i.e., to help them "learn" to be older. They usually learn from one another and from publications directed toward the aged.

Awareness of role loss results in widely divergent modes of adjustment. A successful adjustment is desirable in order to maintain a high level of general life satisfaction, including a positive self-image.

Loss of particular roles presents the opportunities for new roles with which to occupy one's time and to enhance satisfaction and self-realization. The following areas are generally the most affected by aging: retirement and resultant reduction in income, declining health, and altered family structure. The ease of role transitions generally depends on the following factors (Ebersole & Hess, 1985):

- Appropriateness of models
- Supportive environment
- Continuity of some roles
- Appropriate age at time of change
- Cultural and geographic milieu
- Personality and motivation

During these role transitions, it may be helpful for the aging person to participate in a life review for help in interpreting past experiences. Realizing their past achievements and remembering exciting times may help a more passive present life seem more tolerable. Younger people who may share in this reminiscence may gain valuable insight into history as well as their own potential roles.

Family

Aged men and women differ greatly as to marital status and living arrangements. More than 75% of the men are married and live with their wives, and more than 83% of the men live in family settings. However, only 40% of the women are married and live with their husbands, while about 75% of the women live with families (U.S. Bureau of the Census, 1983, p. 21).

The major source of emotional strength for many of the aged is their families, with whom most of them have regular contact. Although few of the aged live with family members other than spouses, contact with the extended family seems to endure. Even though career commitments result in the children of middle-class families living in other than close proximity to their parents, the parents do take pride in their children's accomplishments. Both the children and their aged parents prefer to live separately and maintain independence, but there is a high degree of interaction among these households (Hendricks & Hendricks, 1981).

Although social needs of the aged change, their children often prefer that the parents maintain a more active role than the parents wish. The children may complain about the aged parents' relative passivity during visits and feel bored despite the fact that their interest and presence may be very comforting to the parent(s).

Siblings may play a more important role with increasing age as people often seek to maintain family loyalty and renew old relationships. Other than living with their children, more of the aged live with siblings than with any other persons. The death of a sibling may be even more of a shock than deaths of others (Atchley, 1980).

Conflict may exist within an aged person's family because of anticipated inheritance or perceptions that labor or resources in caring for the aged individual have been unequally distributed. The gerontological nurse practitioner should be in contact with several of the aged individual's relatives in order to obtain a more balanced perspective of the family dynamics.

Late remarriage may be another potential source of family conflict. Such marriages have better chances of enduring if the couple is well acquainted and has an adequate income. Approval by family and friends and the establishment of a new home are also important factors in the success of the marriage. Finally, both members of the couple need to be making a successful adaptation to aging (Ebersole & Hess, 1985).

A parent's role is dynamic throughout life. Parents may feel freed when their children become independent and move out to begin their adult lives; later parents may themselves become dependent, either physically or financially. The parents often feel guilt and anger. The children may feel guilt and resentment, and their spouses may resent the time and/or money being devoted to their in-laws. It has been found that daughters, as opposed to sons, offer more help to aging parents (Hendricks & Hendricks, 1981).

If it becomes necessary for the aged to move in with children and grandchildren, some ground rules can be established. The spouse and grandchildren should be involved in the planning. Plans for privacy and outside activities need to be included for each member of the family (Abrams, 1987).

Most grandparents perceive their role as positive and satisfying. Children progress, with age, from expecting gifts and favors from their grandparents to sharing of fun, to wanting affection and information about family history. Grandchildren think they should visit their grandparents and offer affection and tangible help. Grandparenthood offers compensation for lowered morale and increases the life satisfaction of the aged. It is thought that absence of a meaningful grandparent relationship during one's own childhood may limit the richness of relating to one's own grandchildren (Kivnick, 1982). On the other hand, a positive, meaningful experience with one's own grandparents, especially the association with a favorite grandparent, contributes to a positive outlook on one's own grandparenthood, especially as related to one's own emotional, social, material, and physiological circumstances. (Fig. 1-1).

The kinship network of grandparents has expanded during recent years due to the high incidence of divorce and remarriage. Maintaining contact with grandparents is seen to have a stabilizing effect on grandchildren in a divorced family (Johnson & Barer, 1987).

Class difference plays a large role in the amount of influence grandparents may have. Within families of lower socioeconomic status, grandparents generally provide more needed assistance and live in closer proximity, therefore visiting more frequently, than do grandparents in middle- or upper-class families (Ebersole & Hess, 1985). Frequency of visits, of course, has a direct relation to the development of affectional ties. It is also important to note that widows are more usually involved in mutual assistance with their daughters than are married mothers (Atchley, 1980). The aged may contribute to their families in the following ways: (1) economic, (2) child care, and (3) housekeeping.

Dimensions of grandparenthood are widely varied. Grandparents may be lenient and indulgent and therefore contribute to the "spoiled" child. They may feel a sense of patriarchal/matriarchal responsibility and family im-

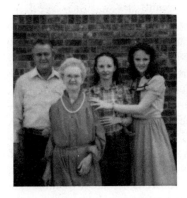

Four
Generations

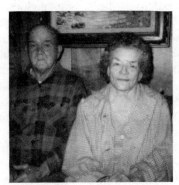

A marriage of
67 years

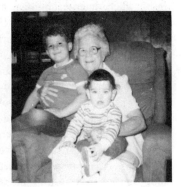

The Joys of
Grandchildren

Figure 1-1. Families

mortality as they see the family continuing through grandchildren into the indefinite future. They may serve as resources to grandchildren and assume the role of the wise, esteemed elder. They may relive experiences from their own childhoods and wonder about their own grandparents. Finally, grandparenthood may become the central factor in one's personal meaning of life (Kivnick, 1982).

Friends

Other human relationships or support systems are important, but less so than those of the aged with their children. Friendships are gratifying to the aged and are a factor in maintaining self-esteem. Intimate friends are a great source of strength, and peer groups continue to serve as socializing agents throughout the aging process. Neighborhood ties are a major reason many of the aged refuse to relocate, even to better housing.

In addition to physical propinquity, potential friends among the aged frequently share similar social characteristics. Friendship patterns also reflect class patterns, and married people more often have good friends than do nonmarried. Women generally have more friends than do men. Those who live in age-segregated environments tend to have more friends than do those where intergenerational proximity is the rule (Hendricks & Hendricks, 1981).

The gerontological nurse practitioner needs to assess an aged client's social network in order to identify persons who would be called in an emergency or upon whom the client can rely to discuss problems or possible loneliness. Many other questions could be asked about contacts maintained with significant others, enjoyment of relationships, etc. It should be remembered that solitary persons are not necessarily lonely and may, indeed, have a high morale. Those who want but have been unable to establish friendships are most at risk for emotional problems, although the aged do tend to have fewer contacts with friends (Hendricks & Hendricks, 1981).

Abuse

The aged have the same basic rights as all persons. However, they are at risk of losing those rights because of their relative inability to defend themselves against abuse.

The ill aged are especially vulnerable and their care is complicated in the current society where most women are employed outside the home. With no caretaker available and mounting expenses, children may resent the imposition on their life-styles and give vent to long suppressed hostility toward their parent(s). In addition to actual violence toward the parents, the children may indulge in denial of the parent's true condition, so that the family system may be maintained. Denial of the violence itself may also be tolerated. Physical abuse may take more subtle forms than actual beatings. A so-called benign neglect may exist in homes where there is no younger person at home during the day to care for the aged. Poor diet or missed meals may be prevalent, along with over- and underuse of medications. Nonambulatory persons may be left unattended for long periods; others may be tied up while the children are gone or busy with household tasks. Medical care may not be obtained when needed.

Verbal abuse and isolation are common forms of psychological abuse. The abuser may not understand the significance of losses to the aged, may not acknowledge the social needs of the aged, or may treat the aged like children. The so-called stubbornness of the aged may actually "be a desperate attempt to hold remaining possessions or lifestyles" (Beck & Ferguson, 1981, p. 336). Theft or misuse of money or property constitutes the all-too-common material abuse.

Research has revealed surprising characteristics of the abused and abusers. "The abused elder is likely to be Protestant, middle class, white, female, to live with relatives—most likely children—and to have some degree of physical or mental impairment. The abuser is likely to be white, female, middle class, and the child of the abused" (Block and Sinnott, 1979, p. 29).

Legal Concerns

The aged have the same legal rights as other people. Aged clients have the right to refuse various medical treatments, to keep personal possessions with them, and to make telephone calls. Gerontological nurse practitioners should see that their clients are aware of their rights and review each one's status appropriately. Gerontological nurse practitioners need to observe and document their clients' actions indicative of abilities or inabilities to manage their own affairs.

Many of the aged need legal help but do not know where to turn. Most attorneys maintain low profiles and are inaccessible to the aged. Sometimes government-sponsored legal aid is available if the aged know where to look. Help may be needed for estate planning, welfare appeals, property management, taxes, and guardianships.

Aged persons may be very concerned about who will inherit their property. Whether a large amount of money or a few objects of sentimental value are involved, the aged person wants to leave his/her possessions to someone who will appreciate them. The gerontological nurse practitioner may facilitate the aged one's peace of mind by helping arrange an appointment with an attorney to handle this matter. The gerontological nurse practitioner may witness signatures on a will or other legal document, if not forbidden to do so by an employer's policy. It is important for the gerontological nurse practitioner to assess and note whether or not the signer appeared alert and oriented at the time or was coerced.

A power of attorney may sometimes be necessary in order that someone else may carry on the aged person's business. The aged individual can grant limited or extended authority on either a temporary or permanent basis. A guardian may be appointed to manage financial affairs and is accountable to the court for actions performed on behalf of the aged. A guardianship may be needed to protect the aged from squandering possessions or from victimization.

The state may initiate an involuntary commitment for someone whose actions threaten or harm another. Also, one can be declared legally incompetent and, thus, lose privileges, such as the right to manage property, drive, marry or divorce, vote, or hold office. These limitations vary among the states, and gerontological nurse practitioners need to know which apply in their own setting. Such an incompetency ruling also eliminates the need to obtain the client's permission for medical treatment and prevents the client from refusing needed treatment.

One's client can prepare a living will to keep one's life from being prolonged by extraordinary means. Specific types of treatment can be specified that one does not wish to receive if he or she becomes incompetent and terminally ill. Two competent adults should witness the client's signature (Paulus, 1987).

Retirement

Retirement causes major role changes for the aging person. Some people have difficulty in adjusting to all the changes in retirement and feel that they have lost much of their identity by no longer being employed. Some dread retirement because of reduced income, reduced contact with job acquaintances, poor health, and death of relatives and friends. However, it should be pointed out that the majority of the aged adjust to retirement easily and look forward to having time to do the things they enjoy (Morgan, 1982).

Preretirement programs are helpful in preparing people for retirement. Such programs ask the future retirees to identify their interests, talents, and achievements in order to remind them of what they have accomplished and what activities they might continue after retirement. Programs on health can focus on preventive aspects such as diet and exercise, accident prevention, stress management and symptoms of health problems for which one should seek care. Financial programs should include information on budgets, investments, taxes, insurance, estate planning, and availability of community services. Plans for leisure activities should be encouraged, along with opportunities for part-time employment and civic involvement. Housing and family and emotional concerns should also be addressed, along with the spouse's needs and interests. The spouse may not yet be ready to retire; conversely, he or she may already be retired, so that the two will be spending much more time together. Their communication pattern, level of intimacy, and decision-making patterns may need adjustment.

The phases of retirement, according to Atchley, are not tied to definite periods of time or specific ages of each retiree. All phases are not experienced by all retirees.

1. *Remote phase:* early in one's career. Knows that retirement will happen some day, but does no planning
2. *Near phase:* looks forward to specific date of retirement. Fantasizes about the new role, prepares to leave job
3. *Honeymoon:* excited about doing all the things one never had time to do before. May be limited by available resources
4. *Disenchantment:* period of letdown or depression. Often dependent on reality of preretirement fantasies
5. *Reorientation:* develops more realistic view of own alternatives
6. *Stability:* more predictable and satisfying life-style. Have criteria that allow one to live in relatively comfortable, routine manner
7. *Termination:* end of retirement role due to return to employment or illness or disability leading to dependency (Atchley, 1980)

During the preretirement phase, a worker can prepare for retirement by developing hobbies and finding meaningful uses for leisure time, thus allowing the worker to substitute new activities for satisfactions lost along with the job. On the other hand, one may cope by accommodation or adaptation to the inevitable changes. Workers who have developed interpersonal networks and intellectual interests seem to deal with retirement more effectively. Adjustment may be more difficult for those who refuse

to retire until forced to do so. Persons who voluntarily retire seem to have more positive attitudes toward themselves and feel more useful (Morgan, 1982). Persons who were active before retirement generally remain so even though one's social position and social role are largely determined by one's occupational identification. The national attitude toward retirement is essentially ambivalent because one is withdrawing from something, but a leisure existence is becoming more acceptable to Americans.

Other roles are changed by retirement—in both positive and negative ways. Organizations may either welcome or reject retired members. Marriages may either be strengthened or fail. Spouses may respond unpredictably, some welcoming and others fearing their partner's retirement. The spouse may not yet be retired or may resent interference with his or her own home routines.

In addition to work, one's identity is closely related to age, health, friendships, and marital status, as well as community involvement. One may enjoy retirement and maintain a strong sense of well-being.

Economics

The problem of income maintenance is a major one for the aged. Lowered life satisfaction is directly related to lowered income. Lengthened retirement periods and low amounts of benefits available to only small numbers of eligible aged contribute to stress and health problems in the aged. Inflation adds to these problems, as aged on fixed budgets find it necessary to adjust their long-accustomed life-styles to accommodate for increases in cost of food, housing, clothing, and other necessities. Traveling and organizational memberships have to be sacrificed, and the aged find it especially difficult to discontinue giving gifts to family and friends. Home maintenance costs and property taxes make it difficult to maintain independent housing.

An absence of sufficient financial resources aggravates the misery of the aged in regard to diet, health, housing, safety, and independence.

Retirement income is usually less than half of that earned while the retiree was fully employed. Less than one fifth of the aged have income from a private pension plan (U.S. Bureau of the Census, 1983, pp. 7–8). Very few have enough assets to feel financially secure.

One of every seven aged persons lives in poverty now, but this has improved since 1959, when more than one in three had incomes below the poverty level. The poverty rate for the aged in 1981 was 18%. Including the ''near poor,'' this figure rose to almost 30%. Highest poverty rates are found among those over 75 years old, women, minorities, those who live alone, the unmarried, the unemployed, those who depend entirely on Social Security benefits, and those living in small towns and rural areas. The highest median incomes are received by white men, who in 1981 had median incomes of $8600. White women and black men each had median incomes of $4900; for black women the comparable figure was $3500. Sources of income for the elderly in 1981 included Social Security (37%), earnings (25%), property (23%), and pensions (13%) (U.S. Bureau of the Census, 1983, pp. 8–11).

There is, however, no consensus regarding what constitutes an adequate level of income. There are wide differences between standard figures and actual expenditures by persons or families. Some people may prefer to spend more while young and less when old, or, conversely, to save for their old age. Alternatively, a compromise approach would allow a comfortable standard of living to be maintained throughout one's life. Research shows, however, that, in the elderly, the drop in real income at retirement is not accompanied by an increased tendency to spend savings (Stoller & Stoller, 1987, p. 314).

In addition to pensions, sources of income to the aged may include wages and salaries, self-employment, supply of property resources, and unearned income. Most of the aged are unable to adjust their incomes to changing economic circumstances and therefore cannot combat declining real income. Important sex, marital status, and race differences exist. The income levels of men, married couples, and whites are more likely to be adequate. Even if the income is adequate at the time of retirement, however, it often becomes inadequate as time passes. If assets are used to supplement the income, then interest, dividend, and/or rental incomes will decline, too. The proportion of income spent on health care and other necessities increases with age while income decreases.

Many businesses are just beginning to note the buying potential of such a large portion of the population. At least one study has been conducted to determine the shopping habits of aged food buyers. Findings include the following. Buying was not the primary reason for shopping in more than half the cases studied. Shopping was considered an enjoyable pastime, made more valuable by the sensory experiences and exercise gained. Informed buying decisions were made after consultation with family and friends, comparison shopping, and media exposure. Businesses which offered discounts to senior citizens usually retained their loyalty. A written budget was not used by 86% of the sample. Most preferred early morning shopping. Only about half of those eligible for food stamps used them, and many of them never used coupons. The aged consumer was found to be less likely to complain about goods or services and to be very trusting (Ebersole & Hess, 1985).

As one means of helping aged people's financial situation, the Housing Annuity Plan (HAP) allows homeowners to trade their equity in a home for disposable cash. The home would not be sold outright, and the homeowner and surviving spouse would have lifetime occupancy rights to the house. Through a trust agreement, the homeowner would have a regular monthly income, with the title to the home being transferred after the owner's and spouse's deaths. Also, home maintenance costs would be covered by this program.

Some problems exist for aged retirees receiving private pension funds. Often the level of benefits is fixed, without adjustments for inflation. Often the pension plan terminates upon the death of the former employee. Such plans are usually immobile when one changes employers.

Government pensions, either military or civil service, are usually more adequate than private pensions and have periodic cost-of-living escalator clauses. Veterans' benefits are of many types, e.g., disability benefits, GI home loans, hospitalization and medical care, burial expense allowances, and vocational rehabilitation.

The Tax Reform Act of 1986 lowered from ten to five years the vesting requirement, but people need to understand that several small pensions will not be as large as a single one accumulated over 20 plus years (Rix, 1987).

Social Security
Social security benefits provide the major source of income for most of the aged, although this program was not designed for that purpose. The benefits are based on the average income for a period of years before retirement, which is the same basis of determining benefits to one's dependents or survivors. The benefits increase automatically with inflation. The plan is financed by deductions of a percentage of an employee's salary. Retirement benefits are normally taken at age 65 but may be taken at age 62 at a reduced level. In 1983, Congress changed the Social Security system by implementing a plan to gradually increase the age of eligibility for full retirement benefits (Rix, 1987). Disability benefits may be paid before age 65 if the person is unable to work and is expected to be disabled at least 12 months or is expected to die. Wives who have worked may receive their own benefits or half of the amount their husbands receive, whichever is greater. Survivors' benefits may be paid to families if an employee entitled to benefits dies before the age of 65.

Medicare
Medicare is a federal health insurance program for people aged 65 and older and specific disabled persons. It is directed by the Health Care Financing Administration. Medicare has two parts—hospital insurance and medical insurance. Hospital insurance helps pay for inpatient hospital care, medically necessary inpatient care

in a skilled nursing facility after a hospital stay, home health care, and hospice care. There is a limit to the number of days of hospital or skilled nursing facility care that Medicare will pay for within each benefit period, but one's hospital insurance protection is renewed each time a new benefit period is started.

Medicare hospital insurance will pay for most of the services received in a hospital or skilled nursing facility or from a home health agency or hospice program. However, it does not pay the full cost of some covered services. The payments are handled by private insurance organizations under contract with the government.

Medical insurance can help pay for medically necessary doctors' services, outpatient hospital services, and a number of other medical services and supplies that are not covered by the hospital insurance part of Medicare. Medical insurance also can pay for home health services.

Medicaid
Medicaid is a program that pays medical bills for low-income people who cannot afford the costs of medical care. Although each state designs its own program, the following basic medical services are covered: inpatient hospital services; outpatient hospital services; outpatient laboratory and x-ray services; rural health clinic services; skilled nursing services; home health services; and physicians' services. Provision of the following items varies from state to state: prescription drugs, dental services, eyeglasses, prosthetic devices, physical therapy, emergency room, optometrists, podiatrists, chiropractors, mental hospitals, ambulance service, and private duty nursing.

Supplemental Security Income (SSI)
Supplemental Security Income (SSI) is a federal program that pays monthly checks to aged, disabled, and blind persons who have limited income and assets. People may be eligible for SSI payments even if they have never worked. People who receive SSI checks may also receive

Social Security checks, if they are eligible for both. Persons may still qualify for SSI even if they have some assets and income. For example, homeownership, if the home is one's main place of residence, does not count against eligibility.

For both the SSI and Social Security programs, it is wise for the recipients to have their checks deposited directly in the bank each month. Potential thieves know that these checks arrive dependably on the third of each month.

Leisure

Leisure activities are traditionally performed on a discretionary basis without concern for financial gain, but as a source of self-expression and autonomy. Most leisure activities include a sense of play and psychological freedom and also provide sources of self-respect, status, interesting experiences, friendships, and pastime. (Fig. 1-2). The proportion of one's time spent in leisure pursuits gradually expands with age. Leisure activities that stimulate the aged person may help prevent mental disorders and may replace prior activities that had to. be abandoned. Idleness is an alternative but may literally be deadly for the aged.

Retired people tend to increase the number of leisure activities that they pursue but generally continue the same types of activities. Life satisfaction is higher for those persons who increase their number of activities after retirement. A wide diversity of leisure roles exists but choices are limited for many aged persons because of physical or financial limitations or lack of transportation. There are a few differences between the leisure activities chosen by the aged as opposed to those chosen by young persons. The aged read fewer books and magazines and attend the theater, concerts, movies, and sporting events less frequently. Most of the aged spend the majority of their leisure time at home (Atchley, 1980).

Housing

One's home fills the need for shelter, security, and a sense of belonging. However, there may also be neighborhood deterioration, rising property taxes, and problems of home and yard maintenance. Most of the aged are quite attached to their houses, and few of them move. Even fewer of them change communities because their environment is the source of deeply rooted friendships and rich memories; and time is necessary to become acquainted with a new community. Social networks appear to be critical to survival and lead to lower mortality. In the absence of such support, diseases such as cancer and car-

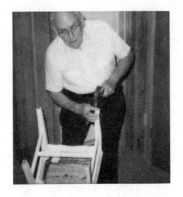
Woodworking

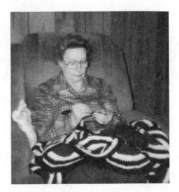
Needlecrafts

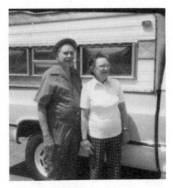
Traveling

Figure 1-2. Leisure Activities

diovascular disorders predominate (Ebersole & Hess, 1985).

The rural aged are at greater risk for isolation and loneliness, as transportation is often a problem, there are few health care services, and age cohorts are less common. Widowhood also contributes to such isolation. On the other hand, urban life has its own problems, including crowding, the rapid pace of life, and anonymity so prevalent that one does not even see an acquaintance on the street.

Most of the aged wish to live independently as long as possible, even though they are so vulnerable to falls, other accidents, and temperature extremes. Proper lighting and noise control are more important in their environments than in those of younger persons. People often judge themselves and are judged by their houses and neighborhoods, so home management and upkeep is significant for several reasons. Also, control of some aspect of one's environment, whether it be decorating or gardening, can give one a needed sense of mastery.

People have a basic need to identify with their environment, whether that is considered a building or town. They also need to interact with other people, either family or friends, and then to have some privacy each day. Psychological stimulation is necessary, for sensory deprivation can lead to a wide variety of mental health problems; so, too, however, can sensory overload.

Aged people have expressed specific needs from their environment. Most importantly, they need nursing or medical care nearby and a safe place to cash checks. It is desirable to have a grocery store, drug store, bus stop, house of worship, library, and social center within six blocks.

Because of economic or sentimental reasons, aged persons may remain in their old homes long past the point of safety. However, one's sense of competence and ability to cope may be enhanced by the services of homemakers, home health aides, social workers, delivery of meals to the home, and hotlines for emergencies. Day care centers often enable the aged to remain longer in their own or children's homes before institutionalization. In addition to meals and opportunities for socialization, day care centers may offer psychosocial services, health screening, family support services, and even transportation to and from the center.

Several programs financed by the U. S. Department of Housing and Urban Development are designed to provide housing for low- and moderate-income families. Each program has different criteria for tenant eligibility. All programs have specific income limits that are set by the department and that vary by location and number of persons in the family.

The "Rent Supplement" program provides funds to private owners, on behalf of eligible families, making it possible to rent to low-income families. Families must be able to pay a minimum based on the unit rent regardless of income. In the Section 236 program, each apartment complex has one fixed basic rent per bedroom size unit. The basic rent is the minimum rent; families with higher income pay more than the basic rent. Depending on a family's income, rents vary between the basic, or minimum, rent and the fair market, or maximum, rent.

"Below market interest rate" apartment complexes operate at fixed unit rents. This rental rate is generally lower than that of most conventional apartments, because of the low interest rate given to the owner. "Section 8" housing is found in some HUD-insured complexes that have a certain number of units that may be rented to low-income families. The government pays a portion of the rent and qualified families pay approximately 30% of their income for rent.

Institutionalization

Although only 5% of the population 65 years and older resides in long-term care institutions at a given time, the possibility of needing to move into one concerns many of the other 95%. It is best for the aged person to have input into the decision for relocation. Visits to the new setting prior to moving are especially helpful. Rapid formation of new friendships after moving is very important to successful adaptation.

Relocation is not without hazard even if the aged person is leaving an unpleasant or dangerous situation. Some risk factors have been identified that may make a person more vulnerable to translocation syndrome. These include depression, anxiety, confusion, and being older than age 85 (Rantz & Egan, 1987). Reducing the impact of relocation is an important consideration.

A more positive outcome of relocation may be expected if the one who moves is in stable health, has few concomitant stresses, and has the support of family or significant other(s). Positive staff attitudes are important. Measures to aid one's adjustment to the new facility include having a compatible roommate, access to legal aid, some choices regarding one's own activities and care, and accurate information about one's condition and environment. One should be allowed to keep personal items and to help decorate one's own room. Contact with pets, plants, and children is encouraged in the most progressive institutions, where there may also be provisions for recording one's life history, attending memorials for residents who have died, and having one's birthday celebrated on that day. The choice of dress is also important because wearing one's daytime clothing, as opposed to nightclothes or institutional gowns, seems to encourage independence and self-esteem (Pensiero & Adams, 1987).

Territoriality and Personal Space

One's adaptation to aging may be eased if previous patterns of privacy and interaction with others are maintained. Most authorities see that personal space contracts with age, even though feelings of separation and distance are caused by decreased sensory perception. Invasion of one's space may engender many reactions—acting out, talkativeness, depression, anger, withdrawal, or confusion.

Ethnicity, mental competence, and educational level influence the patterns of desired closeness, including eye contact and sound. One may claim territory in a day room or dining room by frequent use. Positioning oneself in a particular way invites or discourages company. Manipulation of the environment may be useful in reaching a higher level of therapeutic resident interaction. Gerontological nurse practitioners can enhance a client's sense of territorial security by respecting the arrangement of the client's space and the client's dignity and modesty. The nurse should ask clients whether they prefer their doors and curtains open or shut; the nurse should also remain alert to their reactions to being touched.

Safety

Safety can take many forms—in the neighborhood as a whole, prevention of crime in the home, or home safety related to falls, fire, or food poisoning.

Safety in the neighborhood can also depend on the incline and surface of sidewalks that the elderly must use. Inclines of 5% or less are ideal. Paved sidewalks are most desirable, along with designated crosswalks, and traffic light timing slower than usual. Benches placed at optimal intervals along the walks are helpful if they are in areas of good lighting, regular police surveillance, and enough pedestrian traffic to naturally monitor behavior. Park areas attract the aged if the landscape design is optimal and benches are oriented toward appropriate views and interaction.

Fear of crime may limit pedestrian traffic, especially if the neighbors are known to be hesitant about calling police. Data indicate that there is a decreasing amount of crime and victimization with aging (Fielo, 1987), but fear of such may almost paralyze the aged and cause them to isolate themselves at home. Crime prevention programs that emphasize locks, window bars, and relocation to a safe neighborhood are of slight help to the aged, who have few financial resources and merely become more scared after hearing such warnings.

Freezing weather is another concern because of the high price of heating fuel, the danger of asphyxiation due to escaping fumes, and the possibility of fire. The aged are especially vulnerable to hypothermia, so some heating method is absolutely necessary. Smoke detectors and sprinkling systems are helpful but also expensive.

Home safety has many aspects that a gerontological nurse practitioner may have occasion to assess. Scatter rugs should be firmly anchored. Electrical appliances, including the cords, need to be in good repair. Adequate light, heat, and ventilation, sturdy furniture arranged in a well-organized manner, a clean kitchen, safe storage of food, handrails in the bathroom, stairs in good repair and marked with color, handrails, screen, and more than one exit are also necessary.

Transportation

Lack of transportation often contributes to other problems such as poor nutrition, lack of health care, or social withdrawal. Most of the aged rely on relatives and friends for transportation. The rural aged are especially isolated, and even urban aged may live far from a bus stop or be unable to afford the fare. Moreover, physical disability might prohibit the use of public transportation. The aged who drive their own cars find that insurance is quite costly. Physiological changes may cause them to be overly cautious or unwittingly careless (Ebersole & Hess, 1985). Many aged are afraid of freeways and go far out of the way to reach a destination. Some of the aged realize that their friends no longer drive safely and stop riding with them, thus increasing their own isolation.

Politics

Most of the aged remain interested in and informed about politics. About the same proportions of them vote as did so in middle age. They are rather evenly split in party identification between the Democratic and Republican parties, but their party identification is strong only if they have been members for many years. Some political action coalitions of the aged are beginning to form to influence future legislation. With the growing number of aged and their political mobilization, it is likely that they will become a powerful voting bloc. Consciousness raising is increasing, and the mass media are more involved, so the "gray power" movement may gain more strength. Differences in political outlooks of the various age groups is probably due not to aging, but to a generational bias based on the historical circumstances surrounding each group's life. Viewpoints of the various age groups are influenced by familiarity, experience, and proximity.

Education

There is an inverse relation between age and education, although the proportion of aged people seeking education continues to rise. Educational institutions are beginning to adapt some programs to older people, and, indeed, to attract such students. Reduced tuition fees have also been instituted at many universities to attract older students. It is now believed that attitude characteristics of the aged are due to their education and to the time that has passed since their education was completed (Hendricks & Hendricks, 1981).

Religion

With increasing age, people seem to rely more on their religious faith and beliefs for support. Their involvement in religion usually continues if it began in earlier years.

Women have higher attendance rates at religious services than do men of their age group, and rural people participate more. The working class has few group activities other than religious-related ones. Attendance gradually declines with increasing age, due to disability, immobility, and financial problems. Activities like reading the Bible or books by other religious authorities, praying, and meditating steadily rise with age. Belief in God or a god, belief in immortality, and belief in generally conservative religious doctrines reach highest levels with advanced age.

It may be debated whether good mental health is due to strong religious beliefs or leads to them. Aged persons have been able to deal with loneliness and unhappiness due to their expressed beliefs in God and to the affirmation of individual worth found in the teachings of Judaism and Christianity.

The view of death as a portal to immortality may engender a sense of serenity and lessened fear of death. Fear of the process of dying is apparently worse than the fear of death itself. Also greatly feared are leaving behind unfinished business, leaving one's survivors, and especially social isolation as one is dying.

Ethnicity

Many aged members of minority groups have borne discrimination throughout their entire lives and have been disadvantaged financially, educationally, and in their health. In some cases they may be illiterate, or unable to speak English adequately or at all. The gerontological nurse practitioner must be especially careful to confirm that these clients do in fact understand health teaching and are not nodding their heads merely to be polite.

The minority aged usually turn to family or friends for assistance instead of the health care system, and professional help is sought only in emergencies. The gerontological nurse practitioner must be careful to avoid making generalizations about minority groups. Early immigration patterns evoked ethnic rivalry that still exists among some of the aged groups. Immigrants may still cling to parts, or all, of their original culture. The nurse will need to ascertain which characteristics the aged person seeks to retain and which have been adapted. Food and religious orientation are often most closely based on the original culture (Ochoco, 1987).

STANDARDS OF GERONTOLOGICAL NURSING PRACTICE

Gerontological nurses were held in low esteem by their colleagues for many years. The specialty was very low on the hierarchy of preferred nursing roles, as the nursing students saw mostly negative examples of aging. However, improvement began in 1961 when the American Nurses' Association formed a specialty group for geriatric nurses. Between 1967 and 1969, this group wrote the Standards for Geriatric Nursing. Eventually the name of the group was changed to Gerontological Nursing Division in 1976, and the title of the standards was changed accordingly. In 1987, the standards were revised and entitled Standards and Scope of Gerontological Nursing Practice.

It is assumed that knowledge of the theories and process of aging can be applied to the practice of nursing in order to improve the level of care rendered to the aged. The standards follow the generally accepted outline of the nursing process, namely assessing, planning, implementing, and evaluating. Maximizing independence and maintenance of as high a level of wellness as is congruent with the client's condition are emphasized. The standards follow.

Standard I. Organization Of Gerontological Nursing Services. All gerontological nursing services are planned, organized, and directed by a nurse executive. The nurse executive has baccalaureate of master's preparation and has experience in gerontological nursing and administration of long-term care services or acute care services for older clients.

Standard II. Theory. The nurse participates in the generation and testing of theory as a basis for clinical decisions. The nurse uses theoretical concepts to guide the effective practice of gerontological nursing.

Standard III. Data Collection. The health status of the older person is regularly assessed in a comprehensive, accurate, and systematic manner. The information obtained during the health asssessment is accessible to and shared with appropriate members of the interdisciplinary health care team, including the older person and the family.

Standard IV. Nursing Diagnosis. The nurse uses health assessment data to determine nursing diagnoses.

Standard V. Planning And Continuity Of Care. The nurse develops the plan of care in conjunction with the older person and appropriate others. Mutual goals, priorities, nursing approaches, and measures in the care plan address the therapeutic, preventive, restorative, and rehabilitative needs of the older person. The care plan helps the older person attain and maintain the highest level of health, well-being, and quality of life achievable, as well as a peaceful death. The plan of care facilitates continuity of care over time as the client moves to various care settings, and is revised as necessary.

Standard VI. Intervention. The nurse, guided by the plan of care, intervenes to provide care to restore the older person's functional capabilities and to prevent complications and excess disability. Nursing interventions are derived from nursing diagnoses and are based on gerontological nursing theory.

Standard VII. Evaluation. The nurse continually evaluates the client's and family's responses to interventions in order to determine progress toward goal attainment and to revise the data base, nursing diagnoses, and plan of care.

Standard VIII. Interdisciplinary Collaboration. The nurse collaborates with other members of the health care team in the various settings in which care is given to the older person. The team meets regularly to evaluate the effectiveness of the care plan for the client and family and to adjust the plan of care to accommodate changing needs.

Standard IX. Research. The nurse participates in research designed to generate an organized body of gerontological nursing knowledge, disseminates research findings, and uses them in practice.

Standard X. Ethics. The nurse uses the Code for Nurses established by the American Nurses' Association as a guide for ethical descision making in practice.

Standard XI. Professional Development. The nurse assumes responsibility for professional development and contributes to the professional growth of interdisciplinary team members. The nurse participates in peer review and other means of evaluation to assure the quality of nursing practice.
(American Nurses' Asssociation, 1987, reprinted with permission).

ASSESSMENT

Assessment of all phases of a client's life is necessary in order to establish baseline data against which future progression or regression can be measured. It is necessary for a gerontological nurse practitioner to understand a client's psychosocial background, as well as physical status, in order to be aware of the derivation of the client's self-concept. The nurse may also learn of the client's possible misperceptions regarding her or his own condition and therapy or normal changes with aging and, thus, be able to help the

client with a modification of life-style or an indicated referral.

The holistic approach to assessment clearly reflects the interrelationship of physical well-being, behavior, and emotional state. Physical health, mental health, relationships with family and friends, educational background, financial situation, current environment, activities of daily living, safety, and preventive practices may all be examined in a functional assessment.

Psychosocial assessment may be complicated by the heightened body consciousness of most of the aged. This psychological change may occur because the aged person is found in a world of steadily reduced familiarity. The client's family and friends are dying, the environment begins to lose its meaning, and introversion increases. With the growing inefficiency of sensory receptors, less stimuli reach the aged person; lack of an optimal level of stimulation has been shown to exacerbate cell degeneration and to disrupt the normal integration of sensations, perception, memories, and images (Ernst et al., 1978).

When the gerontological nurse practitioner decides to assess a client, for whatever reason, a quiet location, free from disruptions, should be used. If the client is not able to undergo a complete assessment during one session, the nurse should set priorities early in the interview regarding which aspects are most important to assess at that time. Assessments should be organized so as to conserve the client's energy. Sufficient time must be allotted to prevent rushing clients who may need more time to answer questions or who may move slowly. Resource persons, such as family or friends, may be helpful in providing information to the gerontological nurse practitioner, as well as becoming involved in planning and giving care.

Aspects of the Physical Assessment

Present Status
Basic facts to be investigated are the following:

1. Existence of chronic disease or condition
2. Effects of illness on life-style

3. Presence of pain
4. Sensory changes
5. Medication usage (prescription or over-the-counter)
6. Immunization history

The nurse might follow up with questions such as these: What does health mean to you? Do you regularly perform any practices for health maintenance? Do you provide care for any family member? To what extent do you think your health could be improved?

Past Medical History
The client should be asked about the following:

1. Date of last physical examination
2. Names of physicians seen
3. Previous illnesses (date, duration, treatment, sequelae)
4. Previous hospitalizations
5. Previous x-rays
6. Previous surgeries
7. Blood transfusions

Family History
Genetic predispositions to any disease or condition should be determined. The age and condition or cause of and age at death, along with any other illnesses before death, should be ascertained for a client's parents, siblings, children, and spouse.

Review of Systems
A review of each body system may reveal data on pain, functional disorders, and specific tests or treatments affecting that system. A head-to-toe approach will help organize the interview. The nurse will, of course, obtain specific information on each symptom or dysfunction mentioned by the client. General questions may be asked first before proceeding to each physiological system. Most physical assessment nursing textbooks provide specific guides to such interviews.

Physical Assessment
The reader without physical assessment skills is referred to the many good textbooks on that topic that are available. Because a portion of these books are not specific to the aged person, each chapter in Part Two of this book presents changes that are common to the aging process for the body system discussed in that chapter.

Assessment of Specific Physical Points

Diet
The client should be questioned about the following:

1. Knowledge of nutritional needs
2. Amount of fluids taken
3. Ability to procure and prepare foods
4. Ability to feed self
5. Foods consumed during the previous 24 hours
6. Favorite and most disliked foods
7. Appetite
8. Weight change
9. Use of alcoholic beverages

Mobility/Exercise
The gerontological nurse practitioner should question the client about the following:

1. Ability to get in and out of bed/bathtub, use toilet
2. Ability to walk around room, up and down stairs, around the block
3. Dizziness or falls
4. Coordination
5. Typical type and amount of exercise per week
6. Adherence to a specific exercise program
7. Changes in stamina
8. Use of leisure time
9. Activities of a typical day, week
10. Ability to drive or use public transportation

Sleep/Rest
Patterns of sleep and rest may be assessed as follows:

1. Number of hours of sleep per 24 hours
2. Usual bedtime
3. Any changes in sleep patterns
4. Any insomnia

5. Rituals to facilitate sleep
6. Environment of bedroom

Elimination

Both bowel and bladder elimination should be assessed. These points may be considered:

1. Frequency and characteristics of bowel movements
2. Routines to maintain bowel integrity
3. Flatus
4. Continency
5. Use of assistive devices
6. Fluid intake and output
7. Frequency of urination
8. Characteristics of urine
9. Control of urine stream

Sexuality

Many aged persons are not used to discussing their sexuality. Assurance of privacy will be particularly helpful as the gerontological nurse practitioner asks these questions:

1. Age of onset of sexual activity
2. Present sexual activity; age of partners, if any
3. Age-related changes in ability to have sexual intercourse
4. Satisfaction with present level of sexual activity
5. Use of nongenital forms of sexual expression

For females, the following may be asked:

1. Any sequelae of childbearing
2. Age at and characteristics of menopause
3. Date of last Pap smear
4. Date of last breast self-examination

For males, the following may be asked:

1. Changes in size or anatomical position of genitalia

Personal Care

Points of consideration include the following:

1. Hearing, vision, teeth corrected if necessary
2. Corrective devices fit and function properly
3. Ability to bathe, groom (cut nails, comb hair, shave, brush teeth), and dress
4. Appearance (well-groomed or not)

Tobacco Usage

Previous and/or present usage of tobacco should be addressed:

1. Past use of tobacco
2. Present use, type, frequency
3. Physical changes related to tobacco habit

Drug Usage

Be sure to include alcohol.

1. Past use of drugs
2. Present use, kind, frequency

Communication

This is, of course, the basis for the entire assessment process. The gerontological nurse practitioner needs to learn the client's perception of the present illness and situation. The nurse may need to rephrase the client's statements in order to verify perceptions. It is important, too, to maintain eye contact during the interaction. The following aspects are necessary to assess:

1. Presence of social amenities
2. Language
3. Speech patterns
4. Distinctness of words
5. Mechanical patterns
6. Logical flow of ideas

Financial Situation

The following points should be considered:

1. Amount and sources of income
2. Adequacy of income
3. Insurance coverage
4. Job history
5. Effects of retirement
6. Use of income
7. Management of finances
8. Preparation of will
9. Power of attorney

Education

It is helpful for the gerontological nurse practitioner to know the client's present level of education in order to interact more effectively. Plans for future education may be clues to the client's self-esteem and motivation.

Culture

It is important for the gerontological nurse practitioner to be cognizant of the client's cultural and ethnic background because this has a great influence over one's self-care health practices:

1. Place of birth
2. Ethnic and/or cultural identification
3. Ethnic and/or cultural practices presently in family
4. Language(s) spoken
5. Place considered "home"

Environment

The concept of environment extends from one's clothes to one's immediate surroundings to one's residence. Aspects to be investigated include the following:

1. Clothing
2. Furnishings of room, home
3. Size of bed, wheelchair, etc.
4. Privacy
5. Location of home
6. Pollution
7. Possibility of relocation

Housekeeping

Is the client or another responsible party able to maintain a clean environment?

1. Ability to clean dishes, stove, refrigerator (if any)
2. Ability to dust, wash, iron
3. Ability to vacuum, mop
4. Ability to clean bathroom
5. Ability to do yardwork, including pruning
6. Ability to clean windows, repair screens

Safety

Many aspects of safety have been previously alluded to but need to be summarized here:

1. Slippers and shoes of proper fit, nonskid soles
2. Sleeves and skirts close-fitting (to stay out of fires)
3. Condition of canes, walkers, and wheelchair
4. Medications labeled, taken correctly
5. Ability to use phone

6. Condition of house and furnishings
7. Protection from criminal activity
8. Presence of smoke detector and fire extinguisher

Assessment of Mental Health

Mental health is most commonly assessed according to one's orientation to person, place, and time. Level of consciousness is a gross indication, as is orientation, but more refined measures are needed for many clients. Especially for those wishing to remain in independent settings, it is valuable to evaluate their ability to handle their finances, including making purchases, writing checks, and living within their budget. Recent and intermediate memory should be checked along with the ability to abstract. Appropriate responses to touch, ability to describe one's comfort status, and the absence or presence of hallucinations and delusions also need to be considered.

Self-concept

Clients' self-concept may be assessed by asking them to describe themselves, especially in relation to significant events in their lives, and goal achievement or lack thereof. A description of what the person most enjoys now and any future plans are also good indicators of the degree of satisfaction.

One's attitude toward death and other losses is an important factor for the aged person. "Anniversary reaction" on the date a loved one died is not uncommon. Having clients describe their parents' aging is useful, as are questions to determine their own opinions concerning death. Questions concerning the loss of a spouse or other significant other(s), the client's reactions to these losses, and the client's spiritual preferences provide increased insight to the nurse, as do direct questions regarding loneliness and depression.

A client's relation to family and friends is assessed by questions about the client's family responsibilities, decision-making patterns, amount of family contact, and family activities. Also to be determined are friendship patterns (either longstanding or new), organizational memberships, or presence of any pets in the household.

SUMMARY

The steadily rising number of aged people necessitates that nurses have gerontological preparation and are aware of the social problems facing the aged that impinge on health care. By using the Standards of Gerontological Nursing and basic assessment skills, the gerontological nurse practitioner can effectively care for aged clients. The gerontological nurse practitioner can promote proper treatment modalities for all of the aged and help prevent inappropriate labeling of persons with symptoms.

REFERENCES

Abrams, R. S. (1987). Coping with three generations under one roof: Conflict or cooperation? *Perspectives on Aging 16*(2), 24.

Age, Sex, Race & Spanish Origin of the Population by Regions, Divisions, and States, 1980. (1980). *1980 census of population.* Washington, DC: United States Department of Commerce.

American Nurses' Association. (1987). *Standards and scope of gerontological nursing.* Kansas City, Missouri: Author.

American Psychiatric Association. (1980). *Diagnostic and statistical manual of mental disorders* (3rd ed.). Washington, DC: Author.

Annual Summary of Births, Deaths, Marriages, and Divorces: United States, 1980. (1982, September 17). *Monthly vital statistics report.* Hyattsville, MD: United States Department of Health and Human Services.

Atchley, R. C. (1980). *The social forces in later life* (3rd ed.). Belmont, CA: Wadsworth.

Beck, C., & Ferguson, D. (1981). Aged abuse. *Journal of Gerontological Nursing, 7,* 333–336.

Block, M. R., & Sinnott, J. D. (Eds.). (1979). The battered elder syndrome: An exploratory study, In D. Johnson (1981) Abuse of the Elderly. *Nurse Practitioner, 6*(1), 29–34.

Dolan, M. B. (1987). Meet the chronologically gifted. *Nursing 87, 17*(10), 56–57.

Ebersole, P., & Hess, P. (1985). *Toward healthy aging* (2nd ed.). St. Louis: Mosby.

Ernst, P., Beran, B., Safford, F., & Kleinhauz, M. (1978). Isolation and the symptoms of chronic brain syndrome. *The Gerontologist, 18,* 468–473.

Fielo, S. B. (1987). How does crime affect the elderly? *Geriatric Nursing, 8*(2), 80–83.

Haynes, S., & Feinleib, M. (Eds.). (1980). *Conference on epidemiology of aging.* Washington, DC: United States Department of Health and Human Services.

Hendricks, J., & Hendricks, C. D. (1981). *Aging in mass society: Myths & realities* (2nd ed.). Cambridge, MA: Winthrop.

Johnson, C. L., & Barer, B. M. (1987). Marital instability and the changing kinship networks of grandparents. *The Gerontologist, 27*(3), 330–335.

Kivnick, H. Q. (1982). Grandparenthood: An overview of meaning and mental health. *The Gerontologist, 22,* 59–66.

Levenson, A. J., & Porter, D. M. (1984). *An Introduction to Gerontology and Geriatrics.* Springfield, IL: Thomas.

Morgan, L. A. (1982). Social roles in later life, In C. Eisdorfer (Ed.), *Annual review of gerontology and geriatrics.* New York: Springer.

Ochoco, L. (1987). Group work with the frail ethnic elderly. *Geriatric Nursing, 8*(4), 185–187.

Paulus, S. (1987). If your patient wants to draw up a living will. *RN, 50*(9), 63–66.

Pensiero, M., & Adams, M. (1987). Dress and self-esteem. *Journal of Gerontological Nursing, 13*(10), 11–17.

Rantz, M., & Egan, K. (1987). Reducing death from translocation syndrome. *American Journal of Nursing, 87*(10), 1351–1352.

Rix, S. E. (1987). Pensions, social security gain from longer worklife. *Perspective on Aging, 16*(2), 3–6.

Stoller, E. P., & Stoller, M. A. (1987). The propensity to save among the elderly. *The Gerontologist, 27*(3), 314–320.

Ubell, E. (1984). The population explosion of old people. *Parade Magazine,* November 25.

United States Bureau of the Census, Current Population Reports, Series P-23, No. 128. (1983, September). *America in Transition: An Aging Society.* Washington, DC: United States Government Printing Office.

THEORIES OF AGING

Since the beginning of time, humans have experienced the phenomena of aging. For most of human history, however, aging occurred over a relatively brief time span, for disease, infection, malnutrition, and wars seriously limited life expectancy. One was considered "old" if one reached the age of 40 years, with few people living beyond this age. During the 19th century and especially the 20th century, research efforts brought discoveries and remarkable advances in medicine (e.g., immunizations, antibiotics, and new and improved diagnostic procedures) that have had a dramatic impact on the life expectancy of every man, woman, and child. With immunization available to everyone, and the ill and malnourished being effectively treated, life expectancy began to greatly exceed what had previously been possible. Today, it is not uncommon for one who has successfully survived the many health hazards and life's stressors to surpass the age of 80 years; many people live beyond the age of 100 years.

The increase in the number of older individuals has provided a more visible awareness of the aging process. This awareness has further stimulated the need for investigation to answer the question, Why does one age?

Throughout history there have been speculations about this question. Theories on aging initially were mere speculations or assumptions; one could go so far as to classify some as old wives tales. Research conducted during the past two decades to explore the aging process still has not provided conclusive evidence to answer the question, Why does one age?

This chapter discusses past and present theories related to the aging process. These theories will include the biological, psychosocial and environmental aspects of aging.

A CONCEPTUAL FRAMEWORK

In formulating a framework to conceptualize a theory, or theories, of aging, it is necessary to identify first the contributing factors that have been used in providing rationale for the aging phenomena. Biological, psychosocial, and environmental factors have been recognized to have a major impact on the aging process, either in retarding or accelerating its progress. The acknowledgment that relationships existed between the speculative factors has fostered further scientific inquiry which has provided for a more qualitative approach to the question, Why does one age? Scientific inquiry has been and is now being used to study the aging process, particularly in the area of cellular activity related to aging.

Figure 2–1 offers a conceptualization of how the major categories of contributing factors interact with one another and impact upon the aging process. Theories representative of the major categories may include the following but

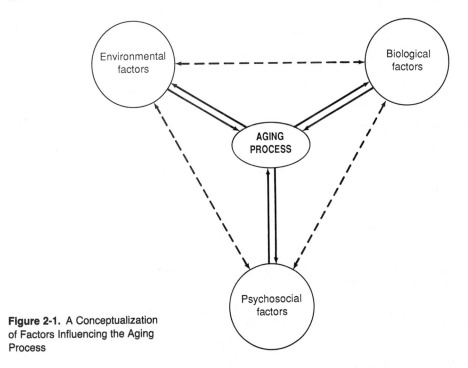

Figure 2-1. A Conceptualization of Factors Influencing the Aging Process

are not inclusive: Biological Theories—Cellular Theory, Genetic Theory, Somatic Mutation Theory, Wear and Tear Theory, Error Theory, Autoimmune Theory, Free-Radical Theory, and Crosslinkage Theory; Psychosocial Theories—Disengagement Theory, Activity Theory, Continuity Theory, and Social Exchange Theory; and Environmental Theories—Radiation Theory, Stress Theory, Pollution Theory, and Exposure Theory.

BIOLOGICAL THEORIES

During the past two decades there has been much interest in the scientific inquiry of aging. Based on their research, scientists have proposed various theories, which have provided additional information to be considered in the understanding of the aging phenomena. It is important for the nurse practitioner to realize that the biological theories, as well as the psychosocial and environmental theories, should be examined for

their applicability to the practice of gerontological nursing. The aging phenomenon is still unknown to scientists; the end result of the aging process, death of the organism, is the only aspect of this phenomenon that is conclusive.

Cell Theory

The cell has been the subject of much scientific inquiry in exploring the aging phenomena. The cell has three definite components that have contributed to the basic foundation of other biological theories. The three cell components include cells that reproduce, cells that do not reproduce, and intercellular substances/materials.

The theory based on cells that reproduce postulates that during reproduction some of the new cells are nonfunctioning or less effective than the other cells that were replaced (Busse, 1971). There are three systems in the human organism where cells are continuously being replaced: the skin (epidermis), the lining of the intestine, and the circulatory system.

The major feature these cells have in common is their vulnerability to injury by the environment, i.e., photo and physical exposure, noxious substances and digestive enzymes, and the roughness and uneven forces that are encountered when being pumped endlessly through the vascular network (Strehler, 1977).

During the aging process the inefficiency or loss of function of the cells being replaced is not noticed at first. However, as the aging process progresses and there is an accumulation of inefficient and nonfunctioning cells, the organism's functional ability becomes apparent. The skin, for example, takes on visible changes during the aging process, namely irregular surface areas (scars, wrinkles), roughness, thin and shiny, dryness, pigmented areas, warts, and moles.

The theory related to cells that do not reproduce postulates that with age the cells progressively wear out and/or are destroyed (Busse, 1971). Therefore, systems that comprise cells that do not reproduce, for example, the central nervous system, gradually develop an accumulation of nonfunctioning cells, which causes the system to become less efficient and unable to handle the usual work load. The kidneys, for example, during the aging process gradually experience a decrease in blood flow, glomerular filtration, and tubular reabsorption (Strehler, 1977), which may result in electrolyte imbalances, albuminuria, edema, and glucosuria.

The theory related to the intercellular substances postulates that there is a gradual deterioration of the intercellular material with aging (Busse, 1971). This reduces the ability of the cells to provide the necessary nutrients and oxygen for the respective tissues, thus directly interfering with the functioning abilities of each system.

Programmed Aging Theory

According to Wilson (1974), aging is obviously programmed because there is a predictable, species-specific pattern of changes that occurs as an organism grows older. Programming is a defi-
nite set or sequence of events that have been built into the organism through selective pressures. Therefore, one may postulate that there are direct or indirect selective advantages to limiting the life-span through aging. The programmed aging theory postulates that the life-span of an organism is programmed within the genes of the organism. The program sets or controls the rate and time that the individual proceeds through the life-span (aging) and dies. If the programmed events are not present, aging would not occur or would occur later when the programmed events are experienced.

Synonymous with the Programmed Aging Theory, the Rate of Living Theory was proposed in 1908 by Max Rubner, a German physiologist (Behnke, Finch, & Momenr, 1978). Rubner hypothesized that the length of life in mammals is a reflection of the rate of physiological living and pointed out that there is a correlation between the total number of calories of energy burned per gram of body weight during the lifetime of mammals of greatly different sizes and life-spans. Although supported by the research findings, the significance of this theory has been questioned, as has its relationship to the aging process.

The Rate of Living Theory postulates that the human species has a programmed amount of energy, entropy, or other properties that are used up as a function of life and living. When the programmed amount is used up, death occurs. The rate by which the programmed amount is used determines the life-span of the individual (Hershey, 1974).

Somatic Mutation Theory

For centuries scientists have been debating whether or not the instability of genetic structures affects the aging process (Strehler, 1977). The Somatic Mutation Theory postulates that during spontaneous mutation there is an alteration of DNA by spontaneous hydrolysis, irradiation, or miscoding of enzymes; if uncorrected by the systems of repair enzymes, the replicated cells will perpetuate the mutation, thus decreasing cellular function and organ efficiency (Rockstein, 1974; Ebersole & Hess, 1981).

To test this theory, the following question is posed: "Do conditions which result in an increased rate of mutation cause a corresponding increase in the rate of aging" (Strehler, 1977)? If gene mutation or chromosomal aberrations within the somatic cells are the source of aging, then the exposure to mutagenic agents such as x-rays or chemical mutagens should increase the rate of aging. The problem inherent in addressing the above question is that there are no means, at present, to measure the rate of mutation of the key somatic cells in which the most prevalent changes clearly occur (Strehler, 1977).

Strehler (1977, p. 274–283) discussed five lines of evidence regarding this theory. It was concluded from these research studies that it is highly improbable that the aging process is generally a consequence of the accumulation of classical somatic mutations or chromosomal aberrations with age.

Sinex (1974) identified three types of mutations: spontaneous hydrolysis, radiation-induced mutation, and aging hits. Each respective type varies qualitatively and quantitatively: spontaneous hydrolysis is rather easily repaired, radiation injury is somewhat less repairable, and both have some significance in aging. Aging hits, however, have a low level of repairability and are highly significant in aging.

Most species that age because of somatic mutation also have cancer, the reason being that the activation of oncogenic virus is associated with efforts to repair aging hits (Sinex, 1974).

Crosslinkage Theory

The Crosslinkage Theory (commonly referred to as the Collagen Theory) postulates that there are chemical reactions between DNA and crosslinking molecules that result in changes in connective tissue. As one ages there is an increase in the number of crosslinks in extracellular components. The extracellular components include the various fibrous and colloidal elements that give texture, elasticity, and form to the aggregate of cells (Gross, 1961).

There are three types of fibers to be considered: (1) collagenous fibers, which are fairly nonelastic in nature; (2) elastic fibers; and (3) reticular fibers. Each fiber type has a defined functional use and a specific location within the body.

The collagenous fibers are found in those situations where a fair amount of rigidity is required. They are the major constituents of tendons and fascia, which are supportive of such functions as transmission of force and locomotion (Strehler, 1977).

The elastic fibers are found in the skin and the large arteries. They have the property of being able to return to their original shapes after deformation, enabling the organism to adapt itself to distorting forces and movements with a minimum of permanent damage. With the increase in the crosslinkage of elastin as one ages, gross changes can be observed in the skin in particular. With the aging process, skin that once appeared smooth, soft, and firm slowly begins to appear dry, saggy, and wrinkled (loss of elasticity). The large blood vessels are also affected by the crosslinkage phenomenon. The replacement by nonelastic fibrous connective tissue during the crosslinkage process decreases the elasticity of the blood vessels, affecting their ability to dilate and contract to their optimum. This could result in blood pressure changes and a decrease in the efficiency with which the work of the heart can be used to perfuse the tissues (Strehler, 1977).

The reticular fibers are much finer than the collagenous and elastic fibers and appear to be involved in the support of the individual cells, especially in areas of continuous membranes such as the so-called basement membranes that underlie the typical epithelium (Strehler, 1977). The complete chemical nature of reticular fibers is still unknown, and investigation continues to explore the function and composition of the reticular fibers.

There has been an observable relationship

of the crosslinkage theory and other principal theories of aging. The immunologic theory, for example, is mutually consistent with the crosslinkage theory. Autoimmunity is considered to be a critically important mechanism in the aging process. The immunologic theory postulates that the immune response deteriorates with aging. The cause of this age-dependent deterioration is considered to be an effect of random uncontrolled crosslinkages that interfere with the functioning of essential molecules, resulting in destruction of sites in DNA that govern immunologic functions (Bjorksten, 1974).

The isolation of enzymes from the organism *Bacillus cereus* have been effective in dissolving crosslinked preparations. The enzyme is being further tested for potential use in humans. Means for production and oral administration of the enzyme are still under study (Bjorksten, 1974).

Free-Radical Theory

Free radicals are highly reactive cellular components derived from atoms or molecules in which an electron pair has been transiently separated into two electrons that exhibit independence of motion (Pryor, 1973). The magnetic moments of these radicals are no longer complementary. They exhibit a large increment of free energy and will oxidatively attack adjacent molecules.

In biological systems, the molecule that most commonly generates free radicals is oxygen (Demopoules, 1973). In 1956, Harman proposed the free radical theory and stressed the importance of the use of oxygen by the cell (Krohn, 1965). Oxygen is a highly reactive element and is necessary for the metabolism (oxidation) of organic materials, namely protein, fat, and carbohydrate, which results in the formation of free radicals and by-product compounds. The free radical end products are not usable and may cause molecular pathology.

One quality that characterizes free radical action is that they do not appear to contain or reflect any useful biological information. Their actions on membranes, therefore, represent the replacement of genetically determined order by randomness (Gordon, 1974).

Because the process of oxidation is continuous within the body, it is reasonable to assume that free radicals are continuously being produced, causing an accumulation of tissue damage. Such accumulation and injury to biological membranes during aging may produce (1) cells with an altered permeability to electrolytes, (2) microsomes and mitochondria that have a greater degree of heterogeneity in function and structure, (3) microsomes deficient in cholesterol, and (4) an accumulation of products of lipid peroxidation within cells and in body fluids, for example, the bloodstream (Gordon, 1974).

It is the view of many scientists that free radical-induced peroxidation of unsaturated fatty acids is a major determinant of biological aging. However, the full importance of free radical–induced pathology is yet to be determined. Experiments have provided evidence that free radical information and free radical–induced pathology are events in the aging process (Gordon, 1974).

There is a growing concern regarding the antioxidant effects in aging. The effects of vitamin E and chemically unrelated antioxidants on the aging process have been studied to explain how antioxidants can suppress the lipid peroxidation of biological membranes (Green, 1972; Milvy, 1973). Scientists are interested in knowing to what degree these antioxidant compounds can retard the aging phenomena.

Studies (Tappel, Fletcher, & Deamer, 1973) have indicated that the accumulation of peroxidized lipofuscin pigments in the central nervous system is interrelated with the aging of this organ in various rodents and dogs. Lipofuscin pigments accumulate in many organs during the aging process and have been determined to be in an abnormally conjugated and crosslinked state and exhibit fluorescence characteristics that can be duplicated by the peroxidation of polyunsaturated lipids. It has not yet been determined whether the accumulation of lipofuscin causes intracellular damage.

It is assumed that lipofuscin is a form of intracellular debris that cannot be metabolized (Gordon, 1974). Studies (Nandy, 1968) have indicated that lipofuscin is not an immutable end product. The injection of the drug Centrophenoxine into guinea pigs aged 6 months to 6 years reduced the disposition of lipofuscin that was accumulated in the guinea pig brain. Effects were noted after 12 weeks of treatment with Centrophenoxine.

These studies indicate that the accumulation of lipofuscin pigment during the aging process can be retarded and even reversed by chemical agents other than antioxidants. The reversal of lipofuscin disposition is an interesting finding and indicates that latent lipofuscin scavenging mechanisms may be activated that would favor the aging organism's life-span.

Another drug, Isoprinosine, has been observed to cause a reversal of lipofuscin pigments in the brains of aged rats. It was noted that Isoprinosine not only caused a partial reversal of the brain ribosomes and increased the brain function for certain learning tasks but also exerted an antiviral effect (Gordon, 1974). Investigation continues with this drug to explore the relationship between aging and viral infections.

Error Theory

The Error Theory hypothesizes that a mistranscription or mistranslation of certain gene products [messenger RNA (mRNA)], especially those coding for enzymes involved in DNA replication and in message transcription and translation, will result in self-amplifying error-producing derangements (Strehler, 1977). The initial error will, most likely, result in further errors of similar types, causing the production of faulty products of other genes which accumulate with aging. Studies that have indicated that enzymes with decreased catalytic activity and/or increased thermal lability accumulate in aging tissues are consistent with the theory. However, other studies tend to question the validity of the error catastrophe theory.

The Error Theory, along with the Somatic Mutation Theory, is not regarded to be as important today in the attempt to understand the aging process. However, both theories have stimulated much thought and question in the investigation and support of other theories regarding aging.

Wear and Tear Theory

The Wear and Tear Theory postulates that an organism "wears out" with use. The man–machine analogy has a long history and has provided a framework for investigating the aging phenomena.

Even though this theory has not been supported consistently by research, in the early 1900s it was observed that by increasing the environmental temperature of poikilothermic animals their life-span was significantly shortened (Loeb & Northrup, 1917). The underlying hypothesis was that an increase in metabolism in the animal accelerated the rate at which it would "wear out."

The man–machine analogy, however, does not take into account that the organism has two important characteristics that do not apply to machines: (1) the organism possesses intrinsic properties (mechanisms) for self-repair that a machine does not possess, and (2) the organism may be improved by use (Shock, 1974). The latter can be in, for example, a physical fitness program that results in increased muscle mass, strength, and cardiovascular function/output.

The Wear and Tear Theory should not be totally discarded, however, as it may be directly associated with other aging theories, for example, the Crosslinkage Theory, Programmed Aging Theory, and Cell Theory.

Autoimmune Theory

The Autoimmune Theory postulates that, with age, the immune system produces auto-antibodies that cause cell death or cell changes that foster the aging process (Walford, 1969). There is an association between age and production of auto-antibodies (Adler, 1974); however, there is no reliable evidence to link the causal relationship to the disease process in aging.

The immune system is the most important body defense against environmental insults. The cells that comprise the immune system produce antibodies that counteract the effect of nonidentifiable materials. The Autoimmune Theory speculates that with aging a defect occurs in the cellular immune system's tolerance, and the system manufactures auto-antibodies to one or more of its own tissues, which causes serious damage to the tissue (Strehler, 1977).

Adler (1974) proposed a series of viral infections to be the unifying event that accounts for a decreased cellular immune function, auto-antibody formation, age-related diseases, and the aging phenomena. He suggests that if the viral infected tissue is not subjected to the lymphocytes, it is attacked by antiviral antibodies or antitissue antibodies that manifest the auto-antibody phenomena. The combination of the virus and antibody results in immune complex disease, and the diseased tissue is not rejected. Repeated viral infections continue to cause normal tissue disease and the formation of tumors. With the decrease or absence of an effective cellular immune system, the tumors are allowed to grow. It is believed (Adler, 1974) that the results of infection, decreased immune function, immune complex disease, and carcinogenesis are all contributors of the Autoimmune Theory to the aging process.

PSYCHOSOCIAL THEORIES

Since the beginning of time there has been much interest in exploring the psychological and sociological aspects of the human organism. Psychologists have studied such areas as personality development, heredity, environmental influences, intelligence, memory, and psychogenic disorders. The sociologists, on the other hand, have devoted their research activities to attitudes, family structures, economic influences, cultural differences, organizations, political influences, and socioeconomic-class differences.

The psychological aspects of aging have centered on a variety of problems encountered with the aging phenomena. Psychologists have attempted to explore the effect of aging on needs and motives, the effect of prior experience in the aging process, the effect of age upon learning, the effect of age on psychomotor performance, the psychodynamics of the emotional life of the elderly, the role and importance of sensory changes in aging, the adjustment of the individual to the aging process, and the emotional needs of the elderly (Geist, 1968). All of these problem areas have been of particular interest to the psychologists who have studied behaviors and the aging process.

The study of the psychology of aging can be traced to the publication, in 1835, of Quetelet's book, *Sur l'Homme et le Developpement des ses Facultes* (Geist, 1968). Other, more objective studies of the psychology of aging followed. The personality theories that resulted from these studies conceptualized the aging process in different contexts. Some of the extant theories include Kretschmer's (1926) constitution theory and aging; Freud's (1904) psychoanalysis and aging; Erikson's (1959) epigenetic theory; Adler's (1971) individual psychology theory; Jung's (1971) theory of the aging process; Lewin's (1951) field theory; the organismic theory of Goldstein (1939) and Scheerer (1954) and Gelb (1929); the role theory of Havighurst and Albrecht (1953) and Tuckman and Lorge (1953); Hull's (1943) and Guthrie's (1935) learning theories and the aging process; communication theory and the aging process; materation–degeneration theory; transfer of training theory and aging; retroactive and proactive inhibition theory; and environmental theories.

Social gerontologists today have been unable to support a general theory of behavior in later years of life that accounts for the social structure of aging and cross-cultural variations in aging behavior. However, there are a variety of concepts that attempt to explain selected aspects of behavior and/or influences of social and cultural contexts in the determination of behavior in later years (Watson & Maxwell, 1977). As a result of these studies, concepts such as societal disengagement, individual disengagement, age grading, activity, and continuity have been identified, and theories in regard to each concept have been presented to assist in the prediction and understanding of behaviors that occur in later years of life.

The gerontological nurse practitioner must critically evaluate the psychosocial theories of aging that have evolved over the past centuries. These theories will provide a foundation for the nurse practitioner to consider when developing a practice framework. It is also imperative that the nurse practitioner have an understanding of these theories and apply them appropriately when caring for the elderly.

The following psychosocial theories are presented: Disengagement Theory, Activity Theory, Continuity Theory, and Social Exchange Theory. These theories are considered helpful in understanding behaviors of the elderly.

Disengagement Theory

A 5-year study by Cumming and Henry culminated in the development of the Disengagement Theory. The theory postulates that with aging there is "an inevitable mutual withdrawal of the individual from society and society from the individual resulting in decreased interaction between the aging person and others in the social systems he belongs to. The process may be initiated by the individual or by others in the situation" (Cumming & Henry, 1961, pp. 14–15).

From the Disengagement Theory the following premises are evident: (1) disengagement is a progressive gradual process; (2) disengagement is inevitable; (3) disengagement is a mutually satisfying process; (4) disengagement is universal to all social systems; and (5) disengagement is the norm (Gubrium, 1973). Cumming

and Henry have questioned these premises and each has provided different viewpoints regarding the Disengagement Theory.

Cumming believes that "disengagement frees the old to die without disrupting vital affairs," whereas, when a fully engaged middle-aged person dies, he leaves many broken ties and disrupted situations (Cumming, 1963, pp. 384–85). Cumming recognized that there are social roles that are "concerned with persistent values" and resist obsolescence because they focus on "timeless values." The acknowledgment of such social roles leaves room for possible lifelong engagement by the elderly. These roles are considered to be primarily socioemotional (Gubrium, 1973).

Henry (1965) revised the original Disengagement Theory. He questions both the evitability of disengagement and its intrinsic character. From the original cases in the Kansas City Study of Adult Life, he noted that signs of withdrawal do not appear for some persons well into old age. As for the intrinsic character, he argues that it depends on how biological the intrinsic nature of disengagement is taken to be. Henry (1965) places the Disengagement Theory in a progressive personality development framework. By taking a developmental approach to aging, he views social behavior as personally emergent over time, implying that whether or not a person disengages in old age is a product of lifelong development (Gubrium, 1973).

There have been recent studies (Kerns, 1980; Watson and Maxwell, 1977) that have challenged the Disengagement Theory of aging. In a study by Kerns (1980), the majority of elderly black Caribs refused to accept the inferior status positions that were assigned to them by the younger generation of their society. They were concerned about remaining active as long as possible and not becoming socially old. Three characteristics designated a member of the black Caribs as socially old. First, there was infertility or reproductive incapacity, that is, menopause in women and impotence in men. Second, there was permanent unemployment, which was viewed by Kerns (1980) to have two different sex-related roles that determined unemployment and old social age: (1) men who became physically disabled were usually permanently unemployed and designated socially old; and (2) women experienced sex discrimination in the labor market after the age of 50, which placed them as being socially older at an earlier chronological age. The third identity marker was their sensitivity to changes in physical appearance that commonly occur with advanced aging, i.e., graying of the hair and wrinkling of the skin (Watson, 1982).

A study by Watson and Maxwell (1977) suggested that there are cross-cultural variations in behavior associated with aging. Their findings indicated that black nurses and nursing assistants demonstrated increasing interaction and caregiving to older black patients who were identified as being severely impaired in mental and physical functioning. This, however, was not found to be the same for nurses caring for the aged Jewish patients that exhibited patterns of disengagement (Watson, 1982).

The outcomes of these recent studies clearly suggests that additional research is needed to explore the behavior of the engagement–disengagement continuum. Gerontological nurse practitioners have unlimited opportunities in the practice arena to collect data to further test the behaviors and characteristics of the Disengagement Theory. By doing so, they can test the postulates in relation to nursing interventions that may result in determining their significance for nursing practice and implications for further study.

The gerontological nurse practitioner must be aware of those clients who are experiencing disengagement and provide the necessary support/guidance required for maintaining a state of equilibrium. Because depression is a major psychological manifestation that commonly occurs with aging, the nurse practitioner must be observant of the signs and symptoms of depression and be able to differentiate depression and disengagement withdrawal.

Activity Theory

The Activity Theory was first recognized as a sociological approach to aging in the publication of *Personal Adjustment in Old Age* (Cavan, Burgess, Havighurst, & Goldhammer, 1949). Aging was conceived by these sociologists as a problem in the personal resolution of strains on self-conception resulting from changes in later life roles. They differentiated two types of conceptions: (1) the social structure aspects of growing old in American society; and (2) personal adjustment, especially the overt behavioral and psychological factors associated with role change (Gubrium, 1973).

The Activity Theory thus postulates that life satisfaction in later years occurs when individuals maintain an optimal level of social activity. Less active older persons were found to be less successful in coping with the demands of everyday life (Watson, 1982). The basic premise of the Activity Theory is that activity promotes well-being and life satisfaction.

The Activity Theory suggests that with aging new roles, new relationships, new hobbies, and new interests should replace those activities that are no longer a part of the individual's social structure.

The gerontological nurse practitioner must recognize those individuals who desire to maintain an active social role. It is the nurse practitioner's responsibility to assess the client's physical and psychological capabilities for the desired activities. The assessment should also include an appraisal of the client's interests, hobbies, and previous and current social activities. It is important to help the client select activities that are of interest, appropriate, and attainable. The client should be the one to select the activities, thus avoiding activities that are not desirable and/or viewed by the client as being degrading or a form of punishment. At times the nurse practitioner must direct the client toward activities that are considered therapeutic rather than simply recreational. It is imperative that the rationale for the therapeutic activity be thoroughly explained, with emphasis placed on the purpose, procedures, and expected outcomes of the activity.

Continuity Theory

The Continuity Theory (Atchley, 1977, 1983; Erickson, 1963; Frenkel-Brunswick, 1968; Neugarten, Havighurst, & Tobin, 1968; and Watson, 1980) is viewed as a manifestation of physiological, psychological, and interpersonal adjustments that the aging person makes in the context of the social and cultural constraints that condition or mold behavior in later years of life. The theory, therefore, postulates that as the individual matures into adulthood certain habits, characteristic traits, personal tastes and preferences, associations, and goals and commitments become a part of the personality. As people grow older, the Continuity Theory suggests that they tend to express through their personal and interpersonal adjustments those behaviors that were conducive to their ability to adjust to past life experiences (Watson, 1982). Given these conditions, the older person's personality does not usually change; there may be, however, conflict between "old ways" and "new demands" and as a result the "old ways" may become suppressed.

Older persons are usually not concerned with everyday demands or trends in living. Instead they are more involved with themselves and tend to display an increasing prominence of certain idiosyncrasies and personal tastes and preferences for action and selectivity in social relations, whether for amusement or assistance in problem solving (Watson, 1982).

The older person's personality behaviors, as viewed by Neugarten and Berkowitz (1964), may change with the aging process. The older person may experience a decrease in ego energy, ego style, and sex-role perception (Neugarten, 1964; Neugarten & Gutman, 1968). Men and women seem to switch roles, with the man assuming a more nurturing, tolerant role, and the woman displaying leadership and a more aggressive role.

The gerontological nurse practitioner's awareness of the Continuity Theory provides a means for understanding existing personality behaviors of the older person. The theory suggests that the nurse practitioner should attempt to assess the developmental and personality behaviors of the older client and plan nursing interventions that are realistic and appropriate for the client's adaptation to aging.

Social Exchange Theory

As one becomes old there is a decrease in social interaction. This assumption is supported by the Activity Theory and the Disengagement Theory. Social interactions primarily exist among individuals and groups because they are personally gratifying. The outcome of social exchange that is expressed as rewarding or self-gratifying usually carries with it a cost factor. Profits derived from social exchange are equal to reward minus cost (Dowd, 1975). The Social Exchange Theory postulates that social interaction between individuals and groups continues as long as everyone profits from the interaction. When there is no longer an equal profit from the social exchange, an imbalance occurs in the interaction and one individual is perceived as having more power than the other.

Power is defined as the ability of an individual or group to influence the actions or intentions of another, irrespective of the preferences for action among the members of the object class (Watson, 1982, p. 76). Historically positions of power were based on age and wisdom. For example, in ancient Greece only elderly and propertied men could belong to the Athenian congress and have voting power (Watson, 1982).

The decrease in social interaction of the aged is the result of exchange relationships/encounters that gradually erode the power of the aged. This usually occurs as the power resources (namely, health, relationships, and income) become diminished. When these power resources are no longer available, the older person has no alternative but to comply with society and the young. This results in an unbalanced exchange relationship. If the older person is unsuccessful in rebalancing the relationship, it is viewed as the expected norm for the situation (Dowd, 1975).

The gerontological nurse practitioner must view this theory as having implications for nursing practice. The nurse practitioner should identify the older person who is experiencing an imbalance in exchange relationships and/or dependency on others. A major goal for the nurse practitioner should be to assist the older person in regaining his or her power resources. During the rebalancing process the older person needs support and encouragement in the attempt to remain involved in previous and develop new exchange relationships.

The nurse practitioner must be aware of the nature of power and power structures in exchange relationships and assist/guide the older person in interpersonal and intergroup relations that are gratifying and provide a means to rebalance the exchange relationships. Examples of power resources in which the nurse practitioner might encourage the older person to become involved are continued group activities, joining new organizations, neighborhood activities, working in child day-care centers, foster grandparenting, political activities, and organizations that represent aging (Gray Panthers; National Caucus on the Black Aged).

THE ENVIRONMENT AND AGING

The elements in the environment have been considered by researchers to have an effect on the aging phenomenon. Biologists have considered the effects of the environment on the cellular structures of the human organism. For example, excessive exposure to the sun's radiation puts the skin at risk during the somatic mutation process. The cumulative effect of repeated exposure to the radiation most likely causes a disruption of the skin and disease. According to other theories (e.g., the Wear and Tear Theory), overexposure to the sun will cause the skin to age faster, be-

coming dry, thin, and wrinkled. According to Perlman (1954), human aging is a "disease syndrome" arising from a struggle between environmental stress and biological resistance and relative adaptation to the effects of stressor agents. These stressor agents might include air pollutants, chemicals, and psychological and sociological events.

Aging has also been associated with the declining ability to adapt to environmental stress. Selye (1970, 1976) suggests that the phenomenon of aging may be due to the cumulative effect of repeated exposure to stress conducive or irreversible "chemical scars" in organs.

The ecological model (Lawton & Nahemow, 1973) suggests that behavior is the product of the interaction between a person and the environment. Ecologists have provided information that should be considered when attempting to understand the interaction between the individual and the environment during the aging process.

SUMMARY

The biological, psychosocial, and environmental theories of aging have guided the research activities to explore the aging phenomenon. These theories have attempted to provide rationales for the physiological, biological, and psychosocial behavioral changes that occur with the aging process.

The biological theories discussed in this chapter have provided some insight into the aging phenomena and can serve as a stimulus to further questions for research on aging. Although the theories are provocative in nature, they have not provided any conclusive facts to answer the question, Why does one age? When this question is answered, the next question to be posed is, How can the aging process be slowed or altered?

The psychosocial theories discussed in this chapter provide a greater understanding of personality development and social interactions of the aged. From these theories, there is a stimulus for further inquiry to better understand the behaviors and social world of the aged.

The gerontological nurse practitioner must be knowledgeable of the theories of aging and critically evaluate each for their appropriateness for support of nursing interventions. Although some of these theories are abstract and nonconclusive, they do provide a foundation for the nurse practitioner in developing a theoretical framework for gerontological nursing. This should ultimately result in an understanding of aging and provide a means for nursing interventions that will promote the health, wellness, and self-gratification of the aged.

REFERENCES

Adler, A. (1971). *The practice and theory of individual psychology* (P. Radin, Trans.). New York: Humanities Press.

Adler, W. H. (1974). An "autoimmune" theory of aging. In M. Rockstein (Ed.), *Theoretical aspects of aging.* New York: Academic Press.

Atchley, R. C. (1977). *The social forces in later life: An introduction to social gerontology.* Belmont, CA: Wadsworth.

Atchley, R. C. (1983). *Aging, continuity and change.* Belmont, CA: Wadsworth.

Behnke, J. A., Finch, C. E., & Moment, G. B. (Eds.). (1978). *The biology of aging.* New York: Plenum.

Bjorksten, J. (1974). Crosslinkage and the aging process. In M. Rockstein (Ed.), *Theoretical aspects of aging.* New York: Academic Press.

Busse, E. W. (1971). Biologic and sociologic changes affecting adaptation in mid and late life. *Annals of Internal Medicine, 15*(7), 115–120.

Cavan, R. S., Burgess, E. W., Havighurst, R. J., & Goldhammer, H. (1949). *Personal adjustment in old age.* Chicago: Science Research Associates.

Collins, R. M. (1982). Toward a theory of gerontological nursing. *Nursing & Health Care, 3,* 550–556.

Cumming, E. (1963). Further thoughts on the theory of disengagement. *International Social Science Journal, 15,* 377–393.

Cumming, E., & Henry, H. (1961). *Growing old: The process of disengagement.* New York: Basic Books.

Decker, D. L. (1980). *Social gerontology: An introduction to the dynamics of aging.* Boston: Little, Brown.

Demopoulos, H. B. (1973). The basis of free radical pathology. *Federation of American Societies for Experimental Biology: Federation Proceedings, 32,* 1859–1861.

Dowd, J. J. (1975). Aging as exchange: A preface to theory. *Journal of Gerontology, 30,* 584–594.

Ebersole, P. & Hess, P. (1981). *Toward healthy aging: Human needs and nursing responses.* St. Louis: Mosby.

Erikson, E. H. (1959). *Identity and the life cycle.* New York: International Press.

Erikson, E. H. (1963). *Childhood and society.* New York: Norton.

Frenkel-Brunswik, E. (1968). Adjustments and reorientation in the course of the life span. In B. L. Neugarten (Ed.), *Middle age and aging: A reader in social psychology.* Chicago: University of Chicago Press.

Freud, S. (1904). *On psychotherapy—Collected papers. Vol. 1.* London: Hogarth Press.

Geist, H. (1968). *The psychological aspects of the aging process with sociological implications.* St. Louis: Warren H. Green.

Gelb, A. (1929). Die "Farbenkostanz" der Sehdinge. In *Handbuch der normalen und pathologischen Physiologic.* Reception-sorgane, II: Photoreceptoren, I Teil. Berlin: Springer-Verlag.

Goldstein, K. (1939). *The organism.* New York: American Book.

Gordon, P. (1974). Free radicals and the aging process. In M. Rockstein (Ed.), *Theoretical aspects of Aging.* New York: Academic Press.

Green, J. (1972). Vitamin E and the biological antioxidant theory. *Annals of New York Academy of Science, 203,* 29–44.

Gross, J. (1961). Collagen. *Scientific American, 204*(5), 121–130.

Gubrium, J. F. (1973). *The myth of the golden years.* Springfield, IL: Thomas.

Guthrie, E. R. (1935). *The psychology of learning.* New York: Harper & Row.

Havighurst, R. L., & Albrecht, R. (1953). *Older people.* New York: Longmans.

Havighurst, R. J., Neugarten, B. L., & Tobin, S. S. (1968). Disengagement and patterns of aging. In B.

L. Neugarten (Ed.), *Middle age and aging*. Chicago: University of Chicago Press.

Hayflick, L. (1968). Human cells and aging. *Scientific American, 218*(3), 32–37.

Hayflick, L. (1975). *Cell biology of aging*. *Bioscience, 25*, 629–637.

Henry, W. E. (1965). Engagement and disengagement: Toward a theory of adult development. In R. Kastenbaum (Ed.), *Contributions to the psychobiology of aging*. New York: Springer.

Hershey, D. (1974). *Lifespan and factors affecting it*. Springfield, IL: Thomas.

Hull, C. L. (1943). *Principles of behavior*. New York: Appleton-Century-Crofts.

Jung, C. (1971). The stages of life. In J. Campbell (Ed.), *The portable Jung, Hull, R.F.C.* New York: Viking Press.

Kerns, V. (1980). Aging and mutual support relations among the black Carib. In C. L. Fry (Ed.), *Aging in culture and society: Comparative viewpoints and strategies*. New York: Bergen.

Kretschmer, E. (1926). *Physique and character*. New Jersey: Harcourt, Brace & World.

Krohn, P. L. (1965). *Topics in the biology of aging*. New York: Wiley.

Lawton, M. P., & Nahemow, L. (1973). Ecology and the aging process. In C. Eisdorfer & M. P. Lawton (Eds.), *The psychology of adult development and aging*. Washington, DC: American Psychological Association.

Lewin, K. (1951). *Field theory in social sciences— Theoretical papers* (D. Cartwright, Ed.). New York: Harper.

Loeb, J., & Northrop, J. H. (1917). On the influence of food and temperature upon the duration of life. *Journal of Biological Chemistry, 32*, 103–121.

Maddox, G. L. (1970). Themes and issues in sociological theories of human aging. *Human Development, 13*, 17–27.

Milvy, P. (1973). Control of free radical mechanisms in nucleic acid systems: Studies in radioprotection and radiosensitization. *Federation of American Societies for Experimental Biology: Federation Proceedings, 32*, 1895–1902.

Nandy, K. (1968). Further studies on the effects of Centrophenoxine on the lipofuscin pigment in the neurons of senile guinea pigs. *Journal of Gerontology, 23*, 82–92.

Neugarten, B. L., & Berkowitz, H. (Eds.). (1964). *Personality in middle and late life*. New York: Atherton Press.

Neugarten, B. L. (1968). *Middle age and aging*. Chicago: University of Chicago Press.

Neugarten, B. L., & Gutmann, D. L. (1968). Age-sex roles and personality in middle age: A thematic apperception study. In B. L. Neugarten (Ed.), *Middle age and aging*. Chicago: University of Chicago Press.

Neugarten, B. L., Havighurst, R. J., & Tobin, S. S. (1968). Personality and patterns of aging. In B. L. Neugarten (Ed.), *Middle age and aging: A reader in social psychology*. Chicago: University of Chicago Press.

Osgood, C. E. (1953). *Method and theory in experimental psychology*. New York: Oxford University Press.

Perlman, R. M. (1954). The aging syndrome. *Journal of American Geriatrics Society, 2*, 123–219.

Pryor, W. A. (1973). Free radical reactions and their importance in biochemical systems. *Federation of American Societies for Experimental Biology: Federation Proceedings, 32*, 1862–1869.

Rockstein, M. (Ed.). (1974). *Theoretical aspects of aging*. New York: Academic Press.

Scheerer, M. (1954). Cognitive theory. In G. Lindzey (Ed.), *Handbook of social psychology*. Cambridge, MA: Addison-Wesley.

Selye, H. (1970). Stress and aging. *Journal of American Geriatrics Society, 18*, 669–680.

Seyle, H. (1976). *Stress in health and disease*. Boston: Butterworths.

Shock, N. W. (1962). The physiology of aging. *Scientific American, 206*(1), 100–110.

Shock, N. W. (1974). Physiological theories of aging. In M. Rockstein (Ed.), *Theoretical aspects of aging*. New York: Academic Press.

Sinex, F. M. (1974). The mutation theory of aging. In M. Rockstein (Ed.), *Theoretical aspects of aging*. New York: Academic Press.

Smith, D. W. (1973). *Biologic ages of man from conception through old age*. Philadelphia: Saunders.

Strehler, B. L. (1977). *Time, cells, and aging*. New York: Academic Press.

Tappel, A. L., Fletcher, B., & Deamer, D. (1973). Effects of antioxidants and nutrients on lipid peroxidation fluorescent products and aging parameters in the mouse. *Journal of Gerontology, 28*, 415–424.

Tuckman, J., & Lorge, I. (1953). Attitudes toward old people. *Journal of Social Psychology, 37,* 249–260.

Walford, L. (1969). *The immunologic theory of aging.* Baltimore, MD: Williams & Wilkins.

Watson, W. H. (1980). *Stress and old age: A case study of black aging and transplantation shock.* New Brunswick, NJ: Transaction Books.

Watson, W. H. (1982). *Aging and social behavior.* Monterey, CA: Wadsworth.

Watson, W. H. & Maxwell, R. J. (1977). *Human aging and dying: A study in sociocultural gerontology.* New York: St. Martin's Press.

Wilson, D. L. (1974). The programmed theory of aging. In M. Rockstein (Ed.), *Theoretical aspects of aging.* New York: Academic Press.

DRUG THERAPY IN THE ELDERLY

Physicians and nurses, as well as their elderly clients, are drug abusers. If this statement sounds dramatic and indicting, it is meant to be. The way the elderly are wittingly and unwittingly cajoled and coerced to ingest large quantities of drugs that have little or no effect on them because of physiological and biochemical limitations is a national disgrace. Ignorance of prescribing for the elderly, ignorance of proper administration, ignorance of drug interactions, insensitivity to the real reasons signs and symptoms of drug-related distress occur, and ignorance of what drugs can do to the body all lead to abuse of drugs.

While recognizing that drugs can be lifesaving and can add both longevity and a better quality of life for individuals, what is intolerable is such abuse of drugs that other drugs must be given to counteract the original drug's side effects or that cause the ingestors to function like zombies, chemically restraining them from participating in any of the activities of daily living. What is needed is drug therapy for the elderly that cures, restores, and rehabilitates, not drug prescriptions that restrain, mask, or cloud older persons' abilities to lead as full a life as they possibly can.

PRACTICES AND BELIEFS ABOUT DRUG THERAPY IN THE ELDERLY

The elevation of geriatric pharmacology to a specialty is a somewhat recent occurrence. In the past, elderly persons needing medication, e.g., for hypertension, received the same standardized dose the physician ordinarily ordered for any other age group. Only the diligent physician or nurse observer would suspect that a lesser drug dose or a change of drug was needed.

The cohort of our present elderly grew up in a time when it was expected that a medication would be given for each and every complaint presented to the doctor. Care was not deemed "good" unless the medication was given. Also, the elderly tended to have such implicit faith in their physicians that they did not dare to question the doctor's authority or refuse the prescription. Because many of the drugs masked the signs and symptoms of the discomfort or distress, often no attempt was made to seek the real etiology of the complaint. The medical model focused on how quickly patients could describe their complaints and be issued prescriptions to mask or alleviate their problems.

Nurses, adhering to their traditions, conscientiously administered drugs as ordered by the physician, never daring to question the orders and rarely observing patients for side effects or adverse interactions. If the patient complained, a medication was given, even though the nurse's therapeutic use of self and psychosomatic comfort measures might have obviated the need to administer a drug.

Some changes are finally beginning to occur. Within the last few years, texts on geriatric pharmacology have been written (Lamy, 1981; Goldberg & Roberts, 1983; and Simonson, 1984), numerous workshops on geriatric drug prescribing and drug interactions have been held, and drug manufacturers are being more explicit in warning about potential dangers of their drugs for the elderly. Further, numerous journal articles have been written describing the age-related changes that influence drug therapy in the elderly and identifying what is necessary to avoid adverse drug interactions. Armed with this knowledge, every nurse can serve as an advocate for the elderly for whom drugs are prescribed or suggested.

What makes drug therapy in the elderly so difficult are the changes that occur with aging. Further complicating the problem are intraindividual as well as interindividual differences of aging and health status changes. Therefore, although general principles of drug therapy must be known and followed, it should be recognized that each prescription for drug therapy for an older person is an experiment and must be monitored closely and accurately.

Drug therapy for older persons results from clinical competence and the conclusion that non-drug interventions are inappropriate or inadequate. Would the depressed older person benefit more from interventions to raise his self-esteem, e.g., new hair style and being taken to a restaurant for dinner, than from a tranquilizer that reduces his ability to function normally? Would the hypertensive patient benefit more from weight reduction, exercise, and a healthy diet than from expensive antihypertensive drugs? Would the older person with non-insulin dependent diabetes benefit more from a diet change and exercise program than from oral diabetic agents? These are the types of questions all primary care-givers must ask themselves when drug therapy is being contemplated. Also, the nonchemical modalities must be tried before the drugs are instituted. Chemicals should be a last resort when therapeutic use of self and clients' self-care assets fail.

The greater possibilities of drug interactions should also be recognized. The risk–benefit ratio should always be weighed before a drug is prescribed (Hussar, 1976). When a person can achieve the same results without chemical intervention, he or she should be encouraged to do so, especially if the drug in question is costly and would reduce the amount of funds available for necessities such as food and shelter.

Because older persons have multiple problems that affect their mental and somatic status, a careful health assessment must be done and the proper interventions performed before drugs are considered. For example, an 86-year-old woman complained of difficulty in falling asleep. A review of her diet pattern showed she was hypoglycemic at bedtime. A correction in her diet, giving her a protein drink in the evening, assisted her to return to her normal sleep pattern. Sleeping pills, which her physician had wanted to prescribe for her, were unnecessary.

GENERAL PRINCIPLES OF DRUG THERAPY IN THE ELDERLY

The decision to manage an older person's complaints with drugs should be based on a knowledge and appreciation of the pharmacokinetics of the chemicals being used. Overall, the effectiveness of any drug treatment depends upon the bioavailability of the right dosage at the site of action and the sensitivity of the target tissue to the drug (Williamson, 1980). Even though far more research is needed in the area of drug kinetics, there is a growing body of information in the areas of drug absorption, distribution, metabolism, excretion, sensitivity of target tissues, and variability of function in old age.

Absorption

Drugs that are absorbed from the gastrointestinal tract may be inhibited in their action due to reduced intestinal blood flow, delayed gastric emptying, and elevation of the gastric pH, all of which can affect the solubility and ionization of certain drugs. When more than one drug is given at the same time, the more (or most) active drug may accelerate or retard absorption of the other(s). For example, Pro-Banthine will increase the absorption of digoxin by increasing the length of time digoxin has contact with the absorbing surface (Williamson, 1980).

Medications, therefore, should be given in an easily absorbed state and without other drugs that can influence absorptive rates.

Distribution

An appropriate transport system is vital to proper distribution of a drug in the body. The elderly tend to drink less fluid, which increases the plasma concentration of drugs, e.g., digoxin plasma levels would rapidly rise. More importantly, the body of the older person tends to be deficient in lean mass with an increase in body fat. This is one reason that drug dosages cannot be calculated using body weight for older persons as they are for younger ones. Drugs that are highly lipid-soluble tend to accumulate in the body fat, which prolongs their period of action.

Protein-binding of drugs is also affected by age-related alterations in serum albumin levels. Because there are fewer places for drugs to bind, those drugs with the strongest affinity for binding sites will attach themselves to the protein molecules, thus causing weaker, but potentially dangerous, unbound drugs to float freely in the plasma, promoting their prolonged and potent actions. On the other hand, the free, active drug

might be excreted before it can act therapeutically. For example, aspirin is a strong binder and would displace warfarin if they were given together.

Metabolism

Breaking down drugs for therapeutic use and subsequent elimination requires a competent liver. However, age-related changes may produce a decline in the liver microsomal enzyme system and blood flow, thus inhibiting this metabolic process. There is a paucity of definite positive research findings to support the belief that a decrease in microsomal enzymes helps to cause drug toxicity in the elderly (Hollister, 1977). Nevertheless, any impairment in liver function has the potential to affect drug therapy in an older person.

Elimination

Ridding the body of most drugs also requires a competent renal system. However, the renal system of the elderly shows physiological decline. There is an approximate 50% loss of nephrons and a decrease in both glomerular and tubular filtration. Excretion through the renal system is further inhibited by the tendency of the elderly not to drink sufficient quantities of water. Any disease process or homeostatic alteration may also affect the kidneys and thus drug excretion. The effect on the renal system may be devastatingly abrupt. If drugs cannot be properly excreted, they can produce toxic effects in the older person. The drug given must be in smaller dosages and plasma drug levels, and overt signs and symptoms of side and toxic effects must be carefully monitored.

Sensitivity of Target Tissues

Persons who have never been sensitive or allergic to a drug before may suddenly find themselves showing increased sensitivity or a frankly allergic reaction to a drug. This is because older persons have more cell/tissue sensitivity to drugs such as barbiturates. There is a decrease in T cells and increased permeability of the blood–brain barrier. Drug dosages overall need to be smaller to avoid confusional, hypotensive, or toxic effects.

DRUG INTERACTIONS

As recently as 5 years ago, there was little emphasis on drug interactions for any age group, much less the elderly. Although a few common interactions were well known and publicized, not much was appreciated in the realm of the polypharmacy of the elderly as it related to their life-style, health beliefs, and food habits. Fortunately, there is now a great deal of interest being shown in drug interactions. The *Physicians' Desk Reference* (1984) is now specifically mentioning alterations in recommended dosages for the elderly, as well as certain possible side effects and interactions that could occur. More importantly, reference texts in geriatric pharmacology devote considerable space to the possible interactions of drugs in older persons' bodies.

It has been estimated that more than one fourth of the prescriptions written today are for persons over the age of 65 (Butler, 1975, p. 174). It has also been estimated that the elderly average more than 13 prescriptions per year (Lamy, 1977). If the older person took only three different medications per day, the potential drug interactions are estimated to be 77 million (Karsh & Karsh, 1978).

Because the number of drug interactions is legion, it is impossible for nurses to know at all times each interaction that could occur. Nurses have a legal and ethical duty to know the principles of drug interactions and the specific ones for drugs they are administering. Nurses must always be alert to the possibility of adverse effects of drug interactions. That is why each nurse

practitioner must always have drug information resources handy.

Hussar (1976) identified eight basic interactive mechanisms that will help nurses to recognize and understand drug interactions:

- *Similar Pharmacological Effects:* Interactions of these drugs may produce similar effects. For example, Lanoxin has a secondary diuretic effect, so that if it is given over a long period of time with a diazide, a low sodium syndrome could occur from the removal of too much sodium from the body.
- *Opposing Pharmacological Effects:* One physician may order a drug for one complaint and another physician may order a drug for another complaint, thus canceling out the effect of the first drug. For example, Coumadin (anticoagulant) may be ordered by a cardiologist while a barbiturate is ordered by an internist, with the latter drug decreasing the potency of the Coumadin.
- *Altered Gastrointestinal Absorption:* An older person may be taking a tetracycline and may also self-prescribe an antacid for heartburn, not realizing that antacids inhibit the absorption of tetracyclines (Friesen, 1983, p. 282).
- *Altered Metabolic Processes:* Certain drugs have the potential for inhibiting the metabolism of other drugs taken in combination. For example, overindulging in alcohol in a short period of time while taking an anticoagulant slows down the metabolism of the anticoagulant, thus prolonging the latter's blood thining effect. On the other hand, prolonged use of an alcohol-based cough syrup while taking an anticoagulant will speed up the rate at which the anticoagulant is metabolized (Larkin, 1978). When the cough syrup is finally stopped, the patient could experience a greater anticoagulant effect and hemorrhage.
- *Altered Urinary Excretion:* Certain drugs like probenecid (Benemid) may be given with penicillin in order to block the rapid tubular excre-

tion of the antibiotic in patients with rheumatic fever. Urinary pH influences the absorption and excretion of drugs because of their acidic or alkaline nature. For example, if an older person is taking ammonium chloride and is also taking aspirin (acetyl-salicylic acid), the effect of the aspirin will be longer, for more will be absorbed into the bloodstream. On the other hand, if the person had taken Alka-Seltzer and then the aspirin, the aspirin would not be absorbed as readily due to the alkalinity of the urine from the sodium bicarbonate in the Alka-Seltzer.

- *Altered Electrolyte Levels:* Certain drugs given in combination may alter the electrolyte balance of the client. As in the first example given above, sodium can be excreted in such large amounts that low sodium syndromes occur. If the client is taking lithium, toxicity can quickly occur if the sodium is depleted. Potassium is wasted in such large quantities by overzealous use of diuretics that cardiac function can be compromised. Drugs that cause vomiting as a side effect, e.g., barbiturates, may cause a chloride depletion.

- *Protein-Binding Site Displacement:* Serum albumin levels tend to be lower in the elderly (Hanan, 1978). If two or more drugs having high protein-binding affinity are given simultaneously, the ones with the most binding power will attach themselves to the limited binding site, leaving the other drugs to circulate in the blood to either act with full power or else be excreted. Either way, the client does not receive the desired mechanism of effect of the drug. Phenylbutazone (Butazolidin) is a stronger binder than warfarin, so if the two drugs are given together, the anticoagulant activity of the warfarin would be increased.

- *Interaction at the Adrenergic Neuron:* Drugs that break down catecholamines, especially norepinephrine, and cause the circulating levels of these catecholamines to increase, can result in a hypertensive crisis. Monamine ox-

idase inhibitors (MAO inhibitors) are one group of drugs that cause this adverse interaction. Tricyclic antidepressants have been reported to antagonize the antihypertensive effect of guanethidine (Hassas, 1976).

ALCOHOL AND DRUG THERAPY IN THE ELDERLY

Alcoholism is not uncommon in the elderly. If older persons drink alcohol and take other drugs at the same time, the potential for severe adverse drug interactions is great (Price & Andrews, 1982). Therefore, knowledge of the amount of alcohol the older person ingests must be a part of the drug history before any drug is prescribed or administered. Some common interactions include alcohol and aspirin. The double irritants to the gastric mucosa can cause bleeding, which may be serious due to the clotting inhibition of the aspirin. The taking of central nervous system (CNS) depressants along with alcohol (also a CNS depressant) can be lethal. If barbiturates are ingested along with alcohol, a paradoxical effect can occur, wherein the client complains of "climbing the wall." The use of other drugs (e.g., tolbutamide, ethacrynic acid) with alcohol causes the alcohol to be metabolized inappropriately or incompletely, producing most unpleasant reactions such as vomiting. Cardiac arrhythmias from low potassium can be produced from ingesting alcohol with digitalis. Pseudo-gout can be produced by the elevation of serum uric acid levels caused by certain diuretics. The client should avoid alcohol while taking these drugs, because alcohol also contributes to the rise in the serum uric acid levels. Older adults should be warned about alcohol content of tonics and syrups they buy over-the-counter, for adverse interactions can occur from this alcohol with any other drug they are taking. A good rule to follow is: If you are taking drugs, don't drink. If you drink, don't take any drugs. No drug can be safely taken if alcohol is ingested. Each person should be informed of this rule and urged to follow it.

DRUG–FOOD INTERACTIONS

One of the least appreciated parts of drug administration is the potential for adverse interaction between drugs and food. In fact, these interactions are so important that a nutritionist should be an active member of each drug therapy team. All nursing care plans should identify foods to be avoided when certain drugs are administered.

Lambert (1975) identified three categories of relationships between drugs and food: (1) drug-induced malabsorption of foods, (2) drug effects on nutritional status, and (3) alterations in drug response by nutrients.

Older adults with chronic disease may be on long-term drug therapy, which eventually interferes with the absorption of needed nutrients. Even when the dietary intake is considered adequate for recommended nutrients, deficiencies may occur. For example, antacids can cause thiamine deficiency, antibiotics and phenytoin (Dilantin) can reduce utilization of folic acid, vitamin B_{12}, calcium, and magnesium can inactivate pyridoxine. Colchicine can cause malabsorption of vitamin B_{12}, fat, and electrolytes. Diuretics have long been known for their potential to cause excess potassium loss. Drugs like naproxefen (Naproxyn) may cause diarrhea, which can result in food passing through the bowel too quickly to allow proper absorption.

Drugs can cause weight loss or weight gain, even though these were not the reasons for giving the drugs. Phenothiazines may improve the appetite so that the person eats more. Estrogens and steroid hormones may also cause weight gain. Methylphenidate (Ritalin) and such over-the-counter drugs as decongestants may act as appetite depressants, so that the older person eats less. Other drugs, like antibiotics and tranquilizers, may alter taste perception to the point

that food tastes so poorly that the person prefers not to eat. Loss of appetite may also be caused by the antacid aluminum hydroxide, as well as by digoxin, colchicine, clonidine, and methyldopa (Cerrato, 1987).

Decreases in various vitamins may be caused by foods. Vitamin K deficiency can develop due to bacteria in the gastrointestinal tract that synthesize it being killed by tetracycline. Absorption of fat-soluble vitamins can be hindered by laxatives containing mineral oil (Cerrato, 1987).

Foods may impair the solubility, ionization, and absorption of certain drugs. Food reduces the absorption of such antibiotics as tetracyclines and penicillin. That is why antibiotics should be given 1 to 2 hours before or after food intake. The absorption of acetominophen is inhibited when it is taken with high carbohydrate foods (Mollen, 1982). Ice cream interferes with the absorption of warfarin, so that the prothrombin time cannot be prolonged (Simon & Likes, 1978).

Food may cause complexation of the chemical elements in foods and drugs given together. For example, tetracycline-type antibiotics, if given with dairy products, almonds, sardines, or salmon, induce the calcium in these foods to precipitate the antibiotics so the calcium cannot be used (Graedon, 1982). Iron supplements should not be taken with tea due to the precipitate formed. Charcoal-broiled beef can lower the blood levels of theophylline, a bronchodilator used in asthma (Rodman, 1980).

Taking aspirin and orange juice for respiratory tract infections reduces the therapeutic effect of erythromycin and penicillin. The acidic nature of the aspirin and orange juice (which gives an alkaline ash later in its metabolism) tears away the protective coat of the antibiotic and causes it to be excreted too quickly for effective therapy. Milk and any alkaline foods will dissolve the enteric coating from Bisacodyl, causing profound gastric irritation. Urinary pH, if altered by excess ingestion of alkaline ash foods, can inhibit the excretion of quinidine, thus causing toxicity (Zinn, 1970).

The deaths reported from taking monoamine oxidase (MAO) inhibitors were really the result of the drugs' interactions with foods containing tyramine, e.g., pickled herring, cheese, Chianti wine, and chicken livers (Bauwens & Clemmons, 1978). Licorice has been implicated in hypertensive crisis, due to its ability to cause severe hypokalemia. Monosodium glutamate, a taste enhancer in foods, may cause hyponatremia, a real hazard if the person is already taking diuretics.

Persons on replacement thyroid therapy should avoid foods containing the goitrogenic agent thio-oxazolidine. Foods containing this agent are cabbage, brussel sprouts, cauliflower, kale, turnips, and rutabaga. Foods high in vitamin K like citrus fruits, egg yolks, vegetable oil, potato chips, and green leafy vegetables, may increase prothrombin time (Bauwens & Clemmons, 1978). Griseofulvin is more completely absorbed if taken with a fatty meal. Levodopa has a reduced therapeutic effect if taken with foods high in pyroxidine, e.g., muscle meat, whole grain cereals, fish, and vegetables.

There are some steps nurse practitioners can take to help prevent adverse drug–food interactions:

- Know the usual drug–food interactions for the drugs that you give. These data can be kept in a handy drug file at your work station, noted in your drug reference books, added to the computer drug data, and listed in standard nursing care plans.
- Be active on a committee on drug interactions where a pharmacist and nutritionist are also active members; exchange of information can help prevent nontherapeutic drug–food events.
- Read labels and inserts of all medications. Instruct clients to do the same. Warn clients to inform their nurse practitioners or physicians of any known adverse drug–food interactions.

- Teach clients to ask their physicians about drug–food interactions when a drug is being prescribed for them. Teach them to ask their pharmacist about drug–food interactions when the prescription is being filled.
- Include the drug–food adverse interactions in the nursing care plan and inform the staff, the client, and anyone staying with clients what foods or drugs to avoid. Check menus and trays for offending foods.
- Be assertive as a concerned, ethical professional when discussing drug–food interactions with the physician, the nutritionist, and the pharmacist.

DRUG–FOOD–LABORATORY VALUES INTERACTIONS

There is a growing knowledge about the effects of foods and drugs on laboratory test values. Not only are patients required to fast for a certain number of hours before blood and urine tests, they should also discontinue certain foods and drugs before testing.

Excessive laxative use may inhibit the absorption of calcium, so calcium values may be low. Vitamin C in large doses may lower the urine glucose output, giving false negatives. Thiazide diuretics may elevate the serum glucose and the uric acid, leading to the false conclusion that the person has diabetes or gout. Fish and other seafoods may give false thyroid function values.

Cigarettes and caffeine may interact with drugs and lead to problems. Caffeine is found in chocolate and many soft drinks, as well as in coffee and tea. It can decrease iron absorption and should, therefore, not be taken at the same time iron is being administered. Gastrointestinal irritation can be increased by caffeine, which also opposes the action of cimetidine. Conversely, estrogen and cimetidine can prolong the half-life of caffeine, leading to insomnia. Caffeine further has a mild hypertensive effect, can cause hypokalemia and contributes to anxiety (Todd, 1987).

Nicotine is known as a CNS stimulant and vasoconstrictor. Many drug dosages need to be adjusted for smokers. Serum levels of aminophylline and theophylline are greatly decreased by smoking, which also shortens the half-life of heparin. Peripheral ischemia that can occur with beta blocker drugs is aggravated by smoking. Insulin dosage must be increased for heavy smokers. Finally, increased fluid retention and lessened effectiveness of diuretics may be due to stimulation by nicotine of antidiuretic hormone secretion (Todd, 1987).

SELF-INDUCED DRUG INTERACTIONS

Very often older clients are accessories to the problems that arise from adverse drug interactions. They may buy over-the-counter drugs to counteract the effects of minor illnesses while they are taking prescription drugs. They may borrow or accept drugs from friends and family without any concern for the adverse interactions that could occur. They may eat indiscriminately or not at all, and yet take medications as prescribed, with resultant adverse effects.

Nurse practitioners can help their clients, especially their older ones, to take medications more wisely. Here are a few tips.

- If you are in an ambulatory setting, have your clients bring all their medications (prescription, over-the-counter, and homemade) with them on each visit. In this way, you can check on how much drug is being taken, the condition of the drugs and containers, and the expiration dates.
- Have your clients make drug profiles and use them for drug counseling (Alford & Moll, 1982). Specifically ask about any adverse interactions.
- If in an institutionalized setting, use nursing measures of prevention, health promotion,

comfort, and psychological support before asking that drugs be ordered.
- Discuss drug interactions and their danger with staff and colleagues and encourage all to make the effort to reduce drug-induced problems. Hold periodic drug reviews of patients.
- Warn clients, families, and friends against using any drug not specifically ordered by the physician.
- Encourage the stoppage of drugs when they are no longer needed.
- Have a heathly respect for any drug, especially when it is being used for the elderly. Although we know a great deal about drug therapy in this age group, much remains unknown.

DRUG ADMINISTRATION

One area of drug therapy for the elderly that remains poorly understood and poorly appreciated is the area of drug administration, especially the time at which the medications should be given. The ambiguity of prescriptions that read qid and HS, take with meals, prn arthritic pain, or qAM can no longer be condoned as safe or even therapeutic.* The practice of giving medications at "routine" times is also to be deplored when current knowledge of geriatric pharmacology has proven the danger and inefficacy of such practice. The nonadherence to the principles of drug administration every nurse learns in fundamentals of nursing is totally unprofessional and legally hazardous.

If nurses are going to administer drugs to the elderly, then the following facts and principles must be utilized.

The physician's order must be legal. The name of the drug, the route of administration, the dosage, and the times it is to be administered must be contained in the order. Of course, the order must be signed by the physician. If any parts of the prescription are missing, the order is

---

*Abbreviations: qid = four times daily; HS = hour of sleep; prn = when required.

then considered illegal. The nurse will then have to ask the physician for additional information. The name of the drug may be either its generic or its proprietary name. The route of administration must be not only its most efficacious route, but one that the older person can utilize. For example, Terramycin is best given intramuscularly rather than by mouth.

The dosage of the drug should be explicitly stated, e.g., 500 mg, 5.0 cc, $\frac{1}{6}$ gr, rather than tab ii or tsp 1, except where compounds are not identified by dosage. Because many drugs come in different dosages, simply identifying the number of tablets to administer may not provide the older person with the amount of drug prescribed or needed. The prescription should state whether the drug is a tablet, a capsule, liquid, etc.

More than any other part of the prescription, the time of administration is the most ambiguous. If a drug is ordered with meals, then the drug must be given at that time. However if the older person eats only two meals a day and one of those is tea and toast, is this an appropriate order? If the person is on continuous drip tube feedings, when should medication be given? If the older person eats six small feedings per day, should medication be given with each of the feedings? Rather than say "at meals," the prescription should say "take with food," or "with full meal."

The order of qid and HS is equally ambiguous. If the older person naps at midmorning and midafternoon, is that not "bedtime?" What about the older person who goes to bed at 9:00 PM and gets up at midnight for a few hours? When he or she is ready to go back to bed, is that not HS? Could this older person not become overmedicated with an order like this? This is a not infrequent occurrence when older persons are forced to place their own interpretation upon prescriptions that are not clearly written.

Is not—in its strictest sense—a nurse's obligation to give drugs as ordered? Definite hours of administration of drugs should be established, so that drugs are spaced out enough to be effective and to take advantage of limited binding

sites. The scheduling of drug administration is an area nurses need to research thoroughly.

Drugs ordered prn pose another problem in administration. How frequently should a prn medication be safely given? What should be the maximum dosage that can be safely given? What should be the maximum dosage that can be safely taken in a 12–24-hour period? If pain is continuous, then how is the appropriate determination made for the administration of the prn drug? Can the drug be safely given at meals or with other drugs? As yet, we have no standards to go by to answer these questions. However, a schedule that takes into account the times prn drugs can generally be administered should be included in the drug therapy plan.

Drug orders qAM may be taken any time between 12:01 AM and 12 noon, if one is to follow this prescription. Because many older persons may have several periods of sleep/wakefulness over the 24-hour cycle, they may elect—with all honesty—to take that particular medication at 3:00 AM or 11:30 AM. They may even elect to take it with other medications, thus creating a hazardous polypharmacy. One elderly woman with Parkinson's disease took her prescribed bid Sinemet at 1:30 PM and 6:00 PM. She could not understand why she was so weak and listless in the mornings. When she was helped to change her schedule to 8:00 AM and 8:00 PM, she felt much better and was able to return to normal activities.

When giving medications to the elderly, the nurse must know when each drug is best given, e.g., half an hour before meals, 2 hours postprandial, q6h, qid, at specific times, etc. Also to be taken into account is what other drugs are being given, what foods are being eaten, and what the activity level and stresses of the individual are. This means that, for every drug that is ordered, a drug schedule must be made for the administration of the particular drug at the times that have been determined pharmacokinetically. No longer can there be routine drug administration times. Dietary services will also have to be notified of foods to make available at the time of drug administration or foods to avoid giving the older person because of his or her drug therapy.

Some other principles of drug administration that apply to the older adult are that drugs should never be crushed if this can be avoided. Often liquid forms of the drug are available and can be used if the older person cannot swallow pills. No enteric coated tablets should ever be crushed. Care should also be taken with the food chosen as a vehicle for administering medications. For example, ice cream may interfere with antibiotics. If at all possible, try to have medications the older person cannot take discontinued, using nursing measures, instead, to relieve pain, anxiety, malaise, etc.

No nurse should ever give medications to someone who is not appropriately identified. The belief that the wearing of identification by older institutionalized elderly is degrading is a poor excuse for safety. There are many ways to identify the person. Identification (ID) bracelets and neck medallions can be worn as part of one's jewelry accessories. The residents of nursing homes, for example, in their activity programs, can make bracelets, pendants, barrettes, pins, and sewn-on identification information. The residents' full names, date of birth, and Social Security numbers should appear on the ID accessory. Before any drug is administered, patients should be asked to tell you their full name as you check it against the medicine card. If they do not give their correct name or if they are unable to comply with the nurse's request, then their ID accessory must be compared with the medication card. Do not presume to know who patients are regardless of how often you have administered the medication to them in the past.

The use of a book of photographs is not a valid means of identifying older persons, as their appearance can change quickly with pathophysiological processes. Often, the photographs are dated, or of poor quality, and sometimes the names do not match the photographs. The only safe ID nurses have at the present time is the continuously worn jewelry.

Before giving any medication to the elderly, the professional nurse should evaluate the effect of prior medication, e.g., has the cough lessened, have rales disappeared, is the blood pressure beginning to stabilize, is a diuretic effect present? The nurse should also observe for adverse effects (e.g., rash, tremors) and side effects (e.g., nausea, diarrhea). In this way nurses closely monitor the drug therapy they are administering and can make intelligent decisions as to whether to question the prudence of continued therapy.

When administering medications to older persons, be sure they are seated in an erect position, or have them stand. Remember, the presbyesophagus tends to be poorly supported and is less motile, so any help to gravity is necessary. Nurses may need to assist older persons to take medications by holding the cup of pills, placing each pill in their mouths, and assisting them to drink enough fluid (water preferably) with the medication. Encourage the intake of at least 3–4 ounces with each pill swallowed. If fluid intake is insufficient, the pill can become stuck in the esophagus, resulting in erosion and possibly bleeding. The more pills older persons take, the longer it will take to administer them and the more energy-depleting the experience will be for them. This is another reason to encourage a decrease in the amount of medication given older patients.

After the drug dosage is administered, nurses should make older persons comfortable, see that they have sufficient water at their bedsides, and that their call light is within easy reach. Nurses should make follow-up observations of patients 30–40 minutes after the drug dosage has been administered to determine if any adverse effects have occurred, so immediate steps can be taken to avert serious consequences.

It is not enough to simply document that a drug was given. The nurses' notes should reflect the status of the patient in regard to the drug therapy, including the effect of the drug by the parameters of efficacy, side or adverse effects (and if present, what was done about them), and any difficulties in the patient's ability to take the drug. A drug flowsheet identifying the data to be obtained and observations made could be used to synthesize this information.

Serum drug levels should be closely monitored in several situations. These include drugs in which the metabolism varies greatly, e.g., theophylline, and when saturation occurs. Other reasons are for drugs in which the therapeutic level is very close to the toxic level or when signs of toxicity are hard to recognize, as in the case of quinidine. Gastrointestinal, hepatic, or renal disease also necessitates serum drug level checks, as does the need to monitor drug interactions (Corbett, 1987).

DRUG INTERVENTIONS

This section discusses some of the concerns, hazards, and methods of administering various selected categories of drugs commonly used for the elderly. The reader is referred to the specific drug literature for details of the pharmacokinetics of chemical therapeutic agents.

In nursing, all practitioners are required to know the cause and effects of any drug they administer. Nurses are required to take the appropriate action if any adverse effect is suspected or observed.

Psychotropic Drugs

One group of drugs overused in treating older persons for functional and affective disorders is the psychotropic group, mainly the phenothiazines and monamine oxidase (MAO) inhibitors. Foerst (1979) reports that, in a survey of skilled nursing facilities, tranquilizers were the third most frequently prescribed drugs, and sedatives/hypnotics were the fifth most frequently prescribed drugs. Eisdorfer (1975) reports that psychotropic agents comprise a major proportion of all drugs prescribed in this country. Ray, Federspiel, and Schaffner (1980), in a study of 5902 Medicaid recipients in Tennessee nursing homes, found that 74% of residents had one or more central nervous system drugs prescribed for them.

The phenothiazine group of drugs has been termed chemical restrainers for the psychotic older person. Because these drugs are cholinergic blocking agents, the older recipient may experience the side effects of anticholinergic agents—dry mouth, blurred vision, urinary retention, and constipation. Imagine the problem the older person would have if he or she were on a quick-acting diuretic! Nursing staffs would also be quick to ask that the physician prescribe a laxative for these clients, perhaps causing markedly severe adverse interactions with other drugs prescribed. Phenothiazines may also interfere with glaucoma therapy because of their anticholinergic effects. Cardiac arrhythmias and hypotension can also occur. Seborrheic dermatitis has also been reported as a side effect of the phenothiazines (Duvic, 1983).

The neurotoxic effects of these drugs may produce severe agitation and confusion, for which there is a tendency to increase the dosage rather than decrease it. The worst side effect of the use of phenothiazines in the elderly is the sometimes irreversible extrapyramidal manifestations of tardive dyskinesia. Muscle tremors, rigidity, spasms, extreme restlessness, and bizarre facial and tongue movements characterize this disorder. The tragedy here is that there is a tendency to prescribe drugs for the effects of the primary drugs, i.e., treating the drug therapy to minimize the iatrogenic effects.

Antidepressant drugs may cause a paradoxical effect or further depress the person, as well as cause cardiovascular crises, Parkinson-like tremors, and confusion. The tricyclic antidepressants may take 1–2 weeks before they show any therapeutic effect; there is a danger of drug overdose if drug administration is increased in order to produce an effect. Older persons with bipolar depressions may be taking lithium carbonate, which can quickly cause toxicity, especially when there is poor renal clearance. Nurses must have and follow detailed nursing care plans for all patients taking lithium, so dangerous toxic effects can be prevented.

Some health professionals still advocate the use of barbiturates for the elderly, but it is good to see others finally concluding that barbiturates have little or no place in the geriatric drug armamentarium (Bachinsky, 1978; Fletcher, 1980). It is this author's opinion that barbiturates have absolutely no place in geriatric drug therapy because they are habituating, tend to cause severe paradoxical reactions, inhibit respiration, inhibit the person's daily functioning, and are accumulative in the body.

Drugs to induce sleep are also overprescribed, and should never be used unless a complete sleep history has been taken and less drastic sleep-inducing measures have been tried and failed (Fletcher, 1980). Older persons can be taught to cope with age-related changes in sleep cycles, and they can benefit from the sleep-inducing professional care and comfort measures of nurses.

Psychotropic drugs, if they must be given, should be administered in as small a dose as possible. More is not better; more may be fatal. These drugs should be discontinued as soon as possible to prevent accumulative side effects.

Cardiac Glycosides

Cardiac glycosides, especially digoxin, are among the most commonly prescribed drugs for the elderly. The potential of these drugs for severe interactions and toxicity is not always appreciated by health professionals. Effective transport and renal systems are crucial to the proper utilization and excretion of the cardiac glycosides, and yet the older person may have a decreased fluid intake, may be forcefully losing fluids from use of diuretics, and may have re-

duced renal function as a normal aging phenomenon. The expected 36-hour half-life of digoxin, for example, may be prolonged excessively in older persons with reduced creatinine clearance (Roffman, 1984). Special care must be taken when giving both loading and maintenance doses of digoxin, as overdoses can easily occur. Nurses have the responsibility for closely monitoring older persons on loading and maintenance doses of this cardiac glycoside. Nurses need to look for confusional states, anorexia (sometimes with nausea and vomiting), and changes in color vision (especially blue and yellow), visual acuity, cardiac rhythm, or any other abnormal patterns. If such adverse effects occur, a digoxin blood level should be determined. The physician may need to adjust the dosage of the drug.

Nurses often become too complacent in administration of maintenance doses of digoxin. Often a medication aide or technician gives the drug day after day with no notation in the nurses' notes ever occurring about the client's response to the drug. These aides are even to take the pulse, usually counted for 15 seconds at the radial artery, before giving the drug. This is often false information. A professional nurse should assess the apical rate and rhythm as well as other characteristics of the heart.

Elderly persons on maintenance dosages of cardiac glycosides need careful monitoring for any change in their daily behaviors or activities that may affect their drug therapy. For example, if they decrease their fluid intake or have a kidney infection, they may readily show toxic manifestations of the drug.

The older the person is, the more likely will be the tendency to retain digoxin in the body. For example, the serum half-life of digoxin in persons who are 80 years and older was found to be 70 hours (Cusack, 1979). This is why digitoxin, which is not dependent on renal function, may be more appropriate for older persons (Johnson, 1983).

Moreover, digoxin loading doses must be

carefully tailored to the individual in relation to the glomerular filtration rate, creatinine clearance, and lean body mass. Appropriately loading an older person on digoxin may take 2 weeks or longer.

Other possible reasons for the high digoxin toxicity rate in the elderly include age-related cardioneural end organ sensitivity to digitalis toxicity, hypokalemia from prolonged use of diuretics, frequent medication errors involving digoxin, a decreased effectiveness of the microsomal system of the liver to clear the drug from the body, the use of quinidine with digoxin, thus inhibiting the renal–nonrenal clearance of digoxin from the body, and the displacement of digoxin by quinidine at binding sites.

In addition to being aware of the above causes of digoxin toxicity, the nurse caring for the elderly on this drug must be continually alert for signs and symptoms of digoxin toxicity. The task is not easy, for the complaints are often the usual ones found in this age group. Confusion is often the first presenting sign of toxicity (Moser, 1982). Anorexia is also one of the prime indicators of toxicity. Older persons taking digoxin whose appetites suddenly diminish need to be investigated for drug toxicity. Visual changes, including spots, blurring, and misperception of color, may also be offered as complaints. A decreasing pulse rate may also warn of digoxin toxicity; therefore, accurate graphs of apical rates taken by the professional nurse practitioner should be kept. Data on the quality of the cardiac rhythm should also be noted.

Although digoxin remains a valid medical therapeutic entity for such conditions as atrial fibrillation and left ventricular failure, there is growing evidence (Vestal, 1982; Stults, 1982) that, once these patients' hearts have returned to a stable normal sinus rhythm, digoxin may no longer be needed. If close monitoring shows the patient to have appropriate cardiac function, then the drug need not be resumed. With the discontinuation of the therapeutic regimen, the potential for drug toxicity is eliminated.

Diuretics

Diuretics are extremely important drugs in the treatment of heart failure and hypertension; however, they are another overly prescribed group of drugs for older persons. Requarth (1979) found that diuretics were the second most commonly used drug group in a study of medication records in two long-term care facilities. Brown, Boosinger, Henderson, Rife, Rustia, Taylor, & Young (1977) found that the most frequent adverse drug–drug interaction in patients in a study of drug prescribing in 20 nursing homes was between digitalis and diuretics. The potassium-depleting effects of diuretics (even when potassium supplements are given) can cause cardiac arrhythmias to the point of fatality.

Besides their effect on the heart, thiazide diuretics also have a hypotensive activity and can potentiate nondiuretic antihypertensive agents. Because they affect electrolyte reabsorption in the renal tubules, sodium and chlorides are more readily excreted, with a concomitant loss of potassium and bicarbonate (Hutchins, 1981).

Potassium-sparing diuretics, such as spironolactone (Aldactone), are useful for older persons with gout and diabetes mellitus. Loop diuretics, such as furosemide (Lasix) are potent diuretics that should be used with caution and yet are prescribed freely. They do have an advantage for older persons in that they effect great diuresis without significantly affecting renal blood flow or glomerular filtration (Hutchins, 1981).

In addition to causing digitalis toxicity, diuretics have the potential for causing swift lithium toxicity. Laxative use at the same time diuretics are taken produces potassium depletion signs and symptoms. Thiazide diuretics may cause hyperglycemia, glucose intolerance (Gottleib & Chidsey, 1976), and symptoms of gout (McFarland & Carr, 1977).

Diuretics can cause severe psychosocial problems for the elderly. Fast-acting diuretics may cause bladder overflow so that the older person is unable to reach the toilet in time. They are then labeled incontinent, which is socially stressful. They may decrease socialization because they are afraid that they will have an "accident," are embarrassed by their incontinence, or afraid restroom facilities will not be available if they venture out. If they must go out they will have a tendency to omit medication and then not start it again until their condition points to the omission. Some older individuals may vary the time of day they take the diuretic, thus ingesting too much too close together. A potassium depletion syndrome could ensue.

Antihypertensives

Nurses should have as one of their goals the reduction of blood pressure in older adults. By helping all older adults to maintain their optimal weight, reduce salt, fats, and cholesterol from the diet, engage in an exercise program, and reduce stress, the mild or moderately elevated blood pressure of many older adults can be reduced to within normal limits. Actually this health promotion should be tried before any drug therapy is initiated (Becker & Warshaw, 1983). A blood pressure taken only once is not reliable. Repeated blood pressure readings taken at random are needed to establish a more valid picture of the range of the client's blood pressure in response to life events. A blood pressure taken in a physician's office, for example, may result in a false reading from the "White Coat Syndrome."

If the older person is unable or unwilling to practice positive health habits, then drug therapy should be carefully considered. Those elderly clients with consistently and markedly elevated blood pressure should definitely be placed on drug therapy.

Because of their potential for causing orthostatic hypotension (methyldopa, clonidine, guanethidine), depression (reserpine), impotence (methyldopa, guanethidine), gynecomastia (methyldopa), bradycardia (propranolol), antihypertensive agents should be used with ex-

treme caution in the elderly (Hammond & Kirkendall, 1979; Lowenthal & Swartz, 1985). Because so many elderly are taking medications for other conditions, the potential for adverse drug interactions is great, e.g., sympathomimetics may raise the blood pressure, nonsteroidal anti-inflammatory drugs may cause sodium retention, and so on. The clients' other diseases and conditions themselves can affect the efficacy of antihypertensive drugs. For example, beta blockers should be avoided or used with caution in older persons with congestive heart failure, diabetes mellitus, or chronic obstructive pulmonary disease (COPD); diuretics affect gout and diabetes mellitus, and hydralazine affects coronary artery disease and tremor conditions (Becker & Warshaw, 1983). If the client's blood pressure remains stabilized within normal limits for at least 6 months, and he or she has been practicing positive habits to lower blood pressure, efforts can be made to begin to reduce medication (Freis, Levinson, & Khatri, 1982). Drugs should not be stopped abruptly, but rather, reduced stepwise. Nurses may need to encourage physicians to begin the decrease in drug therapy.

Nurse practitioners caring for elderly hypertensive clients should learn how to take accurate blood pressure readings with calibrated equipment. The blood pressure needs to be monitored in both arms and in the lying, sitting, and standing positions as recommended in the drug literature. The emotional/activity state of the client should also be considered. Other facets of monitoring the client taking antihypertensives include observing for shortness of breath, dizziness, blurred vision, and edema. Therefore, the monitoring of hypertensive clients receiving drug therapy should be a professional function and not one delegated to aides.

Beta-Blockers

Beta-blockers, especially propranolol (Inderal), are frequently prescribed for older adults for a variety of conditions, e.g., hypertension, angina pectoris, cardiac arrhythmias, hypertrophic car-diomyopathy, post–myocardial infarction, glau-coma, and migraine prophylaxis (Johnson & Johanson, 1983). Beta-blockers block stimuli medicated by beta-receptors, i.e., they com-petitively inhibit catecholamine binding at beta-receptor sites (Johnson & Johanson, 1983). Be-cause of the effects of age on the autonomic nervous system and consequently on drug phar-macokinetics, nurses need to be aware of the potential problems that could occur in older adults taking such agents.

The elderly have higher plasma propranolol levels than younger persons, possibly due to hepatic extraction and metabolism. Vestal (1982) believes the threshold for maximum hepatic extraction may be age-related. He goes on to say that it is "more likely that the elderly are predisposed to toxicity because of more ex-tensive cardiovascular disease, diminished renal function with azotemia, and use of multiple car-diovascular drug therapy."

Beta-blockers may cause glucose intol-erance, and both hypoglycemia and hyper-glycemia are seen. Therefore, one should be extremely cautious when administering these drugs to elderly diabetics, especially those on insulin or sulfonylurea therapy. By inhibiting the breakdown of lipids, beta-blockers may in-crease the levels of circulating free acids or tri-glycerides and reduce the levels of low-density lipoproteins (Johnson & Johanson, 1983). The older adult taking beta-blockers will need to be monitored closely, both by observation of status and response and through laboratory studies such as blood glucose, triglycerides, and LDH levels.

Beta-blockers should be used cautiously in older persons in left ventricular dysfunction or failure, because they inhibit normal compen-satory response to such conditions. Because sinus node activity is depressed by these drugs, bradycardia will ensue, thus causing the fast pulse rate indicative of hypoglycemia or in-creased thyroid function. Beta-blockers can also cause bronchospasm, which is especially seen in persons with COPD. Wheezing is often the indi-cator that the drug must be discontinued.

Calcium-Channel Blockers

A class of drugs newer than beta-blockers are the calcium-channel blockers. These drugs (e.g., Nifedipine, Verapamil, and Diltiazem) hold promise for drug therapy in the elderly. These drugs inhibit the flow of calcium along the slow calcium channels, causing a reduction in myo-cardial oxygen demand. Coronary arteries are thus dilated, reversing coronary artery spasm. Calcium-channel blockers may even be more ef-fective than the nitrates and beta-blockers in re-lief of anginal pain (Butler & Harrison, 1983; Somani & Mayhew, 1985).

Because one of the potential adverse reac-tions to these drugs is hypotension, good base-line data on the older person's blood pressure should be known before the drug is adminis-tered. This means that the blood pressure should be taken in the lying, sitting, and standing posi-tions in both arms on a random basis over a period of several days. When the first dosage of the calcium-channel blocker is given, Butler and Harrison (1983) recommend monitoring the blood pressure at least every 30 minutes for the first 2 or 3 hours. If the drug being administered is Verapamil, the rate must also be monitored, for this particular drug has been known to cause bradycardia, heart block, and arrest.

Older patients receiving calcium-channel blockers will require close monitoring as a gen-eral part of the nursing interventions because age-related changes in hepatic or renal function will inhibit the metabolism and excretion of the drugs, thus causing hyperaction or a toxic reac-tion. These drugs should also be administered to older persons in smaller amounts than the usual dosage recommended.

Verapamil taken with quinidine will in-crease the possibility of hypotension; if taken with digitalis, it will increase the possibility of digitalis toxicity. Serum digoxin levels must be monitored closely. The nurse must also be cognizant of the signs and symptoms of hypotension and digitalis toxicity and must be vigilant for their appearance in older clients.

Nonsteroidal Anti-Inflammatory Drugs

Good old aspirin remains the most effective and most frequently used nonsteroidal anti-inflammatory drug (NSAID). Several other NSAIDs have since appeared, but none are reported to be superior to aspirin. All of the newer NSAIDs inhibit prostaglandin synthesis (Baum, 1979). It has been discovered that the individual arthritic patient may need to use several of these agents to achieve benefits from them. For example, ibuprofen (Motrin) may be given initially, and when its effectiveness wanes, naproxen (Naprosyn) may then be tried, and so on. If, on the other hand, there is little or no response from one drug within 2 or 3 weeks, then another drug should be given a trial.

As a group, the elderly are great users of the NSAIDs, but these drugs should not be given to anyone with aspirin sensitivity, active ulcer disease, nasal polyps, angioedema, and bronchospastic reactivity to aspirin (Miller, 1982). Effectiveness of the NSAIDs depends upon well-functioning hepatic and renal systems; the likelihood of chronic impairment of these systems in the elderly limits the use of these drugs. The potential for side effects of these drugs is also increased in the elderly. The principal side effects are gastrointestinal, so that none of these drugs should be taken on an empty stomach. Aspirin may lodge in the esophagus, causing burning, craters, and eventual scar tissue. That is why drugs, especially aspirin, should be taken while the client is standing and with a full glass (at least 6 ounces) of water. These drugs irritate the gastric mucosa by increasing the acidity of the gastric juices as well as sometimes lodging in the mucosa, causing ulcers. Citrus juices should not be given with these drugs because of the potential for increased gastric irritation. Drugs like naproxen and ibuprofen can cause diarrhea.

Other side effects of the NSAIDs include headache (with indomethacin especially), skin rashes (especially with phenylbutazone), and fluid retention. Blood dyscrasias are sometimes seen, particularly with phenylbutazone. This drug, as well as naproxen, may also potentiate oral hypoglycemia agents, because the NSAIDs are stronger in their binding abilities than the hypoglycemic agents and coumadin-type drugs.

If aspirin is given with indomethacin (Indocin), no added effect has been noted, so a combination of these drugs is discouraged (Physicians' Desk Reference, 1984, p. 1291). Indomethacin has also been found to interfere with the antihypertensive effects of the beta-blockers and to reduce coronary blood flow in patients with coronary artery disease (Brooks, Kean, Kassam, & Buchanan, 1984). Yet, over and over again, older clients will report they are not getting the desired effects from Indocin, so they take aspirin to help relieve the pain. Often, the only result is gastrointestinal bleeding.

As with all other drugs, smaller than usual dosages should be tried initially, with the dosage increased if necessary and if tolerated. For example, naproxen may be well tolerated in dosages of 250 mg, but may cause severe diarrhea with life-threatening consequences if the 500-mg dosage is used. Therapeutic blood levels of these drugs are slow to build in the elderly, so the clients who are really in pain may be impatient for relief and either overdose themselves or report a lack of response. The nurse practitioner, then, has a great challenge in helping older clients to use the NSAIDs appropriately.

Antibiotics

Antibiotics are often prescribed for the elderly "just in case," or because the older patient insists upon such a prescription. The fact that adverse reactions to antibiotics are more frequent and severe in older persons is not sufficiently appreciated by health care professionals (Gleckman & Esposito, 1980). Antibiotics can produce superinfections and severe metabolic and neurologic toxicities in older persons. Penicillins that contain potassium and sodium may severely derange an older person's electrolytes, leading to cardiac arrhythmias and even failure. Oral antibiotics, especially tetracyclines, can reduce digitalis absorption. Because of poor clearance in some older persons, antibiotics may remain in the system longer, with the potential of causing muscular twitching or convulsions. Most often, older persons will complain of dizziness and malaise.

Acid-labile antibiotics may be more fully absorbed because of the decrease in gastric acidity in older persons (Lutwick, 1980). Antibiotics like carbenicillin, when taken with aspirin, may prolong bleeding time. Hepatotoxicity and nephrotoxicity may result from the use of tetracyclines in older persons with impaired liver and renal function. Cephalosporins and aminoglycosides also cause nephrotoxicity. A further side effect of the aminoglycosides is ototoxicity. Acute colitis can result from clindamycin. Bone marrow suppression and aplastic anemia can result from chloramphenicol.

Despite the fact that older persons say they have never been allergic to any drug, nurse practitioners should nevertheless be especially careful in administering powerful drugs to them. The immune systems of older persons may have changed, thus making them highly allergic to an antibiotic. Moreover, older persons may not have been allergic to the antibiotics prescribed years ago but may nevertheless be highly allergic to newer forms and types of antibiotics. Anaphylactic shock, angioneurotic edema, and/or exfoliative dermatitis could occur swiftly. Therefore, older persons taking antibiotics, especially for the first time, should be monitored closely for allergic manifestations.

Gastrointestinal side effects, such as nausea, vomiting, and diarrhea, may inhibit older persons from taking a needed antibiotic. The diarrhea may be caused from the death or inhibition of normal bowel flora. If the client is not taking MAO inhibitors or if it is not otherwise contraindicated, the use of blue cheese in the diet will replace the needed flora.

A superimposed monilial vaginitis may occur in older women taking antibiotics. Nurses should be vigilant for this side effect and should refer these women for appropriate therapy so that other vaginal infections do not occur.

Older persons need to be taught that antibiotics are not a cure-all and must not be taken unless truly necessary. They also need to understand that they must take all of the drug prescribed and not "save" any for later possible infection or stop taking the antibiotic simply because they feel better.

Older diabetics requiring antibiotic therapy, especially if it is being administered intramuscularly, may find that the serum levels of the drug are lowered (Lutwick, 1980). This malabsorption may be due to microvascular impairment produced by the diabetes. If the diabetic is taking a hypoglycemic agent, it can be potentiated by certain antibiotics, such as chloramphenicol. Many of the antibiotics can cause false-positive readings if Clinitest is being used (Moellering, 1978).

Oral Hypoglycemic Agents

Oral hypoglycemic agents have been a boon to persons developing diabetes in their later years. These people generally do not need insulin; they need a stimulus for the pancreatic beta cells to secrete insulin. However, the use of such agents is not without problems, and careful monitoring by both care-givers and patients themselves is essential.

The process of aging, with its "wear and tear" effect of decreasing glucose tolerance and a reduced number of insulin receptors, is thought to be a factor in producing non-insulin dependent diabetes in older persons (Skillman, 1979). Obesity, a common finding in older adults, can also decrease the number of insulin receptors. When laboratory studies on older persons show an elevated serum glucose, there is a tendency to prescribe an oral hypoglycemic agent. Diet therapy should be tried first, with close monitoring of blood glucose. Fortunately, products like

Dextrostix and machines like the Glucometer make this monitoring easier, allowing many older persons to monitor their own progress.

Often, when older persons are placed on a reduction diet or a controlled diet and a sulfonylurea is prescribed, hypoglycemic episodes can occur, as there is less need for the boost that the sulfonylurea gives. Older patients need to be prepared to cope with the signs and symptoms of hypoglycemia should they occur. One common instance is beginning to be called the "Sunday Syndrome," where older persons experience hypoglycemic reactions in church, causing them to faint and disrupt the services. Older adults should receive a dispensation from fasting and thus be able to take communion after eating their prescribed meals. Long-chain carbohydrate snacks (e.g., rice crackers and peanut butter) should be eaten if church services extend into the time the next prescribed meal should be eaten.

Older persons on oral hypoglycemic agents should be warned to avoid taking aspirin, other NSAIDs, Dicumarol, and phenylbutazone (Butazolidin) with those agents, as these drugs potentiate the hypoglycemic effects of these agents.

In 1984, a second generation of sulfonylureas was introduced into the United States, even though these drugs have been used in Europe since 1972. The drugs are glyburide (DiaBeta, Micronase) and glipizide (Glucotrol). These drugs are given once daily and are more efficacious in older persons who conform to prescribed diet and exercise programs and who have a fasting blood sugar of less than 140 mg/dL. There are few side effects, and no adverse drug interactions have been reported (Skillman, 1984).

Analgesics

Older persons experiencing pain from chronic muscle and joint disease, gastrointestinal problems, cancer, headaches, and a variety of other problems self-medicate and overmedicate themselves with pain killers. Added to this may be the analgesics prescribed for them by their physicians.

These clients may present with signs and symptoms of gastrointestinal bleeding, anemia, sleep-pattern disturbances, or other adverse effects. Only by careful history-taking can the abuse of analgesic drugs be uncovered. Therefore, every older person should be warned of the hazards of self-medication for pain.

Problems with the use of analgesics in the elderly may result from their tendency to stay in the body longer, causing toxic reactions or potentiating or diminishing the effects of other prescribed drugs. Drugs such as codeine may depress respiration and cause constipation. Barbiturates may have the paradoxical effect of causing severe agitation and lead to accidental trauma resulting from falls or poor coordination on the part of their client.

Aspirin is an excellent analgesic but is often poorly tolerated in the elderly. Older persons should be instructed to take buffered or enteric-coated aspirin with a full 6-ounce glass of water while standing up. Large doses (e.g., three arthritis strengths) of aspirin should be avoided, for tinnitus can quickly occur. One aspirin tablet will produce an analgesic effect within 30–40 minutes. Aspirin dosages should be spread over the day in 4-hour intervals.

Acetaminophen is another analgesic widely taken by the elderly and is effective for mild pain. Of course, it does not have the anti-inflammatory properties of aspirin. The problem with acetaminophen is that overdosing can quickly occur in older persons with hepatic and renal insufficiency, thus causing failure of these body systems. Hypoglycemia can also occur in acetaminophen overdose (Pfeiffer, 1982).

Propoxyphene (Darvon) is commonly prescribed for older persons, but the adverse effects of the drug outweigh its effectiveness. Confusion (with or without hallucination) and respiratory depression can occur. This drug has also been found to create dependency in its users.

In acute pain situations, where the need to control the pain outweighs the danger of potential adverse side effects, narcotic analgesics may be prescribed. Morphine, codeine, and meperidine hydrochloride (Demerol) are the drugs of choice. The nurse practitioner has the responsibility to be alert for any pathological complication causing increased pain, as well as to prevent the effects of decreased respiration and cough reflex and constipation.

In any pain situation, the nurse should provide comfort measures (e.g., position change, back rub), relaxation techniques, biofeedback, and a warm and caring attitude before any analgesic drug is administered.

Laxatives

In a national study of drug prescribing in skilled nursing facilities, laxatives were the single largest class of drugs prescribed for the largest number of nursing home residents (Foerst, 1979). Add to this the large number of laxatives and related preparations bought over-the-counter by the elderly person living independently, and one can recognize the enormity of the problem of dysfunctional bowels brought on by poor bowel hygienic habits (often lifelong) of the elderly and by the effects of prescribed polypharmacy on the bowel.

Drugs that cause decreased bowel motility (e.g., anticholinergics, phenothiazines, and narcotics) often lead the elderly taking these drugs to resort to stimulant cathartics, which increase bowel motility. The problem with this is that if the older person is taking other drugs, especially those in sustained release form, the increased bowel motility will prevent the absorption of the drugs due to their swift passage through the gastrointestinal tract, e.g., drugs like the sulfonamides.

Stool softeners often create a "fecal glue" that obstructs a bowel that has poor motility. Impactions easily develop. Enemas, especially those containing phosphate laxatives, can cause severe hypocalcemia, hypokalemia, and lead to convulsions and renal failure (Wiberg, Turner, & Nuttall, 1978). The hypokalemia may derange

the glucose tolerance, causing higher readings on laboratory studies (Hansten, 1979).

One of the greatest challenges to nurses working with older adults is to teach them good bowel hygiene so that they can create their own bowel movements and not have to rely on artificial, often expensive and harmful means to evacuate the bowel (see Chap. 6).

Often, older persons will overdose themselves on stimulant laxatives with disastrous results. When taking Dulcolax, for example, they may give themselves severe diarrhea by taking too many pills at once. This laxative, also, can cause gastric irritation if taken with milk or antacids.

Electrolyte imbalance, malabsorption syndromes, "cathartic colons" (i.e., bowels that move only when artificially stimulated), and a condition producing bowel changes similar to ulcerative colitis (Nursing 84 Drug Handbook, 1984) can occur with overuse of laxatives. Many laxatives and stool softeners contain sodium and thus may undo drug and diet regimens that attempt to remove sodium from the body.

Dioctyl calcium sulfonsuccinate (Surfak) if taken with a mineral oil laxative may increase the absorption of mineral oil. If Surfak is taken with aspirin there is a great potential for severe gastric mucosal damage (Nursing 84 Drug Handbook, 1984, pp. 397–398).

Antacids

Another group of drugs often overprescribed or abused by the elderly are the antacids. These drugs are often taken habitually after meals as a preventative for heartburn or may be used when taking drugs that cause gastrointestinal discomfort. These over-the-counter drugs can cause severe side effects like constipation, diarrhea, fluid retention, and renal calculi (mainly calcium). Antacids can adversely interact with other drug therapies. For example, they prevent absorption of tetracycline, Thorazine, oral hematinics, phenylbutazone, and the sulfonamides (Friesen, 1983).

Another type of antacid, cimetidine (Tagamet hydrochloride), which is a histamine H_2 antagonist and which inhibits all phases of gastric acid secretion, has been widely used with good success for gastric/duodenal ulcer therapy and gastroesophageal reflux syndromes. The drug produces many adverse side effects in the elderly, especially in individuals with impaired renal function. Various types of confusional states, seizures, respiratory difficulties, diarrhea, dizziness, arthralgias, and myalgias can occur after ingestion of this drug.

By delaying their elimination and increasing their blood levels, cimetidine may inhibit the hepatic metabolism of warfarin-type anticoagulants, phenytoin, propranolol, chlordiazepoxide, and diazepam (Physicians' Desk Reference, 1984, pp. 1892–1895).

Cimetidine should not be given simultaneously with tranquilizers because the ensuing increased toxicity may aggravate confusional states in elderly on this drug. The drug should not be given to clients with Alzheimer's disease because of the likelihood of these individuals developing central nervous system side effects (Jenike, 1982).

Antidiarrheals

Antidiarrheal drug use in older persons may become a habit, as the medications are sometimes taken prophylactically. Long-term usage of these drugs may cause toxic reactions and lead to confusion. These drugs cause constipation and inhibition of absorption of other therapeutic agents like digoxin, thus decreasing their effectiveness.

Over-the-counter antidiarretics like bismuth subsalicylate (Pepto-Bismol) can affect mental abilities, cause hypotension, constipation, and fecal impaction. Kaolin and pectin mixtures (Kaopectate) decrease the absorption of lincomycin from the gut.

Diphenoxylate hydrochloride (Lomotil) can produce dizziness, sedation, headache, depression, numbness in the extremities, and anticholinergic effects. The drug should not be given with other CNS depressants, nor should it be given with MAO inhibitors because of the potential for hypertensive crises (Nursing 84 Drug Handbook, 1984, p. 389).

Loperamide hydrochloride (Imodium) also produces anticholinergic effects, rashes, and dizziness. This drug should be used cautiously in older men with severe prostatic hypertrophy.

DRUG THERAPY IN SPECIAL CIRCUMSTANCES

The elderly need to be acutely aware of the drugs they take and should be able to identify the contents of their drug profile in case it is unavailable when needed. Disasters, accidents, travel, and relocation all can have an impact on the drug therapy of the elderly. Older adults must have contingency plans to cope with such untoward happenings.

First and foremost, the elderly taking medication should wear Medic-Alert(R) or related jewelry detailing their health problems and their drug therapy. They should also carry this information in their wallets. Older women who no longer carry a purse should be counseled to carry their health information in a small wallet they can put in a jacket or strap to their wrists. Regardless of one's age, proper identification and personal information should be carried on one's person.

Disasters

In the event of a natural disaster, the older person may have to escape from a burning, flooded, or devastated building or vehicle without any professional assistance whatsoever. Injury or shock may occur, so that older persons cannot communicate what their health problems are or what medications they are taking. Here is another situation in which medical information jewelry is invaluable. If older persons have sufficient warning to remove themselves from a hazardous situation, they should take all of their medications with them as a priority. For this reason, medications should be kept together in their original containers in a zippered cosmetic style bag or tote bag for ready transport. A good reason for using a single pharmacy is that a list of current drugs being used by the older person would be on file, so that if the pharmacy was not also affected by the disaster, drug therapy could be easily ascertained.

If older persons are taken to a disaster shelter, they should inform the persons in charge of health care of their drug status and should request assistance in keeping drugs safe and at the right temperature. A list of drugs could also be kept in one's safety deposit box as an added resource. A copy of the list could also be kept by a concerned relative living apart from the older person.

Accidents

If older persons are injured away from home and family, they may not be able to communicate their drug status because of trauma or shock. Again, the medical information jewelry and wallet information are crucial. If older persons are coherent and if they have been taught to be knowledgeable about their drug therapy, they should be able to help give needed drug information. It is of little help to say "I take a green pill before meals and a little white heart pill." Older individuals must learn to be specific about the drugs they take into their bodies. Use of the resources listed above under "Disasters" are also valid here.

Nurses receiving elderly victims of accidents for care in emergency rooms or related facilities should make a particular effort to ascertain what drugs older injured persons are taking. Otherwise the adverse consequences could be severe.

Travel

Drug therapy while traveling can pose considerable problems for unwary and uncaring elderly.

Managing drugs and drug therapy when taking trips requires careful preplanning and equally careful management.

Older persons need to ascertain what drugs and in what amounts (including 3 days extra supply) they will need while traveling. They should have their pharmacist place these drugs in appropriately labeled containers to carry in their purse or briefcase. Medications should never be placed in unmarked containers or mixed with one another. Pillboxes, especially metal ones, should never be used, as the oxidation of the drug and metal may interact adversely. Drugs should never be packed in suitcases, for baggage handling may mean leaving luggage stored in hot areas. Worse still, the luggage could be lost.

Because temperature can very readily affect the chemistry of drugs, care must be taken to avoid one's drug supply being subjected to adverse temperatures. Tetracyclines may become nephrotoxic if left in the heat. This means that, even if one is carrying a drug on one's person or in a purse, care must be taken to avoid the heat of direct sun, hot automobiles, or other forms of excessive heat.

Older diabetics can use a lunch box with a coolant to protect their insulin. Older adults on antibiotics may also need to consider this method of keeping drugs cool while traveling.

A copy of one's drug profile should be carried on one's person or in a purse and a copy should be placed in one's luggage. Prescription number, date of filling, and name and telephone number of the pharmacy should also be on the drug profile.

If the trip is to be an extended one, a set of prescriptions can be obtained from one's physician, along with names of possible health professional referrals in case of need. Most hotels have a house physician on call or have an arrangement with an emergency center.

If traveling to remote areas, information about one's drug therapy should be given to a responsible member of the group in case of an adverse event. If in a tour group, a copy of the drug profile, in a sealed envelope, should be given to the tour leader, who should not open it unless necessary.

When traveling, especially if vacationing, there is the tendency to alter eating patterns and fluid intake. Older travelers must be aware of the effect of food and fluid on their drug therapy. Older adults should avoid overeating and underhydrating while traveling and should avoid eating dishes whose ingredients are unknown to them.

Medical information jewelry should be worn at all times during travel. Care should be taken to avoid excess heat or any exertion that would affect drug metabolism. Hats and sunblocks should be worn if the person is taking tetracyclines or using saccharine.

Constipation is often a problem while traveling because of altered eating habits and other stresses. Older travelers should not indiscriminately take any laxative, but should take the safest one suggested by their physician prior to the trip. In fact, older travelers should beware of taking any over-the-counter drugs while traveling unless specifically recommended by their physicians. The danger of an adverse drug interaction is enormous.

Relocation

Relocation for whatever reason can pose life-threatening hazards for older persons on drug therapy. All too often, the older person is relocated by well-meaning relatives who want their parents or other older relative near them. What they fail to relocate are the medical records, including drug profiles and management protocols. Obtaining such information after the older person moves can be exceedingly difficult. If the older person becomes ill or is hospitalized, the care-givers often are inhibited from giving proper therapy because they are dealing with unknown entities.

Whenever older persons relocate, they should take with them a copy of an updated data base including a drug profile written in the Problem-Oriented format. The names, addresses, and telephone numbers of health professionals, including pharmacists, should also be listed. In this way, if questions arise in the new location, information about the older person's past history is easier to obtain.

In the process of relocation, older persons should take with them at least 1 month's supply of their medications and should establish themselves as quickly as possible with physicians and pharmacists in their new location.

SUMMARY

This chapter gives an overview of the exceedingly complex area of safely, accurately, and ethically providing older persons with therapeutic chemicals to help them to combat disease, ease chronic conditions, and/or to promote comfort.

Nursing responsibilities in the selection, administration, and discontinuance of drug therapy in the elderly are an enormous challenge in nurses' day-to-day work with older people. Therefore, gerontological nurses must consult their drug handbooks frequently and must never give a drug without first knowing its action, interactions, side effects, and therapeutic window. They must develop quality monitoring systems for outcomes of drug therapy and prevention of adverse effects. Gerontological nurses must constantly keep their pharmacological knowledge current by reading the periodical literature, consulting current pharmacology texts, and interacting with their peers and colleagues at workshops and meetings.

Gerontological nurses have within their power, through therapeutic use of self and alternative modalities, the professional task of helping to provide safe, effective drug therapy for older adults.

REFERENCES

Alford, D., & Moll, J. (1982, June). Helping elderly patients in ambulatory settings cope with drug therapy. *Nursing Clinics of North America, 17* (6), 275–282.

Bachinsky, M. (1978, February). Geriatric medications: How psychotropic drugs can go astray. *RN, 41*(2), 50–55.

Baum, J. (1979, June). When to prescribe nonsteroidal anti-inflammatory drugs. *Geriatrics, 34*(6), 51–54.

Bauwens, E., & Clemmons, C. (1978). Foods that foil drugs. *RN, 41*(9), 79–81.

Becker, P., & Warshaw, G. (1983, March). Managing hypertension in elderly patients. *Drug Therapy, 13*(3), 61–63, 67–70.

Brooks, P. M., Kean, W. F., Kassam, Y., & Buchanan, W. (1984, March). Problems of antiarthritic therapy in the elderly. *Journal of the American Geriatrics Society, 32*(3), 229–234.

Brown, M. M., Boosinger, J. K., Henderson, M., Rife, S. S., Rustia, J. K., Taylor, O., & Young, W. W. (1977). Drug–drug interactions among residents in homes for the elderly. *Nursing Research, 26*(1), 47–52.

Butler, J., & Harrison, B. (1983). Keeping pace with calcium channel blockers. *Nursing 83, 13*(7), 38–43.

Butler, R. N. (1975). *Why survive? Being old in America.* New York: Harper & Row.

Cerrato, P. L. (1987). When food and drugs collide. *RN, 50*(4), 85–86.

Corbett, J. V. (2nd ed.). (1987). *Laboratory tests and diagnostic procedures with nursing diagnoses.* New York: Appleton & Lange.

Cusack, B., Kelly, K., O'Malley, K., Noel, J., Lavan, J., & Horgan, J. (1979, June). Digoxin in the elderly: Pharmacokinetic consequences of old age. *Clinical Pharmacology and Therapeutics, 25,* 772.

Duvic, M. (1983, March). How to treat geriatric dermatoses. *Drug Therapy, 13,* 75–82.

Eisdorfer, C. (1975, February). Observations on the psychopharmacology of the aged. *Journal of the American Geriatrics Society, 23,* 53–57.

Fletcher, D. (1982). Helping the elderly to sleep without drugs. *Geriatric Consultant, 1*(6), 11–13.

Foerst, H. (1979). Drug-prescribing patterns in skilled nursing facilities. *American Journal of Nursing, 79*(11), 2002–2003.

Freis, E., Levinson, P. D., & Khatri, I. M. (1982). Persistence of normal BP after withdrawal of drug treatment in mild hypertension. *Archives of Internal Medicine, 142,* 2265–2268.

Friesen, A. (1983). Adverse drug reactions in the geriatric client. In L. Pagliaro & A. Pagliaro (Eds.), *Pharmacologic aspects of aging.* St. Louis: Mosby.

Gleckman, R., & Esposito, A. (1980). Antibiotics in the elderly: Skating on therapeutic thin ice. *Geriatrics, 35*(1), 26–28, 33–37.

Goldberg, P., & Roberts, J. (Eds.) (1983). *Handbook on pharmacology of aging.* Boca Raton, FL: CRC Press.

Gottlieb, T., & Chidsey, C. (1976, January). The clinicians guide to pharmacology of antihypertensive agents. *Geriatrics, 31,* 99–105, 109–110.

Graedon, J. (1982, March 2). Foods, drugs can mix for better or worse. *Dallas Times Herald,* p. 10-K.

Hammond, J., & Kirkendall, W. (1979). Antihypertensive drugs for the aging. *Geriatrics, 34*(6), 27–31, 36.

Hanan, Z. (1978). Geriatric medications: How the aged are hurt by drugs meant to help. *RN, 41*(1), 56–61.

Hansten, P. (1979). *Drug interactions* (4th ed.). Philadelphia: Lea & Febiger.

Hollister, L. (1977). Prescribing drugs for the elderly. *Geriatrics, 32*(8), 71–73.

Hussar, D. (1976). Drug interactions: Good and bad. *Nursing 76, 6*(9), 61–65.

Hutchins, L. (1981, June). Drug treatment of high blood pressure. *Nursing Clinics of North America, 16,* 365–376.

Jenike, M. (1982). Cimetidine in elderly patients: Review and uses and risks. *Journal of the American Geriatrics Society, 30*(3), 170–173.

Johnson, G., & Johanson, B. (1983). B-Blockers. *American Journal of Nursing, 83*(7), 1034–1043.

Johnston, G. D. (1983, January). Clinical and pharmacological considerations in digitalis use in the geriatric patient. *Geriatric Medicine Today, 2,* 59–65.

Karsh, F., & Karsh, A. (1978, June). Clinically important drug interactions. *Nurses Drug Alert, 2,* 25.

Lambert, M. (1975). Drugs and diet interactions. *American Journal of Nursing, 75*(3), 402–406.

Lamy, P. (1977). What the physician should keep in mind when prescribing drugs for an elderly patient. *Geriatrics, 32*(5), 37–38.

Lamy, P. (1981). *Prescribing for the elderly.* Littleton, MS: John Wright PSG.

Larkin, T. (1978, March). Mixing medications? Have a care! *FDA Consumer* (reprint).

Lowenthal, D., & Swartz, C. (1985, March). Hypertension in the 1980s. *Primary Care, 12*(3), 101–115.

Lutwick, L. (1980). Principles of antibiotic use in the elderly. *Geriatrics, 35*(2), 54–56, 58–60.

McFarland, K. F., & Carr, A. A. (1977, January). Changes in fasting blood sugar after hydrochlorthiazide and potassium supplementation. *Journal of Clinical Pharmacology, 17,* 13–17.

Miller, S. (1982). NSAIDs: Examining therapeutic alternatives. *Geriatrics, 37*(3), 70–72, 75, 78.

Moellering, R. (1978). Factors influencing the clinical use of antimicrobal agents in elderly patients. *Geriatrics, 32*(2), 83–85, 89–91.

Mollen, A. (1982, April 11). Food and drug dangers. *Dallas Times Herald.*

Moser, M. (1982). The management of cardiovascular disease in the elderly. *Journal of the American Geriatrics Society, 30*(11), S20–S29.

Nursing 84 Drug Handbook (1984). Springhouse, PA: Springhouse Corporation.

Pfeiffer, R. (1982). Drugs for pain in the elderly. *Geriatrics, 37*(2), 67–69, 73, 76.

Physicians' Desk Reference (38th ed.). (1984). Oradell, NJ: Medical Economics.

Price, J., & Andrews, P. (1982). Alcohol abuse in the elderly. *Journal of Gerontological Nursing, 8*(1), 16–19.

Ray, W., Federspiel, C., & Schaffner, W. (1970, May). Study of antipsychotic drug use in nursing homes: Epidemiologic evidence suggesting misuse. *American Journal of Public Health, 70,* 485–491.

Requarth, C. (1979). Medication usage and interaction in the long-term care elderly. *Journal of Gerontological Nursing, 5*(2), 33–37.

Rodman, M. (1980). The drug interactions we all overlook. *RN, 43*(11), 40–43.

Rodman, M. (1982). First of a new class of antiarrhythmia drug. *RN, 45*(2), 144.

Roffman, D. (1984). Special concerns of digitalis use in elderly patients. *Geriatrics, 39*(6), 97–98, 103–105.

Simon, L., & Likes, K. (1978, February). Hypoprothrombinemic response to ice cream. *Drug Intelligence and Clinical Pharmacology, 12,* 121–122.

Simonson, W. (1984). *Medications and the elderly.* Gaithersburg, MD: Aspen Systems Corporation.

Skillman, T. (1979). Oral agents and the elderly diabetic. *Geriatrics, 34*(12), 41–47.

Skillman, T. (1984). Oral hypoglycemic agents for treatment of NIDDM. *Geriatrics, 39*(9), 77–78, 80–83.

Somani, P., & Mayhew, H. (1985, March). Clinical indications for calcium channel blockers. *Primary Care, 12,* 143–164.

Stults, B. (1982). Digoxin use in the elderly. *Journal of the American Geriatrics Society, 30*(3), 158–164.

The 1984 Report of the Joint National Committee on Detection, Evaluation and Treatment of High Blood Pressure. (1984, May). *Archives of Internal Medicine, 144,* 1045–1057.

Todd, B. (1987). Cigarettes and caffeine in drug interactions. *Geriatric Nursing, 8*(2), 97–98.

Vestal, R. (1982). Pharmacology and aging. *Journal of the American Geriatrics Society, 30*(3), 191–200.

Wiberg, J., Turner, G., & Nuttall, F. (1978, July). Effect of phosphate or magnesium cathartics on serum calcium: Observations in normocalcemic patients. *Archives of Internal Medicine, 138,* 1114–1116.

Williamson, J. (1980). Paving the way to safe prescribing for the elderly. *Geriatrics, 35*(9), 32–39.

Zinn, M. (1970, December). Quinidine intoxication from alkali ingestion. *Texas Medicine, 66,* 64–66.

NEUROLOGICAL/SENSORY CHANGES

As people age, their nervous systems and associated sensory systems age. Some changes are expected in the older adult; however, there are also degenerative neurological and sensory changes that can occur. In this chapter, the major changes in these two systems in the body are discussed, including assessment parameters and related nursing care.

NERVOUS SYSTEM CHANGES

Neurons in the central nervous system, unlike other cells in the body, do not reproduce or regenerate after about 2 years of age. The neurons are then maintained by protein synthesis and biochemical metabolism. As aging occurs, both structural and functional changes become evident. Structural changes include loss of neurons, loss of total brain weight, accumulation of a pigment known as lipofuscin, and development of neurofibrillary tangles (Duara, London, & Rapoport, 1985, pp. 596–600). Functional changes include a decrease in synaptic transmission between neuronal cells and a longer reaction time in the neuromuscular and autonomic nervous systems as well as in higher cortical functions (Stewart, 1982, pp. 70–77; Forbes & Fitzsimons, 1981, pp. 22–23).

A loss of neurons is thought to result from a change in the neuronal metabolism that produces the proteins necessary for the viability of the neuron. Another development is the decreased volume of the extracellular space. Nutrients necessary for neuronal activity are also contained in this space. When these proteins and nutrients are unavailable to the neuron, it atrophies and eventually dies (Stewart, 1982, p. 70).

Another structural change in the aged person involves the loss of brain weight. As the brain ages, it loses volume. This lost volume upsets a balance within the cranium between brain tissue, blood, and cerebrospinal fluid. The aged brain, seen either upon autopsy or via computed tomography (CT) scanning, appears to be shrunken. When the brain tissue loses weight, the ventricular spaces enlarge in order to compensate. These enlarged ventricles can also be observed on CT scan. Associated with the loss of brain volume in the older adult is the thinning of some areas of gray and white matter in the tissue. The areas noted to have the greater amount of thinning include the frontal cortex and the superior temporal gyrus (Stewart, 1982, p. 70).

Another structural change noted in the aged is the deposition of lipofuscin. Lipofuscin is a brown-colored waste material having a lipid base that accumulates within the nerves as well as many other body tissue cells. It has been suggested that lipofuscin is a cause of a neuron's inability to function. Although this is as yet unproven, some research has shown that the more active cells contain less of the lipofuscin deposited (Forbes & Fitzsimons, 1981, p. 22).

Neurofibrillary tangles are abnormal tissue that develop within the cytoplasm of the neuron in the aged. These abnormal fibrillar masses occur in small amounts in the normal older adult. However, a large increase in the amount of the tangles is found in the person with neurological changes, such as senile dementia or Alzheimer's disease (Duara et al., 1985, p. 600). Neurofibrillary tangles appear to interrupt communication within the neuron, causing permanent loss of function (Stewart, 1982, p. 71).

One of the functional changes affecting the aged is a decrease in synaptic transmission. Synaptic transmission is the means by which two neurons communicate within the central nervous system. The process involves a neurotransmitter—the message-carrier that travels across a synaptic cleft from one neuron to another neuron. The transmitter causes the postsynaptic neuron to become excited by reacting on the cell surface with receptors. This neuron then carries the message to the next neuron by intracellular communication and then another synapse (Neatherlin, Kamp, & Guthrie, 1981, pp. 146–149). In the older person, the loss of brain weight leads to a decrease in the amount of neurotransmitter produced. Furthermore, because the neurons shrink and die, there is less cell surface on which the neurotransmitter can react. Both these factors lead to an overall reduction in synaptic transmission (Stewart, 1982, p. 71).

In addition to a decreased amount of synaptic transmission, the neurons are slower in sending these transmissions. The electroencephalogram, (EEG) is a measure of brain wave activity. The EEG of the aged person tends to be slower than in a younger person (Forbes & Fitzsimons, 1981, p. 22). Furthermore, the older adult takes a longer period of time to carry out complex motor and sensory skills, such as speed of hand

and foot movements, coordination and balance, hand and arm tracking, and fine skilled hand movements such as grasping and interfinger manipulation (Potvin, Sndulko, Tourtellotte, Lemmon, & Potvin, 1980, pp. 1–9). Reaction time is lengthened in the older adult (Forbes & Fitzsimons, 1981, p. 23).

Although the aged person may be slower to react to situations and integrate information, learning does not seem to be impaired, although the time involved in learning may be lengthened (Stewart, 1982, p. 71). In one study, no significant differences were observed in learning when related to the retesting of complex motor skills after a period of time from the initial testing (Potvin et al., 1980, p. 6). A related area to learning is observed in the person's memory. Possibly due to decreased efficiency, an aged person's recent memory is diminished. Long-term memory, however, does not seem to be affected. The problems with short-term memory may lead to difficulties in learning new tasks and information. Therefore, the aged are able to learn, but need to be allowed time to absorb, integrate, and remember knowledge at their own pace (Graves, 1981a, p. 23).

Sleep Alterations

Another age-related neurological change is the change in the sleep patterns of the older adult. Sleep can be divided into REM (rapid eye movement) and NREM (nonrapid eye movement) periods, and the cycles are controlled by the brainstem. NREM sleep is the period during which the person is not dreaming, and it comprises the majority of the time a person sleeps. It is composed of four stages, progressing from light sleep in stage I to deep sleep in stage IV when a person is very hard to awaken. REM sleep is the period during which a person dreams. It occurs in approximately 90-minute cycles, recurring at intervals during the night. As a person ages, the total amount of time of sleep decreases, including less stages II and IV sleep. Amounts of REM sleep are maintained until extreme old age. Also, the aged person tends to wake more during sleep time and stay awake more during the night. The frequent wakefulness may be due to the need to use the toilet at intervals during the night; however, it has been found that the elderly have a lower threshold for arousal than do younger subjects (Dement, Richardson, Prinz, Carskadon, Kripke, & Zeisler, 1985, pp. 694–697). The aged person usually compensates for this wakefulness by taking a nap or two during the day.

Some of the sleep disturbances that occur in the aged may be symptoms of more serious problems. These sleep problems include sleep apnea, narcolepsy, insomnia, and periodic leg movement during sleep. Sleep apnea is defined as a cessation of breathing during sleep and is usually due to the obstruction of the upper airway by mechanical means, such as the tongue. It may be a symptom of Pickwickian syndrome, which is a form of hypersomnia. However, other causes of sleep apnea must be ruled out, such as cranial tumor, epilepsy, or metabolic imbalance (Gambert & Duthrie, 1981, pp. 63–64). One study reported that sleep apnea often accompanies life-threatening hemodynamic changes (Coleman, Miles, Guilleminault, Zarcone, Hoed, & Dement, 1981, p. 290). Therefore, it should be investigated carefully.

Narcolepsy is another sleep disturbance that should be investigated. It is characterized by the symptoms of sudden muscle weakness and loss of tone. These symptoms may occur singly or together and may begin for no reason. However, narcolepsy may also be a sign of a more serious problem—brain tumor, encephalitis, cerebral trauma, emotional stress, hypothyroidism, or hypopituitarism may be causes of one or both symptoms of narcolepsy (Gambert & Duthrie, 1981, p. 63).

Insomnia seems to be a fairly common problem among the aged. Most of the time, sleeplessness in the elderly is due to anxiety in some form, such as fear, stress, or depression. However, insomnia may also be due to drug interactions or reactions, hyperthyroidism, or withdrawal from alcohol, though the number of aged suffering from these conditions is relatively small. Regardless of its cause, however, insomnia is very distressing to the older person. Sleeping aids may be prescribed (and are discussed later in this chapter) but must be carefully monitored for abuse and overdosage (Gambert & Duthrie, 1981, p. 63).

The restless legs syndrome (RLS) may also be a disturbance to the aged person since this chronic disorder is more severe and more frequent in this age group. This syndrome is most prevalent when the person is trying to go to sleep. The creeping, crawling sensations are coupled with an urge to move. Rapid pacing or massage may bring temporary relief until the person tries to sleep again. Asymptomatic intervals of weeks to months may occur between episodes (Rossman, 1986, p. 698).

Problems with sleep, therefore, may be very disturbing to the aged person. A complete nursing assessment should be performed and should include questions on sleeping habits, stimuli which cause awakening at night, medications taken for sleep, and effective measures that help induce and maintain sleep. It is important to remember that one's sleeping patterns change as one ages. This is probably due to the aging of the neurons and their inability to regenerate.

COMMON NEUROLOGICAL PROBLEMS

Some common neurological disorders that affect the aged include Parkinson's disease, organic brain syndrome, and Alzheimer's disease.

Parkinson's Disease

Parkinson's disease is a chronic, progressive disorder of the basal ganglia and substantia nigra of the cerebral cortex and brainstem. These areas are part of the extrapyramidal system and influence skeletal muscle movement. Parkinson's disease involves the loss of neurons that secrete dopamine, a major neurotransmitter in this area, and resulting depletion of dopamine. When dopamine, an inhibitory neurotransmitter, is decreased, there is a corresponding increase in acetylcholine, an excitatory neurotransmitter (Neatherlin et al., 1981; Topp, 1987). This results in an overall imbalance of neurotransmitters.

The severity of Parkinson's disease appears to coincide with the amount of neurons destroyed. In addition, many persons with Parkinson's disease are found to have decreased amounts of cerebral cortex tissue as well as the presence of Lewy bodies and neurofibrillary tangles (Adams & Victor, 1977, p. 830). The trigger of Parkinson's disease is not understood, although genetic disposition and viral infections have been implicated.

The assessment process usually reveals a history of Parkinsonism after the age of 50 years and slow deterioration over 15–20 years. Some of the first complaints include weakness and fatigue. Family and social history should be reviewed for any indication of genetic or viral involvement. After a history is obtained, a complete review of systems, with emphasis on the musculoskeletal and nervous systems, should be performed.

In assessing the client, four primary symptoms may be observed—tremor, muscle rigidity, decreased ability to begin motor movement, and imbalance (Brunner & Suddarth, 1984, pp. 1346–1347). The tremor is characteristic of Parkinson's disease because it occurs at rest. It also produces a "pill-rolling" effect between the thumb and forefinger, a rhythmic movement that appears as if the client is moving a pill. Tremor occurs more in the hands and fingers than in the arms and in the feet and lower ankles more than in the thighs.

Rigidity occurs more in flexor muscles than in extensors. It is a result of hypertonicity of the muscles. One classic symptom of rigidity seen in most Parkinsonism clients is a sign known as "cogwheel" rigidity. When range of motion is assessed, with the passive movement of an arm or leg, the muscle will stop movement at a certain point and then suddenly release so the limb may be moved past that point. In addition, some clients may have spastic rigidity.

A decreased or absent ability to initiate voluntary muscle movement is known as bradykinesia or akinesia. In addition, clients with Parkinson's disease may be unable to continue the muscle movements after initiation. The inability to continue voluntary muscle movement may be devastating to the patient in performing activities of daily living. Facial and oral movements, such as swallowing, talking, chewing, blinking, and expressions are diminished. The client typically has a shuffling gait that is further complicated by the inability to swing the arms for the maintenance of balance (Topp, 1987).

Imbalance affects about 5% of clients with Parkinson's disease. It involves a combination of the bradykinesia described above and the sensation that the foot has touched the floor before it actually has. This imbalance results in falls and can be transitory or continuous. The transitory form usually decreases with medication and therapy, whereas the continuous sensation of imbalance usually does not respond to therapy.

In addition to voluntary motor movement problems, the influence of the autonomic nervous system may be affected. The client may have problems in voiding or defecation and suffer from excessive perspiration and seborrhea. An additional problem of depression may occur in the latter course of the disease. A summary of symptoms may be found in Table 4–1.

Nursing care is directed toward the preservation of independence, comfort, and safety, with a major focus on problems in ambulation and activities of daily living. Ambulation should be assessed on a continuous basis in order to adjust the environment to ensure safe ambulatory activities. This may include rearranging of furniture, removal of scatter rugs, and avoidance of waxing floors. The activities of daily living should also be assessed on a continuous basis in order to allow for any necessary alterations in the plan of care. The plan of care should provide

TABLE 4–1. SUMMARY OF SYMPTOMS OF PARKINSONISM

Tremor
    Pill-rolling effect
    Greater in distal muscles
Rigidity
    Cog-wheeling
    Spasticity
Bradykinesia
    Long amount of time for activities of daily living
    Decreased swallowing—resultant drooling
    Increased trouble in talking
    Dysphagia
    Trouble in blinking
    Shuffling gait
    Trouble in swinging arms
Imbalance sensation
Autonomic nervous system involvement
    Difficulty in voiding
    Difficulty in defecation
    Excessive perspiration
    Seborrhea
    Depression

adequate time for the client to carry out these activities. Activities to be considered are exercise, eating, elimination, and hygiene. The client should be encouraged to systematically exercise all extremities, along with facial and oral muscles. The client needs to be observed during mealtime to assess problems in swallowing and to determine adequate nutritional intake. The client should be assessed to determine the frequency and consistency of bowel elimination. Constipation is a common problem. Therefore, the client needs to be assessed to determine whether additional intake of fluids, dietary fiber, fruits, and juices is required. In order to decrease body odor and the chance of seborrhea, personal hygiene is an essential aspect of the nursing care plan.

In addition to observations of activities of daily living, the client should be observed for adverse effects that may be caused by medication. Common adverse reactions may include hypotension when sitting or standing, nausea, changes in mental status, and arrhythmias. The blood pressure should be checked immediately when the client rises to determine the presence of hypotension. Support or elastic stockings should be applied if there is a large difference between the lying and the standing pressure. The client should further be observed for changes in cardiac pulse rate and mental status.

The client and family should be instructed in activities of daily living and observations of adverse effects caused by medication. Emphasis of instruction should be placed on the need for continuous observation, maintaining independence of activities of daily living, and providing a safe environment for ambulation.

Organic Brain Syndrome

Organic brain syndrome (OBS) is a deterioration of the brain that may occur in either an acute or chronic form. OBS should not be confused with senescence or senility. Senescence is defined as the process of aging in which the body does not maintain itself holistically (Adams & Victor, 1977, p. 397), whereas senility is generally used to label any older person who is even slightly confused, and this term is generally misapplied.

Acute OBS

Acute OBS may also be named delirium (Stewart, 1982, p. 72) or acute confusional state (Boss, 1982, pp. 61–68). It is considered to be reversible and is usually due to a disturbance of cerebral function and metabolism. Dysfunction may occur as a result of trauma, hypoxia, exposure to toxins, hypoglycemia, tumor, or other structural or metabolic problems. Acute OBS usually appears suddenly, manifested by memory loss, disorientation, delusions, hallucinations, obsessive–compulsive behavior, anxiety, and impaired high cortical functions (Gomez & Gomez, 1987; Linderborn, 1988).

Nursing assessment should include the historical onset of symptoms and the pattern of occurrence and intensity followed by an adequate neurological assessment. It may be necessary to include a family member when obtaining the client history. Before developing a plan of care, it is important to identify the adaptive behavior(s) that the client is using to cope with the problem(s).

Nursing management must focus on decreasing the amount of stimuli to which the client is subjected while making the best use of the stimuli. The following strategies should be considered when developing and implementing a plan of care for the patient with acute OBS:

1. Provide orientation with written as well as verbal and drawn information
2. Obtain familiar objects from the home environment and place them in the client's room if he or she is institutionalized
3. Present a calm but firm attitude when caring for the client, particularly if he or she is delusional or restless
4. Provide safety in all aspects of care
5. Use effective communication skills, such as eye-to-eye contact, listening, and reinforcement, to teach and counsel the client and family (Boss, 1982, pp. 61–68)

Chronic OBS
Chronic OBS is an irreversible condition and is a form of dementia (Stewart, 1982, p. 72). It affects all of the cerebral functioning in areas of memory, intelligence, expression or affect, judgment, and orientation. The level of consciousness is generally not affected. In contrast to acute OBS, the onset is usually slow and unnoticed for a long period of time. Also, acute OBS may appear concurrently with symptoms of chronic OBS, thus complicating the task of distinguishing between the two syndromes (Stoudemire & Thompson, 1981, pp. 112–120).

Nursing assessment of the chronic OBS client should include a thorough history of changes that have occurred. Memory should be assessed closely, because recent memory is more affected. The family history may become important in distinguishing between chronic and acute OBS. The following questions should be considered when assessing the orientation and memory

of the chronic OBS client: How does the client react to new situations? Does the client change from moment to moment? Does the client show no expression or reaction? Does the client show poor judgment in situations that might prove harmful? Is the client oriented to the environment? Can the client perform activities of daily living? (Stewart, 1982, p. 72; Stoudemire & Thompson, 1981, p. 115).

In addition to the aspects of care already described in caring for the acute OBS patient, the following should be considered in the individualized plan of care for the chronic OBS client:

1. Verbal communication should be in simple short sentences presented in a calm and slow manner. This will aid in minimizing the stimuli to be perceived
2. Gestures should be used to help the client understand words. Clients' personal effects that have been placed in closets and/or drawers should be labeled for easy access. In addition, rooms used, such as the bathroom or bedroom, should be identified by signs
3. The client's emotions and reaction to change must be considered in any deviation from usual companions, routine daily activities, or arrangement of personal items
4. The client should be provided choices in activities that have been determined to be appropriate and safe

The nursing care plan should be realistic and provide an opportunity for the family and/or significant others to participate in the teaching and care of the client.

Alzheimer's Disease

Alzheimer's disease, a degenerative disease of cortical tissue, may be called presenile dementia, senile dementia, or Alzheimer type dementia. All forms show similar pathology (Greer, 1982) and therefore are considered together in this section under the term *Alzheimer's disease*.

Alzheimer's disease is caused by the accumulation of neurofibrillary tangles and senile plaques within the cortex. Small numbers of these tangles begin to appear between 50 and 60 years of age and progressively become more apparent as the person ages (Adams & Victor, 1977). There seems to be a biochemical imbalance in the brain tissue of clients affected with this disease. There is a decrease of acetylcholine and choline acetyltransferase and somatostatin, a neurohormone. It is also common to find an increased amount of heavy metal concentrations, such as aluminum, in the brain tissue. All of the mentioned pathological findings in the brain tissue of Alzheimer's disease clients may be a cause of or aggravate the cause of the disease (Greer, 1982). There are also indications that Alzheimer's disease tends to be familial. Recent research using positron emission tomography (PET) has demonstrated that subjects with Alzheimer's disease have "reduced metabolism of glucose in the temporal-parietal cortex" (Research Advances, 1984, p. 5).

Among the symptoms that may be observed when assessing the client with Alzheimer's disease are memory loss and forgetfulness, speech and naming difficulties, arithmetic miscalculation, visual and spatial difficulties, and behavioral changes. Memory loss may involve recall and recent memory. Omitting medications, repeating questions over and over, misplacing items, and forgetting schedules and appointments are all signs of forgetfulness.

Alterations in memory may be insidious at first and become more prominent as the disease progresses. Speech and naming difficulties also appear slowly and increase in frequency and severity as Alzheimer's disease progresses. Initially, the client may be unable to recall a specific word or have difficulty in naming specific objects. As the disease progresses, the client becomes unable to speak in complete sentences or interpret a full sentence. As the disease advances further, the client may become stuck on a single word, repeating that word many times.

At the same time speech and naming difficulties occur, the client begins to experience in-

creased problems in performing calculations. This may be manifested by errors in figuring correct change, adding or subtracting amounts in a checkbook, paying the correct amount of money for purchases, and properly calculating medication amounts.

Visual and spatial difficulties are very damaging, especially when an individual is living independently. Common examples of visual and spatial difficulties are exhibited by the inability of the client to place a pen upon writing paper, the inability to dress alone, the inability to maintain a sense of direction, causing one to become lost when leaving the home environment, and the inability to guide a fork or spoon to the mouth, thus making it impossible to feed oneself.

As the disease progresses to its final stage, behavioral changes are noted. These changes become visible when the client becomes neglectful of hygienic practices. The client may become restless and agitated and alternate these behaviors with somnolence and placidity. The client may display paranoia in personal relationships and business affairs.

Recent studies have shown that behavior patterns of people with Alzheimer's exhibit a continuity from before onset, with the frequency and intensity of past habits apparently increasing. However, the manner of expression has usually been altered (Shomaker, 1987).

Nursing care should be directed toward maintaining independence safely, developing support systems, and education. As with the chronic OBS client, items and places can be labeled for easy access and comprehension. Increasing assistance with activities of daily living will most likely be required. The gerontological nurse practitioner should encourage verbal communication and allow adequate time for responses. The use of pictures and gestures by the gerontological nurse practitioner may be necessary to communicate with the client as the disease progresses. The nursing care plan should provide for assistance in ambulatory activities that will ensure safety and orientation. The client should be discouraged from driving due to perceptual difficulties and loss of sense of direction. Plans for dealing with behavior problems should provide consistency, firmness, and understanding. Should the client exhibit delusions and/or hallucinations, the gerontological nurse practitioner should avoid reinforcing these phenomena by agreeing with the client. The client should be encouraged to continue practicing daily hygiene. The gerontological nurse practitioner should observe for overeating habits that may necessitate the client's being placed on a diet. The gerontological nurse practitioner should observe for behavioral changes that may occur and react accordingly in a compassionate and understanding manner.

Educating the family and/or significant others about the process of Alzheimer's disease is essential in the development of support systems. The educational process allows those individuals involved with the client to explore feelings and gain understanding of the disease. The educational process should be adapted to the different stages of the disease, thus providing the families information necessary to understand the various stages and their development. It is important for the family not to confuse Alzheimer's disease with other illnesses such as alcoholism and psychosis.

It has been found that participation in family support groups may slow the deterioration of patient behavior and enhance the coping of caregivers (Winogrond, Fisk, Kirsling, & Keyes, 1987).

The gerontological nurse practitioner must also realize that in some situations the client has little or no family or significant others. For such a client, other support systems, such as visiting nurses, community resources, and homebound programs, should be used. When planning care for a client with no support systems, the gerontological nurse practitioner should consider all resources available through social service departments, chaplain services, community agencies, and counseling services.

Additional support should be provided to the family when they visit an institutionalized client. If possible, the gerontological nurse practitioner should provide individualized teaching at the bedside. On-site teaching can offer the family an opportunity to observe and obtain the necessary information for caring for the client with Alzheimer's disease.

Families may write to the Alzheimer's Disease Association for further information. Family support groups are being formed in many localities.

SENSORY CHANGES

As a person ages, changes in sensory perception and function develop. In this section, changes in vision, hearing, taste, smell, and touch are examined, with related nursing care discussed.

Vision

Several physical and chemical changes occur in the eye as the person ages. The eye becomes less accommodating because the lens does not change shape in order to see objects and written material at close range. The lens also becomes more opaque with age. The pupil becomes smaller. Light does not filter in as well so that colors are not distinguished as easily, especially blues and greens, and acuity is diminished. More light is needed for the aged person to see the same objects that a younger person visualizes in normal or subdued light. Furthermore, the rods and cones in the retina undergo neurological deterioration, further decreasing acuity and color discrimination. Finally, the cells in and around the eye lose water and shrink. Pockets of skin, or bags, appear around the eyes. The eye itself may become smaller, thus decreasing the surface area that light can affect, further diminishing acuity. The lacrimal glands, which keep the eye moist, produce less fluid, thus leading to the drying of the eye and increased irritation. These expected changes should be considered when assessing and planning care for the aged (Graves, 1981a; Pastalan, 1977).

To accommodate for these reductions in the visual acuity of the aged client, the gerontological nurse practitioner should ensure that written materials are in large print, indirect lighting rather than one large central light is provided, as the latter tends to produce a glare, and that bright contrasting colors, such as red and yellow, are used in the client's environment. Contrasting colors are especially helpful where floor levels change in the environment and doors appear. Low-tone colors, such as blues and greens, cannot be seen well in dim light. Bright light from windows may also be diminished by using sheer curtains.

Senile Macular Degeneration

This retinal disease may be dry (atrophic) or neovascular (exudative). The dry or atrophic form progresses slowly, but the neovascular or exudative type is more rapid. Deterioration occurs in the membrane between the retina and underlying blood vessels. Neovascularization progresses toward the macula. Treatment involves use of lasers to cause photocoagulation (Brunner & Suddarth, 1984).

Narrowed Field

One visual problem associated with the expected changes of age is a narrowed visual field; this may be attributed to the decreased number of rods and cones, decreased accommodation, and decreased light filtering into the retina. It may also be due to other problems, such as an intracranial tumor or glaucoma.

The gerontological nurse practitioner may test the client's field of vision by moving an object, such as a finger or pencil, from outside to into the person's field of vision. One eye is tested at a time, and all four quadrants are assessed—nasal, temporal, upward, and downward. While the client is looking straight ahead, bring the object in slowly and have the client respond when the object becomes visible. When the client states that the object is visible, notice the angle between the object and the eye's straightforward gaze. The visual fields in a younger person will have approximate angles of 60 degrees in the nasal field, 90 degrees in the temporal field, 50 degrees in the upward field, and 70 degrees in the downward field. The physician may also map out visual fields with a perimeter or a tangent screen if additional testing is required (Luckmann & Sorenson, 1980). Careful assessment is necessary because the visual fields of an aged client may be greatly reduced from these values.

Nursing care for a client with a narrowed visual field includes placing items within the client's field, instructing the client . .t the location of objects that he cannot visualize, and speaking to the client when stepping into the room. When speaking to the person, step into the line of vision so the client will know who is speaking. Finally, the client's family and/or significant others should be instructed in rearranging the home so that injuries do not result from a narrowed field. Obstacles that could cause tripping should be removed. Spaces between furniture should be widened. Objects that could cause chest or abdominal injuries should be rearranged to keep the person from accidentally striking them. The family should also be instructed to move into the person's field of vision when conversing and to put objects in his or her visual field.

Night Blindness

Because of decreased light filtration and resulting color discrimination problems, the aged person may develop night blindness. Night blindness may also be due to decreased numbers of rods and cones in the retina. In addition to difficulty in seeing at night, the aged person will experience problems in moving from a bright to a dark environment and vice versa (Stewart, 1982).

Assessment of the person for night blindness should be made carefully, as injury is a potential risk factor. The person should be observed while moving in dark areas or very subdued light. In an unfamiliar environment, the person is more likely to run into objects and have difficulty performing activities of daily living, especially at night. Light–dark accommodation can be tested by observing the client's reaction to moving from a brightly lit area to a dimly lit area. During the observation period, instruct the client to acknowledge when he or she can see again, while timing the length of the client's inability to see. The time required for light–dark accommodation can be shared with the client and considered in the planning of nursing care and homebound care.

Nursing care should focus on maintaining the aged person's safety and on client–family awareness of the presence of night blindness. If the person still drives, discourage driving at night. The availability of family members and/or friends should be identified to provide transportation during night hours. The individual should be encouraged to plan personal and social activities during the daylight hours if possible. The person should be made aware of the importance to pause for a few moments when entering a dark or dimly lit room from a bright area. If there are stairs present, handrails should be installed; and the client should be encouraged to use them. Potential safety hazards in the home, such as loose rugs, electric cords, and/or exposed wires, should be corrected.

Cataracts

A cataract is defined as an opaque lens. Cataracts are the most common visual disorder of the aged. It is unclear why cataracts form; however, research has shown that the lens of the eye is the only organ to grow continuously. As the fibers are produced, they form on the periphery of the lens and compress the older fibers into the center or nucleus. As the nucleus continues to age, it turns from crystal clear to a yellowish-brown and then becomes sclerosed, thus causing a cataract (Kornzweig & Klapper, 1977).

When a bright light is directed into the person's eyes, a cloudy film in the lens indicates a fully mature cataract. The history will usually reveal an increasing loss and blurring of vision over a period ranging from months to years.

Usually there is no associated pain or redness of the eyes. The visual loss becomes more noticeable when cataracts develop bilaterally. In addition, the client will complain of discomfort when exposed to bright lights and glare (Brunner & Suddarth, 1984).

Surgical removal of the cataract is presently the treatment of choice. Among the forms of surgery currently available are intracapsular extraction, extracapsular extraction, cryosurgery, or phaecoemulsification. Intracapsular extraction involves the removal of the lens and its surrounding capsule. Extracapsular extraction is the removal of the lens after anterior capsule rupture with the posterior capsule being left intact. In cryosurgery, the metal probe tip reaches a temperature of $-30°$ to $-40°C$ and is positioned to adhere directly to the lens capsule in order to deliver the lens. In phaecoemulsification, the lens is ultrasonically fragmented and then removed from the eye by aspiration. In addition to having the cataract removed, artificial lenses may be implanted. The prosthetic intraocular implant can be inserted after any type of extraction. It is attached to the iris and causes minimal distortion of the image. It is especially recommended for clients older than 65 years who may be handicapped and therefore unable to manage contact lenses (Brunner & Suddarth, 1984).

Preoperative and postoperative care of the client with cataracts and cataract surgery are essentially the same regardless of which type of surgery has been performed. Preoperative preparation includes education of the client and family regarding postoperative expectations. Generally cataract extraction is done under local anesthesia. Usually the physician prescribes medications preoperatively to induce general relaxation and eyedrops that induce vasoconstriction and pupillary constriction. Clients should be oriented to their environment, such as bedrails, tables, call light, and hospital routines. Assistance should be given to the client when moving from bed to chair and ambulating.

Postoperatively, the involved eye will be

covered with a dressing and a metal shield. The metal shield will guard and protect the eye. Rapid movements and strains to the eye, such as Valsalva maneuver and sneezing, need to be avoided. Therefore, it is important to prevent and observe for constipation and upper respiratory infections. The client may use a small pillow and have the head of the bed at a 30–45-degree angle. Some physicians now allow the client to get out of bed later on the day of surgery. Mild pain is to be expected postoperatively; however, sharp or severe pain should be reported to the physician (Brunner & Suddarth, 1984).

After acute surgical recovery, the client who did not have implant(s) will probably receive temporary cataract glasses with thick convex lenses. These glasses require adjustment by the client before they can be used efficiently. The client should look through the center of the glasses and turn the head to see items in the periphery. The glasses are initially used while sitting; as the person gets used to seeing through the glasses, progressive ambulation may begin. After about 8 weeks, the client usually obtains permanent glasses.

Contact lenses may be used by some select postsurgical clients. These clients must be taught how to insert, remove, and care for the lenses.

Usually eyedrop medications are given postoperatively for an extended period of time. The client and/or family should be taught before discharge how to instill the eyedrops and have a basic understanding of their purpose(s). These eye medications are usually prescribed to relax muscles, keep the eye moist, and prevent infection.

Glaucoma

Glaucoma, a condition in which the intraocular pressure increases, is the second most common visual problem in the aged. Intraocular pressure is the pressure within the anterior and posterior chambers of the eye and normally measures 11 to 22 mm Hg. This pressure within the chamber is maintained by the aqueous humor, which also provides nutrients to the lens. The aqueous humor is produced in the ciliary processes in the posterior chamber, flows through the pupil into the anterior chamber, and then flows through the trabecular meshwork and the canal of Schlemm to be reabsorbed by the anterior ciliary veins. When this flow is obstructed, intraocular pressure builds because the production of aqueous humor occurs without reabsorption. If left untreated, glaucoma leads to blindness.

Glaucoma occurs in both an acute and a chronic form. Acute glaucoma involves the sudden closure of the angle of the anterior chamber where the cornea and iris meet, thus interfering with reabsorption and causing an increase in intraocular pressure. The client will complain of a severe headache, eye pain, nausea, vomiting, blurred vision, and seeing halos around lights. Other observable signs include dilated pupil, edematous ciliary body, and an increased intraocular pressure as measured by a tonometer. Treatment consists of medication to decrease intraocular pressure and eventual surgery to prevent further attacks.

Chronic glaucoma occurs due to an obstruction of the canal of Schlemm and flow pathways. This obstruction occurs over time and is generally insidious, and signs and symptoms usually do not occur until permanent damage has already begun. This is the more common of the two forms of glaucoma. Chronic glaucoma affects peripheral vision first and then central vision. Clients complain of their eyes feeling tired, headaches, halos around lights, and blurred vision. The symptoms seem to be more evident upon arising in the morning. One eye is usually affected; however, both eyes may eventually be involved. Treatment consists of medication to keep the pupil constricted (if the pupil is dilated, further obstruction occurs) and decrease production of aqueous humor. If medication becomes ineffective, surgery may be performed to provide new channels for flow and reabsorption.

Nursing care of the client should focus primarily on client education to prevent further damage to the optic nerve. The client must be taught about medications—their purpose, actions, and proper administration. It should be stressed that the medications must not be skipped even though the client is feeling better. The client must be instructed to avoid any stressful activity—straining, heavy lifting, emotional or physical stress—that will increase intraocular pressure. Medications that cause pupillary dilation and an increase in blood pressure, such as atropine and Neosynephrine, respectively, should be avoided. The client should be instructed that medications may impair night vision, therefore necessitating caution with activities performed during the night or in a dark room. Clients should also be advised to obtain and wear identification explaining their condition in the event that they are unable to speak as a result of a medical problem or accident. It is important to stress to the client the need for regular examinations and progress checks by an ophthalmologist (Kornzweig & Klapper, 1977; Luckmann & Sorenson, 1980).

Detached Retina

A detached retina occurs when a portion of the retina tears away from the choroid to which it is loosely attached. Once the retina detaches in any given area, it may progressively detach; therefore, prompt treatment is necessary. Nursing assessment should include a history of client activities prior to the visual changes as well as the visual problems themselves. This will assist in determining whether the cause was traumatic or pathological. The client may complain of floating spots and flashes of light, and blurred and black areas of vision that give a coating or veiling sensation of sight. If not treated promptly, retinal detachment will become permanent and may lead to blindness.

Bed rest and bilateral eye patches are recommended in order to allow the portion of detached retina to "float" back to the portion of choroid from which it detached. Eye patches are used to allow complete rest for the eyes. However, surgery is usually required to reattach the retina. Different types of surgery exist—electrodiathermy, cryosurgery, scleral buckling,

photocoagulation, and intravitreal injections. Electrodiathermy and cryosurgery cause adhesion between the retina and choroid. Scleral buckling and photocoagulation decrease the diameter of the sclera and interior vitreous humor, thus pushing the sclera and choroid toward the detached retina (Brunner & Suddarth, 1984).

Regardless of the treatment method, nursing care should be directed toward reducing stress, maintaining comfort, and promoting healing. Due to the eye patches, clients should be oriented to their surroundings and nursing care procedures prior to implementation. The client should be made aware of the presence of others in the room. The client's position is extremely important postoperatively; physicians' orders should be followed implicitly. The client should be instructed regarding allowable positions. It is important that the client not assume a prone position or bend over. Any sudden movements and/or conditions that cause added stress on the eye, such as straining, emotional stress, coughing, or sneezing, should be avoided. When first ambulating postoperatively, the client should be assisted and observed for any discomfort. The dressing and patches are usually removed the first postoperative day. The client may watch television but should not read for about 3 weeks. The client should be instructed to be careful in head movement and avoid all heavy work involving lifting for at least 6 weeks postoperatively (Luckmann & Sorenson, 1980).

Corneal Ulcers

A corneal ulcer develops when the cornea becomes inflamed and then deteriorates. Perforation of the cornea may then occur, which may lead to infection and visual loss. Inflammation may be due to previous trauma or bacterial, viral, or fungal infection. Bacterial infections may be treated with local antibiotics and sulfa drugs. The most common viral infection is herpes simplex.

This problem is difficult to treat, and so early detection is important. The gerontological nurse practitioner should gather a history, including past infections, particularly around the eye, eye irritation, nutrition deficiencies, and cerebral vascular accident. The corneal ulcer may be seen by fluoroscopy. Medications to dilate the eye to relieve pain and allow the ciliary body to rest are usually given, as are antibiotics to decrease the infection. The physician may decide to cleanse and cauterize the ulcer. Hot compresses will help the client feel more comfortable. Also, the client should be advised to wear sunglasses to ease discomfort when outside or in brightly lit rooms. The client should also be instructed to seek medical attention immediately if the vision worsens, as it may indicate perforation (Luckmann & Sorenson, 1980).

Hearing

As a person ages, changes in hearing occur. The ear has three basic divisions—external, middle, and internal. The external ear provides an avenue for mediation of sound. The middle ear conducts that sound into the inner ear, which has the nerves for interpretation. As a person ages, the external ear does not change dramatically, though cerumen is produced in lesser quantities. The middle ear may become hardened or atrophied in any one of its parts—tympanic membrane, malleus, incus, or stapes. In the inner ear, however, the nerve degeneration and resulting loss of hearing for high-frequency sounds occur with aging.

Environmental and medical factors may increase the susceptibility to hearing loss. High levels of noise in the person's environment—airplanes, traffic, construction work, and factory assembly lines—can actually cause cell damage. Ear infections, trauma, cerumen impaction, and some drugs may also induce hearing loss. Diabetes and otosclerosis should also be considered as potential causes of hearing loss.

There are two types of hearing deficits, both of which may be occurring in the aged person. Conduction deafness is an interruption in the transmission of sound waves. Otosclerosis and a buildup of ear wax are two examples of this type, which can be easily corrected. Perception deafness is an interruption in the interpretation of sound. Conditions that cause damage to the cochlea and/or auditory nerve lead to this form of deafness.

Presbycusis is defined as the progressive loss of hearing due to the aging process. There is a loss of nerve cells in the eighth cranial nerve, which results in a loss of hearing high-frequency sounds. This is followed by a loss of middle-frequency hearing and finally a loss of low-frequency hearing.

Assessment should include a hearing test by a physician or audiometrist. The gerontological nurse practitioner can test for hearing loss by observing the client's understanding of consonants such as s, z, t, f, and g, which are high-frequency consonants. It is important to consider the setting for the assessment to avoid any background noise that may distract or disturb the client and interfere with communication. With an otoscope, the gerontological nurse practitioner should examine the external ear canals for cerumen buildup and the condition of the tympanic membrane.

Nursing care is directed toward client education and reorganization of life-style. The family should be aware of the aged person's possible reactions to hearing loss. Confusion, suspicion, anger, withdrawal, insecurity, and inappropriate behavior are among the variety of possible reactions. Once a diagnosis has been made, compensation for the hearing loss may be planned. Interventions such as a telephone receiver with increased amplification will enable the person to participate in phone conversations. Speaking slowly, distinctly, and in a low voice tone will facilitate face-to-face conversations. Gestures may also be used to enhance and clarify conversations. One should avoid shouting or speaking in high-pitched tones and avoid using simplistic language with the aged person experiencing hearing problems. These means of communication will only increase that person's self-consciousness and add to his or her insecurity.

Individuals who have hearing loss due to

conduction deficits may desire to use a hearing aid to compensate for the loss. The aged person should consult an otologist to determine if a hearing aid is beneficial before purchasing one. Once a hearing aid is bought, it will take a period of time for the person to adapt to wearing one since *all* sound is amplified. The client should be informed that if the hearing aid is turned on too loudly sounds may be somewhat distorted. Also, it should be noted that reverberations increase the distortion. The nurse should instruct the client in the proper method of using, caring for, and maintaining the hearing aid. The ear mold may be washed in soap and water and dried, and the cannula may be cleaned with a small cotton-tipped applicator (Brunner & Suddarth, 1984).

Taste

As a person ages, changes in the sensation of taste also occur. Structurally, fewer taste buds are functioning. In the aged, taste buds at the back of the tongue that perceive sour and bitter flavors function more effectively and for more years than do the taste buds at the front of the tongue where sweet and salty flavors are perceived (Shore, 1976). Also, the mouth and lips decrease in elasticity, and the amount of saliva is decreased. These gustatory changes, plus an overall decrease in the rate of metabolism, probably account for a decrease in appetite.

Assessment of the client's taste is rather limited, but the gerontological nurse practitioner can touch a client's tongue in different places with a cotton-tipped applicator which has been dipped in various flavors and liquids. The gerontological nurse practitioner can ask questions about the need to add more sugar or salt to foods in order to be tasted, as well as changes in food preference.

Nursing care is related to helping the person adapt to his or her decreased sensation of taste while maintaining adequate nutritional intake. Foods of different colors and aromas should be placed together in order to make the meal appear more appetizing. Different spices may be used to enhance flavor as long as they are not used in overabundance. Persons should also be taught not to oversweeten or oversalt their food, particularly if they have medical problems such as diabetes or heart disease.

Smell

An aged person may also have a decreased sensitivity to smell, although very little research has been done. The receptors in the nose that perceive smell tend to atrophy in the aging process, and the person is unable to smell odors from cooking, cleaning, and the environment. Since smell also plays a large role in taste, a loss of appetite may also result.

Nursing assessment involves interview and observation of the client. Questions that may be asked could be related to complaints the client has about inability to smell certain odors, reactions the client has when walking or driving by a factory, bakery, or dump site, and the client's nutritional intake. The gerontological nurse practitioner may also be able to observe the reaction of the client when certain smells permeate his or her room, such as the smells of excrement or coffee.

As with taste, nursing care should be directed toward compensation as well as stimulation. Foods that have a pleasant odor should be served. Different fragrances from flowers, perfumes, room sprays, and candles can stimulate the olfactory nerves remaining in the nose. If the person is at home or in a nursing home, the family or staff can offer stimulation of the olfactory sense by providing pleasant food smells, such as coffee or freshly baked cookies, cakes, and breads, which should increase the person's appetite. Unpleasant odors should be avoided when attempting to use the sense of smell to stimulate appetite (Stewart, 1982). Clients should be assessed for the ability to smell hazardous gases and/or smoke. Fire detectors can be installed as a safety measure for all aged persons.

It is also important to periodically have the gas company inspect for leaks and ensure proper ventilation.

Touch

Touch is also affected by the aging process. It becomes difficult to discriminate temperatures. A decrease in tactile sensations also affects fine motor discrimination for hand-to-eye coordination. Therefore, the aged person may have trouble in turning pages, tying shoe laces, opening cans and bottles, squeezing oranges and scissors, or turning dials. It has been shown that the tactile sensitivity of the palate diminishes with age, thus increasing one's risk of aspiration (Newman, 1979).

Hot–warm discrimination as well as a sharp–dull and two-point discriminations may be assessed by the gerontological nurse practitioner. Hot–warm discrimination may be tested by using two bowls of water at different temperatures, noting whether or not the person feels the difference. Sharp–dull determination may be made with a paper clip or safety pin. The gerontological nurse practitioner has the client close his or her eyes and then tests in different areas with the sharp or dull edge, having the client express whether or not the point is sharp or dull. Two-point discrimination is performed by having the client discern between being touched by one and two points. All these tests will give an indication of a decrease in tactile sensitivity.

Nursing care should be planned to provide stimulation as well as safety. To provide safety, careful consideration should be given to avoid extremely hot temperatures of bathwater, foods, and serving dishes. When using burners, heaters, and hot water spouts, the aged person should develop a mechanism to remember that these items may cause injury before sensing that a burn is occurring. For stimulation, different weaves and textures of fabric may be used to help the client identify clothing, particularly if the client has trouble with vision.

One aspect of touch to be considered is that of pain. Pain is a nebulous term, one that has different meanings for different people. However, pain does carry the connotation of hurt or discomfort and indicates that something is wrong inside or on the body. In the aged person, pain is diminished because both the sense of touch and the number of neurons are diminished. The decreased ability to sense pain can affect the client's safety. If an aged person with decreased pain perception touches a hot stove or hot water, the degree of thermal injury could easily become more severe. Also, a cut or bruise could bleed considerably before being noticed and treated. A "minor" fall could actually result in major damage, such as a hip fracture, without being felt. Clients should be encouraged to inspect their hands and feet frequently for possible injury and to be examined after any falls that occur. These preventive measures may help in decreasing the chance of complications in the aged person.

COMMON MEDICATIONS

There are many types of medications that are used by the aged person with neurological/sensory changes. Sleeping aids (both prescription and nonprescription), psychotropics, anti-Parkinson drugs, and eye medications (prescription and nonprescription) may be used by the client with the previously mentioned problems. These classes of medications are discussed with regard to their action, interactions, adverse reactions, and nursing implications.

Prescription Medications

Prescription drugs are probably the more commonly used drugs by clients with neurological/sensory problems. Sleeping pills are often prescribed for insomnia and other sleeping problems. Hypnotics promote drowsiness and aid in maintaining sleep (Gilman, Goodman, &

Gilman, 1980). They interact with alcohol, which potentiates side effects, and tend to lead to daytime drowsiness. They do not appear to interfere with REM sleep, but tolerance to the medication may develop. Nursing implications include observing the client for expected effects as well as overdosage, for ataxia or dizziness, which could indicate daytime drowsiness, and for nausea and vomiting. Antihistamines act as sedatives in the body, producing a calming effect by blocking the action of histamine. They interact with and potentiate other central nervous system depressants and anticholinergic drugs. Side effects include dizziness, drowsiness, hypotension, dryness of the mouth and throat, nausea and vomiting, and nervousness. The antihistamines are possibly not as effective as the hypnotics; however, they are safe to use in the aged person (Gambert & Duthrie, 1981; Patterson, Gustafson, & Sheridan, 1980). Nursing implications are essentially the same as for the hypnotics.

Sleeping aids that should be avoided with the aged person are the barbiturates, such as pentobarbital (Nembutal) and phenobarbital (Luminal). These drugs can lead to addiction, adverse reactions, and contrary effects, such as delirium or restlessness. They may also lead to liver damage. Therefore, the individual must be carefully screened and observed for reactions (Gambert & Duthrie, 1981).

The half-life of sleeping medications should be considered when choices are made. The half-life is the length of time necessary for the concentration of a specific drug in the body or plasma to be decreased to one half of its original level. This determines how long the effect of that drug will last; the half-lives of various medications may range from a few hours to 1 week (Simonson, 1984).

Psychotropic drugs, specifically antidepressants and tranquilizers, are used to aid in the treatment of clients with organic brain syndrome and Alzheimer's disease, as well as to help in relieving anxiety associated with these changes. Antidepressants act by blocking various neurotransmitters from being returned into the cycle for use. They also influence anticholinergic activity and potentiate the effects or increase the amount of serotonin and norepinephrine. There are two classes of antidepressants: tricyclics and monoamine oxidase (MAO) inhibitors. The tricyclic antidepressants interact with central nervous system depressants and tend to cause convulsions when used in combination with MAO inhibitors. Adverse reactions include atropine-like effects (dry mouth, pupil dilation, tachycardia, urinary retention, and decreased gastrointestinal mobility), hypotension, facial perspiration, and tremor. Nursing implications for the tricyclic drugs include decreasing the dosage slowly rather than abruptly discontinuing their use, administering them in a single dose, and observing the client for suicidal tendencies. Clients who have had a recent myocardial infarction or severe cardiovascular disease should not receive tricyclics because of their potentiation of cardiovascular effects. The MAO inhibitors interact with certain types of foods, specifically foods containing tyramine, such as ripe cheese, avocados, chocolate, beer, chicken livers, bologna, or canned figs, and may lead to hypertensive crises and/or convulsions. Other side effects include hypotension, restlessness, insomnia, dry mouth, anorexia, nausea, tremors, and paresthesias. The nurse should be observant for interactions and be careful that foods containing tyramine are eliminated from the client's diet. The physician should be consulted as to the advisability of the client receiving tricyclics and MAO inhibitors concurrently before administering such a regimen (Patterson et al., 1980).

Tranquilizers, especially phenothiazine derivatives, are used to calm the client and relieve combative and psychotic behavior. They act by depressing certain portions of the central nervous system (depending on the specific drug used). These drugs interact with barbiturates, causing a potential increase in effects that may lead to hypotension, especially when the client is standing. Other adverse effects include drowsiness, delayed reflexes, tremors or spasticity, blurred vision, constipation, photophobia, and decreased hypothalmic control, which interferes with the client's ability to regulate the body temperature. Gerontological nurse practitioners should be observant for these adverse effects, as well as keeping room temperatures stable, decreasing light in the client's room, assisting the client in walking or sitting down, and maintaining adequate nutritional intake with an increase in fiber and fluids (Graves, 1981b; Patterson et al., 1980).

Antiparkinsonism drugs are given to counteract the symptoms of Parkinson's disease. Though not curative, the drugs ameliorate the effects of Parkinsonism. Drugs used for Parkinson's disease include levodopa, anticholinergic drugs, and dopamine agonists, in addition to antihistamines and major tranquilizers (phenothiazine derivatives).

Probably the most important drug currently being used in the treatment of Parkinson's disease is levodopa (L-dopa). It is a precursor to dopamine, the neurotransmitter that is decreased or absent in Parkinson's disease. Because dopamine does not cross the blood–brain barrier, L-dopa is used. It crosses the barrier and then converts to dopamine for use in the basal ganglia. L-dopa is usually given concurrently with carbidopa, a dopa decarboxylase inhibitor, which decreases the chance of L-dopa conversion in peripheral tissue. L-dopa interacts with MAO inhibitors and phenothiazines. Side effects include nausea and vomiting, cardiac arrhythmias, orthostatic hypotension, anemia, choreiform movements, and periodic return of Parkinsonism. The client must be observed carefully because dosages must be individualized. Gerontological nurse practitioners should give L-dopa with meals and control the amount of protein in the diet. The family should be instructed in the observation of symptoms. The client should not have a vitamin B_6 supplement, as this vitamin assists in converting L-dopa in the peripheral system. It is also important to observe the client for severe depression, which may potentiate suicidal tendencies.

Anticholinergic drugs, such as Artane, Akineton, and Cogentin, are also used in the treatment of Parkinson's disease. These drugs block acetylcholine, thus decreasing muscle cramps, spasm, tremor, and rigidity. One drug may be more effective than another, so they should be given one at a time, increasing the dosage slowly. Side effects include blurred vision, dry mouth, mental changes, hallucinations, agitation, and gastrointestinal upset. These drugs should not be given to clients with glaucoma, tachycardia, or urinary retention. Nursing responsibilities include giving the drug prescribed with food and reporting side effects.

Dopamine agonists, amantadine hydrochloride (Symmetrel) and bromocriptine mesylate (Parlodel), cause the release of dopamine from storage areas and stimulate the dopamine receptors, respectively. They are often given in conjunction with other drugs used to treat Parkinson's disease. Side effects of amantadine hydrochloride include nervousness, insomnia, ataxia, depression, dry mouth, and nausea. Side effects of bromocriptine mesylate include hypotension, nausea, dry mouth, drowsiness, cardiac arrhythmias, dizziness, auditory and visual hallucinations, and delusions. Gerontological nurse practitioners should not administer these drugs if the client has an upper respiratory infection. Side effects should be noted and reported promptly to the physician.

The purpose of antihistamines and tranquilizers is to decrease muscle rigidity and tremors, thus improving speech and voluntary coordination. However, they may cause degrees of depression and should be used with caution (Hickey, 1981; Hoehn, 1981; Perlik, Koller, Weiner, Nausieda, & Klawans, 1980).

Eye medications, such as local anesthetics, antibiotics, antiviral agents, steroids, and autonomic drugs, are used in a variety of conditions.

Local anesthetics are generally used by the ophthalmologist in order to perform procedures on the eye, such as removing stitches after cataract surgery. The client should be advised not to rub the eye for a period of time after a local anesthetic is applied, thus preventing injury to the eye.

Antibiotics are generally used for conjunctivitis. However, it is advisable to rule out glaucoma prior to using ophthalmic antibiotics.

Antiviral agents are used to treat herpes simplex, which may cause corneal ulcers. On the other hand, corneal ulcers may mimic areas of severe herpes infection; therefore, careful assessment of the cornea is necessary to differentiate between the two conditions if the client is receiving antiviral ophthalmic drugs.

Intraocular corticosteroids are used to decrease inflammation and scarring on the surface of the eye. However, if the client has glaucoma or a predisposition to glaucoma, these drugs may cause an increase in intraocular pressure.

Autonomic drugs are widely used for ophthalmic conditions. They are divided into three classes: parasympathomimetics, parasympatholytics, and sympathomimetics. Parasympathomimetics are drugs that cause pupillary constriction and contraction of the ciliary muscles. They act by either directly reacting with cholinergic receptors or indirectly destroying acetylcholinesterase to increase the concentration of acetylcholine. This action allows the free flow of aqueous humor around the lens and cornea. These drugs are used for the treatment of glaucoma. Pilocarpine is the most common drug in this class. Side effects are generally systemic in nature and include nausea, sweating, weakness, bradycardia, hypotension, and bronchial constriction. Because the client will probably need to receive these medications for the remainder of his or her life, the gerontological nurse practitioner must teach the client about these drugs and their administration. The client should also be observed for desired effects and adverse reactions.

Parasympatholytic drugs, on the other hand, prevent acetylcholine from reacting with its receptors. This leads to dilation of the pupil and paralysis of the ciliary muscles. These drugs, the most common of which are atropine, cyclopentolate, and tropicamide, are useful in treating inflammation of the anterior eye, particularly following cataract surgery. Side effects are often systemic and include dry mouth, dry skin, flushing, increased heart rate, and mental disturbances. The gerontological nurse practitioner should not give these drugs to a client with glaucoma unless specifically ordered to do so by the ophthalmologist. The client and family should be taught to give these medications, even though they may be needed only on a short-term basis.

Sympathomimetic agents have alpha- and beta-adrenergic stimulation capabilities, depending on the specific drugs. Some drugs, such as epinephrine hydrochloride, are used to treat chronic glaucoma, whereas others are used strictly for diagnosis. Side effects include headache, conjunctival hyperemia, hypertension, tachycardia, and cardiac arrhythmias. The gerontological nurse practitioner should monitor heart rate and blood pressure frequently. Before the client is discharged, the gerontological nurse practitioner should teach the client and family how to monitor the pulse rate and blood pressure and properly instill the eye medications.

Nonprescription Medications

The two most common nonprescription medication categories used by clients with neurological–sensory problems are sleeping aids and eyedrops. The client should be cautioned that these drugs could be harmful and should consult a physician before taking them. Nonprescription drugs may interact with prescription drugs either synergistically or antagonistically. The gerontological nurse practitioner should teach the client the importance of keeping a record of medications currently used and times taken to prevent an overdose.

Eyedrops such as Visine or Murine are generally not needed and most often will not be beneficial to the client. If the client complains of dry eyes and expresses a need for drops, normal saline drops are the same solution as body fluid and can probably be used safely. However, the client should check with the physician before purchasing and using these drops.

SUMMARY

There are many neurological and sensory changes that may affect the aged person. These changes can become very distressing and debilitating to the client and must be dealt with accordingly. Specific medications are frequently prescribed for these changes but require close monitoring as they commonly have side effects that interfere with effective treatment.

Nursing care should focus on teaching and assisting the individual and family to adapt to the neurological or sensory change. The family should be encouraged to provide the necessary support to assist the individual during the various stages of these changes. It is important that the family visit frequently in the home to give not only emotional support but to assist in providing a safe environment.

REFERENCES

Adams, R., & Victor, M. (1977). *Principles of neurology*. New York: McGraw-Hill.

Boss, B. (1982, April). Acute mood and behavior disturbances of neurological origin: Acute confusional states. *Journal of Neurosurgical Nursing, 14* (2), 61–68.

Brunner, L. S., & Suddarth, D. S. (1984). *Textbook of medical–surgical nursing* (5th ed.). Philadelphia: Lippincott.

Coleman, R., Miles, L., Guilleminault, C., Zarcone, V., Hoed, J. V., & Dement, W. (1981). Sleep–wake disorders in the elderly: A polysommographic analysis. *Journal of the American Geriatric Society, 20* (7), 289–296.

Dement, W., Richardson, G., Prinz, P., Carskadon, M., Kripke, D., & Zeisler, C. (1985). Changes of sleep and wakefulness with age. In C. E. Finch & E. L. Schneider (Eds.), *Handbook of the biology of aging* (2nd ed.). New York: Van Nostrand Reinhold.

Duara, R., London, E. D., & Rapoport, S. I. (1985). Changes in structure and energy metabolism of the aging brain. In C. E. Finch & E. L. Schneider (Eds.), *Handbook of the biology of aging* (2nd ed.). New York: Van Nostrand Reinhold.

Forbes, E. J., & Fitzsimons, V. M. (1981). *The older adult: A process for wellness*. St. Louis: Mosby.

Gambert, S., & Duthrie, E. (1981). Sleep disorders: Coping with a waking nightmare. *Geriatrics, 18* (9), 61–65.

Gilman, A. G., Goodman, L., & Gilman, A. (Eds.). (1980). *Goodman and Gilman's the pharmacological basis of therapeutics* (6th ed.). New York: Macmillan.

Gomez, G. E., & Gomez, E. A. (1987). Delirium. *Geriatric Nursing, 8*(6), 330–332.

Graves, M. (1981a). Physiologic changes and major diseases in the older adult. In M. O. Hogstel (Ed.), *Nursing care of the older adult: In the hospital, nursing home and community*. New York: Wiley.

Graves, M. (1981b). Drug use and abuse among the elderly. In M. O. Hogstel (Ed.), *Nursing care of the older adult: In the hospital, nursing home and community*. New York: Wiley.

Greer, M. (1982). Dementia: A major disease of aging. *Geriatrics, 37* (4), 101–107.

Hickey, J. (1981). *The clinical practice of neurological and neurosurgical nursing*. Philadelphia: Lippincott.

Hoehn, M. (1981). Bromocriptine and its use in Parkinsonism. *Journal of the American Geriatrics Society, 29* (6), 251–258.

Kornzweig, A., & Klapper, R. (1977). Visual processes and aging. In *Sensory processes and aging: Proceedings of a conference at the Dallas Geriatric Research Institute*. Denton, TX: University Center for Community Services for the Center for Studies in Aging, School of Community Services, North Texas State University.

Linderborn, K. M. (1988). The need to assess dementia. *Journal of Gerontological Nursing, 14*(1), 35–39.

Luckmann, J., & Sorenson, K. C. (1980). *Medical–surgical nursing: A psychophysiologic approach*. Philadelphia: Saunders.

Neatherlin, J. S., Kamp, C. W., & Guthrie, M. D. (1981, June). Synaptic transmission within the central nervous system. *Journal of Neurosurgical Nursing, 13* (3), 146–149.

Newman, H. (1979). Palatal sensitivity to touch: Correlation with age. *Journal of the American Geriatrics Society, 28* (7), 319.

Pastalan, L. (1977). Aging and sensory changes: An update and some practical suggestions. In *Sensory Processes and Aging: Proceedings of a conference at the Dallas Geriatric Research Institute.* Denton, TX: University Center for Community Services for the Center for Studies in Aging, School of Community Services, North Texas State University.

Patterson, H. R., Gustafson, E., & Sheridan, E. (1980). *Falconer's Current Drug Handbook 1980–1982.* Philadelphia: Saunders.

Perlik, S. J., Koller, W. C., Weiner, W. J., Nausieda, P., & Klawans, H. L. (1980). Parkinsonism: Is your treatment appropriate? *Geriatrics, 35* (11), 65–70.

Potvin, A. R., Sndulko, K., Tourtellotte, W. W., Lemmon, J. A., & Potvin, J. H. (1980). Human neurologic function and the aging process. *Journal of the American Geriatrics Society, 28,* (1), 1–9.

Prinz, P., Peskind, E., Vitaliano, P., Raskind, M., Eisdorfer, C., Zemcuznikov, N., & Gerber, C. (1982). Changes in the sleep and waking EEGs of nondemented and demented elderly subjects. *Journal of the American Geriatrics Society, 20* (2), 86–93.

Research Advances (1984, December). *Aging Program Letter, 1* (8), 5.

Rossman, Isadore (Ed.). (1986). *Clinical geriatrics* (3rd ed.). Philadelphia: Lippincott.

Shomaker, D. (1987). Problematic behavior and the Alzheimer patient: Retrospection as a method of understanding and counseling. *The Gerontologist, 27* (3), 370–375.

Shore, H. (1976, April). Designing a training program for understanding sensory losses in aging. *The Gerontologist, 16* (2), 157–165.

Simonson, W. (1984). *Medications and the elderly.* Rockville, MD: Aspen.

Stewart, C. M. (1982, April). Age-related changes in the nervous system. *Journal of Neurosurgical Nursing, 14* (2), 69–73.

Stoudemire, A., & Thompson, T. (1981). Recognizing and treating dementia. *Geriatrics, 36* (10), 112–120.

Topp, B. (1987). Toward a better understanding of Parkinson's disease. *Geriatric Nursing, 8* (4), 180–182.

Winogrond, I. R., Fisk, A. A., Kirsling, R. A., & Keyes, B. (1987). The relationship of caregiver burden and morale to Alzheimer's disease patient function in a therapeutic setting. *The Gerontologist, 27* (3), 336–339.

5

INTEGUMENTARY CHANGES

As the body's outermost layer of tissue, the skin serves to protect the inner organs and plays an important role in the client's overall self-image. The effects of trauma, sun, chemicals, burns, and internal problems are readily manifested on the skin. The skin often reflects the client's general well-being and may be the first indicator that something is wrong.

The skin is subjected to much abuse during a lifetime. Much abuse can be prevented or diminished by teaching clients the proper self-care of the skin, thus affording them the opportunity of learning to value and preserve their most visible organ and one of the greatest contributors to their overall body image.

Many common and normal changes occur with aging skin. Older clients may hold many myths about their skin because they lack knowledge and understanding of these changes. The media and society contribute to many myths by spending millions on advertisements to promote products and treatments that purport to remove these normal signs of aging. These prevalent attitudes contribute to an older person's decline in self-image and self-esteem. Therefore, the nurse must assume a role in educating clients regarding the normal aging changes and in promoting clients' acceptance of their aging skin. This acceptance is easier if clients are taught how to properly care for their skin. Knowledge of signs of normal aging assist the nurse in recognition of

abnormalities, therefore expediting referrals to the proper health professional.

AGE-RELATED CHANGES

The aging skin exhibits a thinning of all layers of skin and a general loss of subcutaneous fat. These changes contribute to thinner, looser, and more fragile skin. The older person becomes more prone to manifesting signs of trauma such as purpura or ecchymosis due to this loss of padding. Years of gravitational force and changes in collagen and elastic fibers contribute to the appearance of wrinkles and the sagging of such areas of skin as the chin and jawline, neck, breasts, and upper arms.

The skin becomes drier due to a decrease in sebaceous gland and sweat gland activity. Spontaneous sweating is diminished by approximately 30% in older adults due to a reduction in the number of sweat glands and a decrease in the activity of those that remain. Sebaceous gland activity diminishes in males and females related to a decrease of androgens.

Aging or liver spots, called senile lentignes, become apparent on parts of the skin chronically exposed to the sun, such as the forearms and hands. Senile lentignes develop from localized abnormal proliferations of melanocytes, resulting in a spotty, uneven pigmentation.

Hair

Several factors influence the quantity, quality, and distribution of hair in the older adult. Among these factors are general health, nutrition, and heredity.

The characteristic age-related change noted in the hair is graying. Hair pigment decreases with aging because of the replacement of fully pigmented hairs with depigmented or lightly pigmented hairs. This depigmentation is due to a decrease in tyrosinaise-positive-melanocytes in the hair bulbs of depigmented hairs. The scalp hair often becomes sparse. Facial hair generally decreases in men. Facial hair in women increases, particularly on the upper lip and chin, due to decreased estrogen production to oppose androgens. The eyebrows may become thicker and longer.

Nails

The nails are simply a modification of the integument and reflect age-related changes. The growth rate of the nails progressively slows with age. The nails often become thicker and tougher, thus more difficult to trim.

A common disorder of the aged nail is onychomycosis, a fungal infection. This condition is more prevalent in the toenails and results in very thick, hard nails, often preventing the client from trimming the nail and making it painful to wear shoes.

PROMOTION OF HEALTHY SKIN IN THE OLDER ADULT

Basic Skin Care

The gerontological nurse practitioner must be cognizant of the characteristics of aging skin when providing care or teaching the older person to care for their skin. Two areas that require teaching self-care practices are bathing and the use of skin care products including cosmetics.

The older person should be encouraged to avoid bathing on a daily basis, as this may rob the skin of its natural oils. Bathing should be based on a need for cleanliness, not on habit. A washcloth or loofah sponge should be used gently in bathing to encourage removal of dead skin cells. Use of harsh or deodorant soaps should be avoided. A light covering of an oil or lotion should be applied after bathing, unless the client has oily skin. Older persons who swim or desire to bathe daily can prevent dryness by lubricating their skin daily.

The nurse practitioner may also suggest makeup techniques to the female. The older woman should be encouraged to use a light tone, liquid makeup with a sunscreen. Powders and cake foundations have a drying effect on the skin and accentuate wrinkles. Rouges or blushers should be light tones, as should eyebrow pencils. The older woman should be encouraged to apply light eye makeup and lipstick as this provides facial color and expression. Cosmetics and skin care products that are allergy-tested and unscented are preferable for use on aging skin (Palmer, 1982).

The older woman may be applying makeup too heavily or using too dark an application of lipstick or rouge. This may occur for several reasons. The woman may be continuing to use bright, dark makeup simply out of habit. Diminished visual acuity may also cause overly heavy application of makeup. In addition, the color vision of older adults is affected with aging due to yellowing of the lens, causing reds and yellows to be well visualized and blues and greens difficult to see.

The nurse may also be in the role of educating the client about the use of over-the-counter products to fade dark spots. These products have been reported to have limited effectiveness and require persistent conscientious application for even the slightest change in a dark spot to occur (Engasser & Maiback, 1981). Yet, many women persist in using these products in order to obtain even the slightest improvement.

Chronic Effect of Sun and Preventive Measures

America is filled with sun worshippers who are beginning to manifest the chronic effect of the sun on their skin. The chronic effects of the sun on the skin include:

- Wrinkling of varying degrees
- Thinning and thickening of skin
- Yellowing, graying, reddening of skin
- Scaling
- Liver spots and brown pigmented patches

Chronic exposure to the sun is the most common cause of premature aging of the skin in Caucasians. Susceptibility to premature aging of the skin and skin cancer is greater in persons with red hair and light complexions or with blond hair and blue eyes than in individuals of the same race who have a darker complexion. Blacks are least susceptable, regardless of skin tone (Willis, 1978).

The areas most affected by the chronic effects of the sun are the face, ears, neck, forearms, and hands. Skin changes commonly precede and may provide an environment for the development of premalignant lesions. Premalignant lesions may be flat or raised, hard, dry, adherent scales on a red base. Approximately 25% of persons with multiple lesions of this type (actinic or senile keratoses) develop squamous cell cancer in one or more of the lesions (Willis, 1978).

Preventive measures include avoiding the sun between 10 AM and 3 PM, solar time, as this is the period of greatest risk of harmful solar effects. Sunscreening agents that include para-aminobenzoic acid (PABA) can help protect against the most harmful ultraviolet rays during this time. The sun reflecting from snow, white sand, concrete, and shiny metals increases the amount of harmful ultraviolet rays reaching the skin. White fabric, particularly when wet, also transmits large amounts of ultraviolet light (Willis, 1978).

ASSESSMENT OF THE AGING SKIN

A history of the older person's skin, including past and present problems, routine skin care, and makeup used, is important in both the ambulatory and inpatient setting. This information assists the nurse practitioner in identifying areas where the client needs teaching, assistance with skin care, or referral to a specialist.

The use of a form for history-taking standardizes the information to be obtained and identifies the signs and symptoms to screen for in the older adult (Fig. 5–1). A yes/no checklist format assists the nurse practitioner in readily identifying positive findings. Positive findings are explored and described in further detail. A similar standardized format can be used in documenting the physical examination findings (Fig. 5–2). A drawing of a body, front and back, can be used to locate and describe lesions.

An accurate description of a skin lesion should include the type of lesion (primary or secondary) and its size, shape, color, location, and configuration (isolated or grouped). Primary lesions appear first in response to some change internally or externally. Secondary lesions are the result of some modification of the primary lesion. Table 5–1 identifies the classification of primary and secondary lesions.

PROBLEMS OF AGING SKIN

Pruritus

Itching of the skin is a common concern of the older adult. There are several possible causes when pruritus occurs with a primary lesion. Some internal causes of pruritus are chronic renal disease, hyperthyroidism, drug reactions, and emotional disturbances. However, dry skin is the most common cause of pruritus in the older adult. Scabies and lice should be ruled out as a cause of pruritus especially in persons residing in nursing homes (Thorne, 1978).

Integument		Problem
Yes	No	
		Color Changes
		Pruritus
		Infections
		Dermatosis
		Tumor
		Nevus
		Hair Changes
		Nail Changes

Describe positive findings:

Describe skin care:

Describe cosmetics used:

Figure 5–1. History-Taking Tool.

Integument

	N	A
Turgor		
Texture		
Pigmentation		
Color		
Hair		
Nails		
Temperature		
Hair Distribution		

N = Normal
A = Abnormal

Describe in detail *positive* examination findings:

	A	P
Telangectasia		
Petechiae		
Purpura		
Ecchymoses		
Infections		
Lesions		
Dermatoses		
Corns/Callouses		
Ulceration		
Edema		
Stasis		

A = Absent
P = Present

Figure 5–2. Physical Exam Findings.

The skin can become dry from excessive bathing, use of harsh soaps, overly vigorous towel drying, air-conditioning, and dry heat. The objective signs of dry skin are minute cracking and scaling patches, eczema, and hemorrhagic fissures of the legs (Thorne, 1978).

Dry skin can be readily treated after systemic causes have been ruled out or treated. The nursing care of dry skin in the older adult consists of hydrating the skin. Bathing can further dry the skin and should be done only when required to clean the body. A mild superfatted bath soap should be used and the bath water should be warm, not hot. A washcloth or loofah mitt should be used gently to slough off dead skin cells. The skin should be gently patted dry; vigorous over-toweling should be avoided. A moisturizing agent should be gently massaged into the skin after bathing. Petroleum jelly is the most lubricating and is best for very dry skin (Hanifin, 1979). A cream or lotion can be used. Lotions with high water or alcohol content and perfuming agents should be avoided. Bath oils should not be added to the bath water because of the risk that the older person may slip in the bathtub.

TABLE 5–1. PRIMARY AND SECONDARY LESIONS.

Primary		Secondary	
Macule:	flat, circumscribed change in skin color (freckle)	*Scale:*	flaking of the skin (psoriasis)
Papule:	solid, elevated area less than 0.5 cm in diameter (wart)	*Crust:*	dried serum, blood or purulent exudate (impetigo)
Nodule:	small solid elevation, less than 1 cm in diameter (gouty tophi)	*Erosion:*	circumscribed, moist, loss of superficial epidermis (ulcer)
Tumor:	solid mass larger than 1 cm in diameter	*Scar:*	production of excess collagen due to healing of an injury extending into the dermis (vaccination)
Vesicle:	circumscribed, elevated lesion containing serous fluid, less than 5 mm in diameter (smallpox)	*Fissure:*	cracks in the skin (chapped skin)
Bullae:	vesicle larger than 5 mm in diameter (second-degree burn)		
Pustule:	vesicle containing purulent exudate (acne)		
Wheal:	circumscribed flat-topped elevation of the skin with a defined margin (hives)		
Cyst:	encapsulated, fluid-filled mass in the dermis or subcutaneous layer		

Tumors

New growths may become apparent on the skin of the older adult. These growths may be benign, premalignant, or malignant. The most common growths are benign, posing no threat to the person's health physically, but may concern the person emotionally.

Benign Lesions

Seborrheic Keratoses. Seborrheic keratoses are the most common tumors seen in middle-aged and elderly persons. They appear as a raised lesion 2–3 centimeters in diameter, light tan to black in color, with sharply demarcated borders. They are found most frequently on the head, neck and trunk, especially the back and under pendulous breasts (Wright, 1978).

Sebaceous Hyperplasia. Sebaceous hyperplasia is manifested as small yellow papular to nodular lesions that occur most commonly on the forehead, nose, and cheeks. These growths are seen most often in men (Wright, 1978).

Skin Tags (Acrochordons). Skin tags are common papillomatous lesions that begin in middle or later life. They appear as multiple filiform, smooth, soft papules on the face, neck, and axillary folds (Wright, 1978).

Cherry Angiomas. Cherry angiomas are benign vascular tumors that are small pinpoint to slightly larger red lesions. They occur most frequently on the chest and back.

Seborrheic keratoses, sebaceous hyperplasia, skin tags, and cherry angiomas are all benign lesions that are frequently seen in older adults. They may be removed for cosmetic reasons. The usual treatments for removal are electrodesiccation and curettage or freezing procedures. The side effects of therapy may be temporary depigmentation or hypopigmentation (Wright, 1978).

Premalignant Lesions

Actinic (Solar) Keratoses. Actinic keratoses, also called senile or solar keratoses, are the most common premalignant lesion of the older adult.

The lesion is a slightly elevated, scaly papule, light brown or black in color with a flat, round, or warty surface. They commonly appear on sun-exposed areas such as the face, ears, hands, and forearms. Prevention of actinic keratoses has been discussed previously under "Chronic Effect of Sun and Preventive Measures." Treatment requires a dermatologist and involves removal of the lesion. Removal can be accomplished by electrodesiccation, cryosurgery, cauterization, or topical application of 5-fluorouracil.

Leukoplakia. Leukoplakia is also a premalignant lesion. It is manifested as white plaques that may be smooth or warty and occur on the mucosa. Leukoplakias may be seen on the lips, buccal mucosa, the tongue, or the vaginal area. Predisposing irritating factors include smoking, poor dentition, and infections. Treatment by a physician consists of biopsy and destruction of the lesion. The nurse practitioner must work with the client to alleviate or remove any existing irritating factors that may contribute to the development of leukoplakias. The nurse practitioner should also teach the client to screen for future appearance of leukoplakias.

Malignant Lesions

Malignant lesions of the skin include basal-cell carcinoma, squamous-cell carcinoma, and malignant melanoma. These lesions require prompt identification in order that the client may receive immediate and proper treatment.

Basal-Cell Carcinoma. Early lesions of basal-cell carcinoma appear as small nodular or cystic growths covered by a smooth translucent epidermis progressing to an ulcer with a rolled or flat border. Some lesions may appear as whitish lesions with indistinct margins, whereas other lesions appear as superficial erythematous areas. An occasional basal-cell carcinoma may be pigmented. Basal-cell carcinoma occurs most often between the sixth and eighth decades of life.

Basal-cell carcinomas rarely metastasize (Vargo, 1987).

The best prevention against basal-cell carcinoma is avoidance of the sun. Treatment is handled by a dermatologist and usually consists of surgical excision.

Squamous-Cell Carcinoma. Several precancerous lesions, including actinic or solar keratoses, have been associated with squamous-cell carcinoma. The early lesion of squamous-cell carcinoma appears as a single, hard, cone-shaped nodule. As the lesion grows it becomes attached to the underlying tissues, and is therefore fixed and firm to the touch. The border of the ulcer is often indistinct and raised. Squamous-cell carcinoma most frequently occurs between the sixth and eighth decades of life and is characterized as a slow growing neoplasm that can metastasize.

The client should be referred to a dermatologist. The treatment of choice for squamous-cell carcinoma of the skin is excision of the lesion. The recurrence rate following adequate surgical excision is low (Vargo, 1987).

Malignant Melanoma. Malignant melanoma tends to occur most commonly in adults in their fourth, fifth, and sixth decades. Malignant melanoma is a pigmented lesion with a high rate of metastasis. Most often the melanoma arises from an area free of an identifiable lesion. The client should be referred to a dermatologist, where treatment usually consists of surgical excision, with deep tissue removal and skin grafting (Prigel, 1987).

Infections of the Skin

Several skin infections are prevalent in the older adult, including herpes zoster, moniliasis, perleche, scabies, and cellulitis.

Herpes Zoster

Herpes zoster (shingles) is most common in the fifth to seventh decades of life and is caused by the varicella zoster virus. This is the same virus that causes chickenpox in children. The virus remains dormant unless a secondary reactivation of the infection occurs and produces shingles. The cause of the exacerbation is not clearly understood (Raimer & Pursley, 1981).

The lesions initially appear as erythematous papules that become edematous, eventually showing erosion and crusting. The lesions follow a linear distribution on the skin, usually of the thoracic area. Pain or burning is present for 1–10 days before the lesions appear and is usually present throughout the course of the disease. The disease usually lasts 3–4 weeks. Treatment is largely aimed toward relief of the symptoms. Systemic analgesics and cool, wet compresses or calamine lotion applied to the lesions help to relieve discomfort in most cases.

The most common complications are postherpetic neuralgia and scarring. Steroids may be prescribed with caution in some cases to prevent postherpetic neuralgia (Raimer & Pursley, 1981).

Moniliasis

Moniliasis (candidiasis) is the most common fungal infection of the older adult and is typified by erythema, pruritus, and macerated skin. Erythema is often present beyond the intertrigo area. The most common sites are the groin, folds of the buttocks, under the breasts, and the axillae. Persons with a debilitating disease, particularly diabetes, are at risk, as are persons on antibiotics. Prevention includes keeping areas of skin folds dry, as moisture encourages growth of the organism. Cotton underwear and clothing that allows air to circulate should be worn. Polyester or synthetic materials should be avoided. Treatment consists of heat lamps and application of antimonilial agents until the signs and symptoms have disappeared (Raimer & Pursley, 1981).

Perleche

Perleche is an inflammation that is found at the corner of the mouth. This area is very prone to a monilial infection. It appears as erythematous areas and scaling at the angles of the upper and lower lips. Chronic moisture is an aggravating factor, as is laxness of tissue due to aging and loss of teeth. Proper fitting of dentures prevents this laxness, and antimonilial antibacterial steroid medications are used to treat the infection (Walther & Harber, 1984).

Scabies

Sarcoptes scabiei is the mite that causes scabies. The organism burrows under the skin, appearing as a dark line under the skin and causing pruritus. The lesions are generally symmetrical and commonly involve intertrigo areas such as the wrists, fingers, elbows, umbilicus, buttocks, upper thighs, and genital area (Tschen, 1982). Poor hygiene and infrequent bathing predispose to the infestation, although lack of personal cleanliness need not play a role in the development of the condition. This condition can occur in epidemic proportions in nursing home situations because of the close contact and should be suspected when pruritus is a common complaint. Treatment is accomplished by bathing the infected person, using a brush on the skin followed with Benzyl Benzoate emulsion (25%) applied to the skin. Calamine lotion may be applied to relieve itching (Raimer & Pursley, 1981). Treatment should also be given to persons sharing sleeping quarters (Tschen, 1982). All bedding or clothing in contact with the infected person should be laundered.

Cellulitis

Bacterial infections may also be seen in the elderly. Cellulitis is an inflammation of the dermis and subcutaneous tissue, often caused by streptococcal organisms. Erythema and swelling occur, often with vesicles and bullae at the site. The area is painful, and the older adult may have fever and malaise. Treatment consists of antibiotic therapy and application of warm, wet compresses to the area, rest, and elevation of the affected area.

Other Problems

Corns and Callouses

Corns and callouses are hyperkeratotic lesions appearing over bony areas. Chronic pressure and friction are usually the cause, due to poorly fitting shoes or foot disorders. If untreated, they become painful and sometimes infected. The older adult should be taught or assisted with proper foot care and shoe selection. Referral should be made to a podiatrist, or foot specialist, for treatment of foot disorders and painful corns.

Proper foot care includes

- Monthly trimming of nails straight across, filed until smooth
- Soaking of the feet in warm water if nails are hard or thick
- Use of a special foot emory file on rough areas of the heel and foot
- Daily application of a moisturizing lotion to the feet, including the area around the nails

Proper shoe selection includes

- Measurement of the feet each time shoes are purchased
- Standing on the foot being measured
- Checking for a bend in the shoe at the ball of the foot
- Snug fitting heel
- Finger's width of space at the toe of the shoe
- Selecting leather rather than manmade materials because of leather's ability to mold to the foot and breathe
- Avoidance of high-heeled shoes

Stasis Dermatitis

Many factors may contribute to the development of stasis dermatitis in the older adult: chronic venous insufficiency, venous stasis, and atherosclerosis. Therefore, it becomes important to treat the underlying disorder as well as the secondary dermatoses (Walther & Harber, 1984). Signs of stasis dermatitis consist of erythema, edema and vesicular lesions, and thin, dry skin. The skin may develop a brownish discoloration due to the deposits of hemosiderin in the tissue. The skin is easily traumatized and ulcers may form. The ischemia of the lower extremities leads to poor healing and potential secondary infection.

Swelling is reduced by elevating the legs and application of elastic bandages or pressure stockings. These work best if applied when the client arises, before the appearance of dependent edema (Walther & Harber, 1984). Oral antibiotics are used to treat infection and topical steroid creams to decrease inflammation. Ulcers may be treated with cool, wet dressings of normal saline or topical antibiotic ointments.

Seborrheic Dermatitis

Seborrheic dermatitis is a common skin disorder of the scalp of the older adult. It consists of a fine scaling of the scalp and may extend to the eyebrows and nose. Erythema of involved areas may occur. Antiseborrheic shampoos usually control the condition of the scalp. The shampoo should be used each time the hair is washed, such as twice a week initially and then periodically if the dermatitis recurs. Once the scalp is cleared, facial involvement ceases. Occasionally mild steroid creams are applied to heal the lesions.

Drug-induced Skin Eruptions

Drugs should always be suspected as a cause of an older person's rash. A rash caused by a drug will usually occur within 1 week after ingestion of the causative drug (Fisher, 1979). The most common rash caused by ingestion of a drug is a maculopapular rash. The rash is generalized and pruritic. Hives or vesicular and bullos eruptions may occur. Discontinuation of the causative drug is necessary; symptomatic relief with oral antihistamines may be needed until symptoms disappear (Fisher, 1979).

Decubitus Ulcers

Decubitus ulcers, or pressure sores, are ulcerations of skin over bony prominences. The older adult with limited mobility is at high risk for this condition. Other factors, such as poor overall health, low body weight, atherosclerosis, and incontinence, may contribute to the development of decubiti (Sebern, 1987).

The best treatment for decubiti is prevention. A program for prevention of decubiti must include mobilization of the person, alleviation of pressure, proper skin care, controlling incontinence, and promotion of adequate nutrition (Sebern, 1987).

The client should be repositioned frequently; motorized turning beds are useful in shifting weight. Clients may be taught to periodically redistribute their weight by rocking, rolling, or lifting themselves. Range-of-motion exercises also promote circulation and relieve pressure. Flotation devices, such as water mattresses, or alternating pressure mattresses, and the strategic placement of pillows help to relieve pressure (Taylor, 1980).

The skin should be kept dry, soft, and warm. Incontinence must be prevented by the use of bowel and bladder regimes or external devices. Lotions should be applied frequently to the skin and drying soaps should be avoided.

Adequate nutrition is essential in preventing skin breakdown. A balanced diet with sufficient protein and calories is vital in promoting healthy skin.

Common sites for decubiti are the buttocks, sacrum, heels, and elbows. When the older adult stays in one position for a prolonged period, blood flow is blocked and the stages of skin breakdown begin.

In stage 1, the skin appears pink, red, or mottled and blanches to the touch. The skin feels firm and warm. Further breakdown can usually be prevented by massaging the area. The nurse practitioner should review the plan for prevention of decubiti to ensure that all steps are being taken.

In stage 2, the skin appears cracked, blistered, and broken, and the surrounding skin is reddened. In this stage, an antiseptic cleansing agent should be used followed by irrigation with normal saline solution.

In stage 3 there is a deep pressure sore and tissue involvement. Usually the area must be treated with a debriding agent, or surgical debridement of necrotic tissue may be needed. The area should be cleansed with an antiseptic followed by irrigation with normal saline solution.

Bone and muscle involvement in the deep pressure sore typifies stage 4. The same treatment format as outlined in stage 3 is followed in stage 4. Stage 4 pressure sores are so extensive that the client's general health can be adversely affected.

All immobilized clients should have their skin evaluated on a routine basis for the development of pressure sores. If a pressure area or sore is noted, the location of the involved area should be described in detail on the client's record; the description should include the appearance and measurement of the size of the lesion.

SUMMARY

Assessment and care of the skin in the older adult is a challenging and rewarding aspect of nursing. The gerontological nurse practitioner must be knowledgeable about normal aging skin changes and vigilant for signs of abnormal changes. Thus, the nurse practitioner can promote optimum health of the older adult's skin.

REFERENCES

Engasser, P., & Maibach, H. (1981). Cosmetics and dermatology: Bleaching creams. *Journal of the American Academy of Dermatology, 5,* 143–147.

Fisher, A. A. (1979). Drug induced skin eruptions: Typical treatments for topical problems. *Geriatrics, 34*(2), 45–51, 56–58, 63–64.

Hanifin, J. M. (1979). Eczematous conditions in the elderly: Common and curable. *Geriatrics, 34*(1), 29–38.

Palmer, M. H. (1982). Assisting the older woman with cosmetics. *Journal of Gerontological Nursing, 8*(6), 340–342.

Prigel, C. L. (1987). How to spot melanoma. *Nursing 87, 17*(6), 60–62.

Raimer, S. S., & Pursley, T. V. (1981). Office management of viral skin infections in the elderly. *Geriatrics, 36*(2), 53–63.

Sebern, M. (1987). Home-team strategies for treating pressure sores. *Nursing 87, 17*(4), 50–53.

Taylor, V. E. (1980). Decubitus prevention through early assessment. *Journal of Gerontological Nursing, 6*(7), 389–391.

Thorne, E. G. (1978). Coping with pruritus—A common geriatric complaint. *Geriatrics, 33*(7), 47–49.

Tschen, E. (1982). What treatment for skin infestations in the elderly? *Geriatrics, 37*(8), 38–44.

Vargo, N. L. (1987). The skin cancer success story. *RN, 50*(7), 50–57.

Walther, R., & Harber, L. (1984). Expected skin complaints of the geriatric patient. *Geriatrics, 39*(12), 67–80.

Willis, I. (1978). Sunlight, aging, and skin cancer. *Geriatrics, 33*(8), 33–36.

Wright, E. T. (1978). Identifying and treating common benign skin tumors. *Geriatrics, 33*(6), 37–44.

6

GASTROINTESTINAL CHANGES

Health promotion and health maintenance of the gastrointestinal (GI) tract offer a tremendous challenge to the gerontological nurse practitioner. Many of the problems of the GI system are preventable. Nurse practitioners must devote a good deal of their energy to helping the elderly cope with GI problems that have resulted from the aging process, improper use of laxatives, and, frequently, poor dietary habits. Nurse practitioners also need to help the elderly deal with the consequences of these problems and correct those that can be corrected.

The effects of age on the upper GI tract involve primarily a decrease in peristalsis and a delay in esophageal emptying (Reynolds, Ouyang, & Cohen, 1982). The symptoms due to these changes generally do not seriously limit the function of the upper GI tract.

Previously held concepts that the aging gut fails as one grows older is now incorrect. The GI tract maintains its anatomical and physiological abilities more than adequately throughout the life-span, although, admittedly, secretive and absorptive abilities do decline (Berman & Kirsner, 1972). Therefore, if aging individuals eat prudently, maintain sufficient fluid intake, and practice proper bowel hygiene, they should have no problems with the digestive process. Because, however, many people have been imprudent in their health habits related to the GI tract, this part of the anatomy has become big

business for laxatives, antacids with simethicone, and hemorrhoid preparations.

THE UPPER GI TRACT

Mouth

As is true of all the body's systems, the mouth manifests signs of aging. These signs include progressive changes in dentition, the bone structure of the teeth, the oral mucosa, and salivary secretion, temporomandibular joint abnormalities, and an increase in the rate of malignancy (Langer, 1976).

Dentition

Heredity and environmental factors, which include cultural and socioeconomic standards, may contribute to the retention or loss of teeth in older persons (Langer, 1976). Caries and periodontal disease are the primary contributions to the loss of teeth. The flow of saliva is diminished in older persons, therefore decreasing both the lubrication in the mouth and the ability to protect against caries.

The ability to adequately brush the teeth may be a problem. Individuals with arthritis, Parkinson's disease, or neuromuscular disease may be unable to hold the handle of a toothbrush. Modifications can be applied to toothbrushes

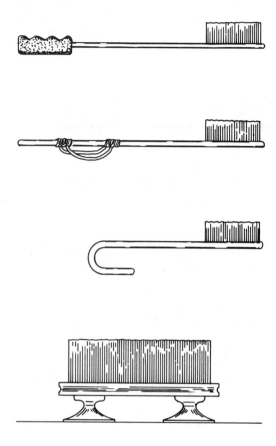

Figure 6-1. Oral Health Care Aids for the Handi-capped. *(Courtesy of Nanci Moll Jones, R.D.H.)*

and floss holders to allow self-administered dental care (Fig. 6–1). Ingestible toothpaste is available (Nasadent) for the individual unable to use ordinary dentifrice products. This toothpaste can be swallowed safely by individuals unable to expectorate adequately.

As the teeth become useless in mastication or as anchorage for prosthetic devices, they may be extracted, therefore preparing the mouth for dentures. Teeth serve not only as a means of mastication, but affect facial expression and appearance. For this reason, teeth contribute to the older person's self-image, and dental restoration and treatment should be promoted.

Another problem is the atrophy of the bone structure supporting the teeth—the alveolar bone. Atrophy of the alveolar bone contributes to a weakening of the teeth's support system and may eventually lead to their loss. The atrophy may continue following loss of the teeth, so that there is insufficient bone structure to support dentures.

Ill-fitting dentures due to bone loss may cause irritation and even painful lesions of the mucosa. Wearing the dentures becomes bothersome or even unbearable (Langer, 1976). There is evidence that tooth-grinding transfers pressure through the denture plates and is harmful to the bone structures and mucous membranes. Persons with dentures should be advised to remove their teeth while sleeping at night.

Oral Mucosa

As a person ages, the oral mucosa becomes more prone to inflammatory, degenerative, and pathological processes due to atrophy of the tissues and the decrease in capillary blood supply. This decrease in capillary blood supply impairs the ability of the oral tissue to regenerate, contributing to the development of leukoplakia (Langer, 1976). Common sites of occurrence are the cheeks, angle of the lips, and tongue. The lips and oral mucosa should be screened for the presence of these white patches; if present, the client should be referred to a dentist. The tongue is also affected by aging changes. The development of atrophic glossitis, with atrophy of the papillary structures of the tongue, may be a result of nutritional deficiencies, especially vitamin B complex (Langer, 1976).

Angular cheilosis is a condition characterized by inflamed, painful fissures located in the corners of the mouth. Cheilosis occurs primarily due to a lack of lip support as a result of loss of teeth and alveolar bone. Iron deficiency and candidiasis may complicate this condition (Pathy, 1985). Recognition and correction of dietary deficiencies, infections, and dental disorders can correct this condition (Schramm, 1980).

Dry Mouth (Xerostomia)

Production of saliva diminishes as a part of the aging process and may produce the complaint of dry mouth, known as xerostomia. Drugs used in Parkinson's disease (trihexyphenidyl and procyclidine) may also decrease the salivary flow. Phenylbutazone, antihistamines, and anticholinergics may also produce dry mouth. Atrophy of the salivary glands may occur due to radiation therapy for head and neck carcinoma (Johns, 1980).

Discontinuation of the causative drug may clear up the complaint of dry mouth. Use of an artificial saliva formula is also beneficial (Ham, 1987). Johns (1980) reports excellent relief of symptoms using 1000 ml of normal saline, 98 ml of Calogel, and 110 ml of glycerine swirled in the mouth every 3–4 hours and swallowed. Chewing gum also promotes salivation and can be beneficial.

Oral Disease

Drugs such as mouthwash, antibiotics, diuretics, and antidepressants may cause an inflammation of the mucous membranes of the mouth. Drug-induced mucositis causes a burning pain, often associated with mouth dryness, changes in taste, and problems wearing dentures. Symptoms improve upon discontinuation of the causative medication (Schramm, 1980). A burning tongue and pharynx with taste disturbances may also be symptoms of diabetes or hypothyroidism. These two diseases should be ruled out when these symptoms are present.

Sjögren's syndrome is an obscure systemic disorder primarily affecting postmenopausal women. A breakdown in the autoimmune mechanism is suspected as a contributory cause (Robbins & Angell, 1971). Symptoms include dryness of the mouth (xerostomia) and pain and a burning sensation in the mouth and on the palate and tongue (glossopyrosis). The pain may be so severe that dental appliances are unable to be worn (Langer, 1976). Langer (1976) reports that dentistry is unable to successfully treat and re-

habilitate clients with Sjögren's syndrome. The use of artificial saliva formulas may help in relieving the symptom of dry mouth (Teutsch & Hill, 1987).

Temporomandibular Joint

The temporomandibular joint may become dislocated when the mouth is opened wide as a result of loss of elasticity of the joint ligaments and muscles with aging. Pain in the temporomandibular joint and surrounding areas may be due to a number of factors. Malocclusion of teeth, or poorly fitting dentures, overclosure due to unopposed molars, and habits such as teeth clenching or grinding are all possible causes. Local applications of moist heat, administration of analgesics, dental care, and exercises to strengthen and relax the surrounding muscles are useful treatments (Schramm, 1980).

Many older persons have evidence of degenerative joint disease (osteoarthritis) which can affect the temporomandibular joint. Symptoms include pain, tenderness, and reduced mobility (Langer, 1976). Aspirin or antiarthritis medications and local applications of moist heat are helpful in this condition.

Esophagus

Degenerative changes due to the aging process alter the structure and function of the older person's esophagus in several ways. Goekas and Haverback (1969) report that predominant cineradiographic findings include a reduced or absent peristalsis, dilation of the esophagus, and delayed esophageal emptying. The older person with esophageal problems may present with symptoms of dysphagia (difficulty in swallowing), heartburn, regurgitation, and nonspecific chest pain (Reynolds et al., 1982).

A thorough history of the complaint should always be taken, including date of onset, frequency, aggravating and alleviating factors, location, radiation, and severity of any pain, and any associated symptoms. The effect of therapy, whether prescription or nonprescription, should be recorded. The gerontological nurse practitioner should also remember that many drugs cause GI symptoms that mimic disease. The medications the older person is taking should be thoroughly reviewed for possible side effects and adverse reactions in order to preclude this possibility.

Attention should also be given to assessment of the older person's psychological state. The symptoms of dysphagia, heartburn, and regurgitation frequently frighten clients, especially as these symptoms may also mimic cardiac problems, and an older person will naturally be concerned about heart trouble (Brandt, 1986). The gerontological nurse practitioner must assure that time is given for clients to express their concerns and to receive support.

Further diagnostic studies are often necessary, and the gerontological nurse practitioner should be prepared to explain these procedures and answer any questions. Endoscopy and GI series are two commonly performed procedures. Endoscopy is a valuable tool in diagnosing and treating gastroenterological disorders. The conditions that require viewing the esophagus are common in the older person. A study by Jacobson and Levy (1977) reported both the feasibility and safety of endoscopy in 215 clients aged 60–102 years.

Once a diagnosis has been established, the gerontological nurse practitioner should assess the older person's readiness for teaching. Instruction should include an explanation of the condition, using drawings or pictures if feasible. Clients should be instructed about the medications they are taking. Clients should learn to identify them by their proper names (rather than as "the blue pill" or "the red and white capsule"). Clients should also understand the purpose and action of medications and be alert to side effects or adverse reactions. If medications require special instructions—for example, they must be taken on a full stomach—clients should be provided with these instructions. Self-care should be taught.

Motility Disorders

The age-related changes that occur in the esophagus alter motility even in the absence of esophageal disease (Goekas & Haverback, 1969). Disordered esophageal motility in the aged is termed *presbyesophagus*. The lack of esophageal peristalsis is termed *achalasia* and is characterized by dysphagia, regurgitation on recumbency, and pulmonary complaints such as nocturnal cough, wheezing, and choking (Reynolds et al., 1982). Problems of esophageal emptying are an important nursing concern because of the possibility of aspiration pneumonitis if older persons are fed in the supine position.

Motility disorders of the esophagus can also be due to systemic diseases and neuromuscular disorders (Reynolds et al., 1982). The presenting symptom is most frequently dysphagia but may also include hoarseness and a depressed gag reflex. Some of these conditions are cerebrovascular disease, Parkinson's disease, hypothyroidism, and hyperthyroidism.

Gastroesophageal Reflux

The lower esophageal sphincter must be competent in order to prevent caustic gastric contents from the abdomen from being expelled into the esophagus (Reynolds et al., 1982). The condition is most often idiopathic, although other factors decreasing the competency of the lower esophageal sphincter may include caffeine, smoking, fatty foods, smooth muscle disorders (e.g., scleroderma), and anticholinergic medication (Reynolds et al., 1982).

An upper GI series or endoscopy are diagnostic tools utilized. The treatment of gastroesophageal reflux usually consists of elevating the head of the bed, taking antacids, reducing excess weight, and avoiding coffee, smoking, fatty foods, tight garments, and anticholinergics (Reynolds et al., 1982). Babka and Castell (1973) studied the effects of certain foods on the lower esophageal sphincter. Based on their study, they recommended drinking nonfat milk rather than whole milk and avoiding chocolate, spicy foods, and citrus juices to assist in increasing the pressure of the lower esophageal sphincter.

Antacids decrease the corrosiveness of the refluxed matter and increase the lower esophageal sphincter pressure. Other medications utilized include H_2 antagonists to decrease volume and acidity of refluxed matter, and bethanechol chloride and metoclopramide hydrochloride to enhance lower esophageal sphincter competence and gastric emptying.

If a medical regimen is not successful in relieving symptoms, surgery may be necessary. Surgery will relieve symptoms in a majority of clients (Reynolds et al., 1982). Repair of a hiatal hernia alone is insufficient; a procedure such as a Nissen fundoplication to increase the tone of the gastroesophageal junction is necessary. Peptic stricture can be treated with medical regimen and dilation (Reynolds et al., 1982).

Hiatal Hernia

The frequency of demonstrable hiatal hernia increases with advancing age to 60–90% by the age of 70 years (Reynolds et al., 1982). Rossman (1986) classifies hernias as two types: type I, the sliding hernia; and type II, the paraesophageal hernia. In type I, the junction of the esophagus and stomach moves above its normal position at the diaphragm, allowing reflux. In type II, the junction remains at the diaphragm, and part of the stomach moves up beside the esophagus and above the diaphragm. Symptoms of hiatal hernia are heartburn, dysphagia, and pain in the area of the sternum, with reflux esophagitis in persons with type I hernia. Bleeding may be massive and may be overt or occult. A hiatal hernia should be ruled out in the presence of iron-deficiency anemia in the older person (Rossman, 1986).

Hiatal hernia may be diagnosed by chest x-ray, upper GI series, or endoscopy. Treatment is aimed at alleviating the symptoms. Obesity can be a contributing factor; therefore, weight reduction is beneficial. Meals should be taken in smaller portions and more frequently. Food should be avoided before bedtime and prior to lying down. Elevating the head of the bed is useful, as are antacids (Rossman, 1986). Surgery is rarely indicated.

Esophageal Carcinoma

Reynolds and colleagues (1982) report that carcinoma of the esophagus occurs most commonly in persons over the age of 60, being responsible for 1% of all carcinomas and 2% of carcinoma deaths in the United States. Dysphagia is the most common presenting complaint but is often manifested late in the disease. More subtle early symptoms are substernal distress and odynophagia (Unger & McGregor, 1976).

Methods of detection of esophageal carcinoma include endoscopy and computed tomography (CT). Early detection may be enhanced through screening for epidemiologic risk factors: smoking, alcohol abuse, poor dental hygiene, and achalasia (Reynolds et al., 1982). The treatment of this condition is esophagogastric bypass or resection. Surgery provides relief of dysphagia in 95% of survivors, and radiation therapy is usually reserved for disease recurrence, nonoperable clients, and palliative relief (Reynolds et al., 1982).

THE LOWER GI TRACT

Most problems occurring in the lower GI tract are not age related, and yet according to one study (Geboes & Bossaert, 1977), these problems comprise 27% of acute medical admissions of persons 65 years and older and 42% of the elderly with chronic illness (Bustin & Iber, 1983). Conditions and diseases such as adynamic ileus, irritable bowel syndrome, and constipation can occur at almost any time during the life-span. Lower GI complaints of young adulthood can be carried into old age; in other instances, a stressor that occurs later in life may exacerbate a previously controlled and long dormant condition. Improper health habits in later life may also produce ailments of the bowel and biliary system requiring medical intervention.

Unfortunately, all too often, the elderly demand and physicians prefer to use medications for presented problems, rather than identifying the reason for and eliminating the cause.

Disorders of the Aging Bowel

Diverticulosis

After the age of 40, diverticular disease of the colon increases. The risk of diverticulosis in older persons is now approximately 50% (Burakoff, 1981). Small stiff stools, resulting from long-term ingestion of a low residue diet, strain the colon. Diverticulosis (a condition of feces-filled multiple pouches found in the bowel mucosa) can then occur anywhere in the bowel, but are found primarily in the sigmoid colon (Painter, 1976). Diverticulitis, a complication of diverticulosis, is often called *left-sided appendicitis,* as the signs and symptoms are similar, even though the etiologies are different.

A history of prolonged poor health practices related to the bowel can eventually result in diverticulosis. These individuals often complain only of constipation. The degree of pain perception varies, even though cramping may be present. Sometimes, the first recognition that something is wrong occurs when colonic hemorrhage is manifested. The diagnosis is made by x-ray findings.

Diverticulitis presents with severe cramping pain over the sigmoid colon or wherever the infected area may be. The older person may also complain of chills and fever, nausea, or vomiting. If any of the diverticuli rupture through the bowel mucosa, peritonitis can occur.

Because the gerontological nurse practitioner may be the first health professional to see the client, a careful assessment of the abdomen is required. Palpation of the abdomen should begin away from and proceed to the site of the localized pain, e.g., starting in the right lower quadrant and carefully moving to the painful left lower quadrant, which may be exquisitely tender and give some rebound. A test for occult blood in the stool should always be done at the rectal examination, as the diverticuli may chronically bleed.

Medical management of diverticulosis will most likely include drugs, e.g., anticholinergics, bulk additives, and stool softeners. Nursing approaches to managing clients with diverticulosis are much more holistic. Nursing care is directed toward encouraging older persons to maintain a high-fiber diet. Much patience on the part of the nurse practitioner is needed, for if older persons have had a long-standing diagnosis of diverticulosis, they had probably been told to eat bland, low-residue foods. Older persons may not be comfortable in drastically changing their diets. They may give numerous excuses for not eating foods high in fiber. The best ways to help these older persons change their diets is to provide high-fiber foods in social settings, e.g., covered dish luncheons, family dinners, and the serving of high-fiber tea cakes or fruit breads with coffee or tea.

One must be careful to avoid including in the diet foods to which older persons are allergic or to which they express an intolerance. For example, in this author's experience, older clients consistently report an intolerance to iceberg lettuce, stating that it causes indigestion and gas. Cabbage is also an offending food for the elderly.

In one of this author's clinics, the elderly were reluctant to utilize bran, believing it to be unpalatable. In order to show them that bran could be delicious, blueberry bran muffins were served as refreshments in a health teaching program. The muffins were well received, and the group was surprised that something so good could contain bran. To further emphasize the importance and use of bran, one of the participants received a door prize of bran muffin mix. The winner was urged by participants to be sure to share with them the muffins that would be made with the prize.

Constipation

Constipation and aging have been stereotyped as occurring together. This is not necessarily true, for many of the health beliefs and poor health habits of the constipated elderly began early in life and have been carried over into late adulthood. Hopefully, as gerontological nurse practitioners fulfill their teaching roles, the elderly can learn proper bowel hygiene so that constipation will eventually be rare, rather than excessively common.

The term *constipation* may mean different things to different people. For example, the nurse practitioner may define constipation as abnormally infrequent stools and abnormally hard, dry stools (Brunner & Suddarth, 1984, p. 806). A client may define the term as "infrequent action (sometimes meaning less than daily) of the bowels or difficulty in passing feces, even though they are passed regularly" (Brocklehurst, 1977).

Constipation occupies a tremendous amount of older persons' time and energies, as well as their money. The problem is apparently as old as mankind itself, for it is one of the oldest discomforts known to humans, and there have been few revolutionary advances in its management over the centuries. In fact, the remedies and relief of this problem seem to be cyclic. Lorand (1912), an early geriatrician, stated "in order to have good bowel movements, we must create them." He advocated high-fiber diets, good nutrition, and plenty of fluids. He did lament the fact that many persons would not follow such healthful advice.

The elderly today come from a cohort that believed that a daily bowel movement was essential to prevent the body from becoming poisoned. They were indoctrinated with the idea of periodic purgings to rid the body of noxious substances. They grew up at a time when *locked bowels* was almost always fatal, so every effort to keep the bowel cleansed and open was imperative.

Constipation is a preventable condition. However, a lifetime of bad habits promote bowel malfunction. Poor diet, lack of exercise, poor bowel hygiene, inadequate fluid intake, and poor emotional health all tend to promote constipation (Borda, 1987).

The immobile elderly, e.g., the bed-bound or chair-bound elderly, are at high risk for *terminal reservoir syndrome,* whereby feces accumulate in the left side of the colon and in the rectum (Brocklehurst, 1980). Further, many elderly have a drug-induced constipation due to the side effects of peristaltic inhibitions and dehydration that these drugs produce. Many frail or handicapped elderly in institutional settings are prevented from practicing good bowel habits because of the poor diet offered, a lack of encouragement and help to drink enough fluids, a lack of help in getting to the toilet on a planned, regular basis, a lack of exercise, and a sense of depersonalization caused by an uncaring staff.

These staffs are then quick to give laxatives, cathartics, and enemas. Enemas are especially hazardous in the elderly. After many years of poor bowel habits, age-related or drug-induced hypotonicity of the bowel, long retention of feces in the rectum, and decreasing age-related structural support of the colon, the rectum may enlarge and droop. Attempts to insert an enema nozzle into the rectum of an older person may perforate the rectal mucosa rather than stay within the rectal lumen. A thorough assessment of the bowel should be made by a competent professional nurse practitioner who can appreciate the physiology of the aged bowel; only then, only if truly necessary, and only by this competent professional should an enema be given.

The older adult suffering from a cathartic colon or laxative dependency might be able to be weaned away from such drugs. Unfortunately, however, some continued use of laxatives might be necessary because of worn-out and nonfunctioning innervations of the bowel.

There should be strict policies against the indiscriminate use of laxatives in situations for the elderly. Inservice programs on proper bowel hygiene should be provided periodically in every geriatric facility. Included in the inservice program should be instruction on the interactions of laxatives with other drugs and foods. Actions and side effects of the multitude of laxatives on the market should also be discussed.

In assessing bowel evacuation, it is necessary to know the usual bowel pattern of the older person, so this pattern—if appropriate—can be maintained. Assessment includes inspection, auscultation, percussion, and palpation of the abdomen, as well as a rectal examination. When examining for constipation, all staff must understand that constipation does not mean that *no* feces are evacuated. Fecal material and water may leak out around an impaction. If this is recorded as a bowel movement, the real problem may not be uncovered. Obstipation (no bowel movement) may then occur. Often the first time that constipation is noted is when a *mass* is discovered in the abdomen. Costly x-rays reveal the fecal obstruction.

If the assessment uncovers acute constipation, a serious problem, the physician should be notified immediately, so that the cause of the problem, e.g., an inflammatory process, can be ascertained. Laxatives, cathartics, and enemas should be withheld until the medical evaluation has been completed.

The rectal examination will give data on the size and condition of the rectum, as well as on the amount and consistency of stool in the rectum. Often a dilated, hypotonic sigmoid colon and rectum become increasingly filled with stool. This is especially true for elderly clients who use stool softeners which make *fecal glue,* thus compounding the constipation problem. Poor perception of anorectal reflexes also promotes this terminal reservoir syndrome (Bulmash, 1981), thus causing the older person to retain stool in the rectum.

If an older person does develop a fecal impaction, the nursing staff faces 7–10 days of hard work. Care must be taken to prevent rectal wall injury as well as shock from manipulation and fluid–electrolyte imbalance when clearing out the impaction.

Manual removal of as much feces in the rectum as possible should be attempted first. Once the rectum is reasonably cleared, an oil retention enema can be given, especially if the feces are very hard. Otherwise, a phosphate enema (if the person does not have a cardiac condition) can be given. Soapsud enemas should be avoided, as they are too harsh and can cause mucosal injury. This process is repeated twice daily until the impaction is cleared. A bowel hygiene program must be implemented for prevention of further impactions.

Characteristically, older persons with constipation are sedentary, eat a low residue diet, drink little water, have irregular bowel habits, and tense their gut when angry or otherwise stressed. There are many variations to this description; for example, some older persons may take care of their physical health but are so emotionally stressed that they literally ''lock'' their bowels. It is not uncommon to find residents of nursing homes expressing their anger toward the staff by refusing to have a bowel movement.

Because, in most cases, constipation can be prevented, gerontological nurse practitioners must teach the elderly the positive health habits necessary for proper bowel hygiene. This teaching is not easy, for older adults are being asked to give up long-cherished beliefs and practices. Kindness and concern expressed by the nurse practitioner for the welfare of the older person, coupled with patience and reinforcement, will allow success in the majority of cases.

Elements of the health teaching plan should include:

1. *Dispelling myths.* Explain to clients that they will not become toxic within 24–36 hours if they do not have a daily bowel movement.
2. *Diet.* Discuss how to correct the diet to include high-fiber and natural laxative foods. Sprinkling a few teaspoons of unprocessed bran into orange juice is quick and easy. With older clients, however, it may be necessary to teach the creative use of bran. For example, bran can be mixed with herbs and spices and used as a salad topping. Bran is easily mixed into cereal, meat loaves, and casseroles.

Another facet of diet that needs correcting

pertains to eating foods that offer a natural laxative effect, e.g., whole grains, raw fruits, and vegetables. Older persons must be encouraged to eat these foods and to refrain from eating refined flours and sugar and other foods that offer little bulk. Peelings, such as from apples and potatoes, are excellent sources of roughage.

3. *Hydration.* Older persons need to be taught to drink at least six to ten 8-ounce glasses of water daily. If activities cause increased water loss, then additional fluids must be consumed. The elderly need to remember that certain drugs they take may cause dehydration. A cup of hot water, hot lemonade, tea, or coffee taken before breakfast is a good peristaltic stimulant and will begin to meet their daily hydration needs.

4. *Establishing regularity.* Older persons need to strive for a regular time to have their bowel movements. The best time would be approximately one-half hour after breakfast daily, every other day, or whenever their normal bowel pattern has been set.

5. *Exercise.* The metabolism is already slowed in the elderly; a sedentary existence further slows body processes, including elimination. Taking a brisk 1–2-mile walk before breakfast, riding a stationary bicycle, or engaging in other exercise can stimulate peristalsis effectively in the ambulatory elderly. Range-of-motion exercises, leg lifts, and abdominal massage, both active and passive, are recommended for the bed-bound elderly.

6. *Stimulating the gastrocolic reflex.* The older person should respond as quickly as possible to the urge (gastrocolic reflex) to have a bowel movement, which is generally initiated by the first morning ingestion of food or hot fluids. After sitting on the toilet, older persons should be taught to prop their feet on a small stool and to thrust the body forward a little. Massaging the abdomen around the natural progression of the colon will also help induce the gastrocolic reflex. If at all possible, the bed-bound older person should be placed in as normal a position as possible for bowel evacuation. This may take a little longer to do, but it could prevent a stroke or other vascular damage (Bustin & Iber, 1983).

Hemorrhoids

Both men and women may bring the long-standing chronic complaint of hemorrhoids to their later life. These individuals often complain of concomitant constipation. The principal cause of hemorrhoids is the pressure exerted by stool pressing on the anal vessels. If a person fails to heed the urge to defecate, the weighty stool causes the distal vessels of the anus to engorge and become painful. Straining at stool is also a major contributory factor in the development of hemorrhoids (Smith, 1978).

Older persons should be taught to develop regular bowel habits, defecating as soon as possible after the urge occurs. All the factors helpful in preventing constipation and diverticulosis are valid for preventing hemorrhoids.

Relief of acute hemorrhoidal discomfort can be provided by very warm compresses. Hot sitz baths in a tub are to be discouraged due to depleting the brain and the upper body of blood. Over-the-counter hemorrhoidal drugs are often effective in small amounts used for brief periods. If more than two or three applications of the drug are needed, a physician should be consulted.

Gerontological nurse practitioners should assess the anus of the elderly for engorged, irritated, or infected hemorrhoids, especially in those elderly complaining of constipation. If rectal bleeding is noted, the nurse practitioner should not assume that the cause is solely hemorrhoids. Further investigation of the rectum is needed to rule out more serious rectal disorders.

Sometimes hemorrhoids become so engorged and painful that surgery may be the only recourse. Therefore, nurse practitioners need to facilitate the elderly's efforts to prevent flare-ups of hemorrhoidal discomfort through positive health habits, thus obviating the need for surgery or other forms of medical therapy.

Diarrhea

Diarrhea in the elderly should be treated with care. Although some causes of diarrhea are self-limiting infections or reactions to stress, the presence of diarrhea may be a warning of more ominous problems. Therefore, the nurse practitioner should use all the nursing process to investigate and manage the elderly with this problem.

Diarrhea may be defined as the passage of three or more watery, loose stools per day which are different from the normal bowel pattern (Bond, 1982). Diarrhea may be acute (such as in bacterial infections) or chronic (as in Crohn's disease). Age may reduce the competency of older persons' immune systems, thus leaving them vulnerable to enteric infections. Another vulnerable group are those elderly with achlorhydria, as there is insufficient stomach acid to kill pathogens entering the stomach. Older persons who have had GI surgery, who have diabetic neuropathy, or who are taking certain drugs (e.g., antibiotics, naproxen, or large doses of antacids) are also at increased risk for diarrhea.

The older traveler to areas where hygenic practices are poor is also at risk (Ravdin & Guerrant, 1983). Poor hand washing on the part of the older person may also contribute to infection. Poor refrigeration and improper cooking of foods at home or in institutions may be a cause of infectious diarrhea. Ingestion of an excess of wheat flour (which is incompletely digested in the small intestines but readily metabolized in the colon) and certain fruits (e.g., pears) containing long-chain carbohydrates may also produce a self-limiting diarrhea with flatulence (Bond, 1982). Elderly persons should ingest these offending foods in moderation or, if necessary, omit them from the diet.

Gerontological nurse practitioners should be alert for a sudden onset of diarrhea in older clients, for they can quickly dehydrate. Fever, abdominal pain, and confusion may accompany the diarrhea. The physician should be notified after the third stool or earlier if the client is prostrate. Stool specimens may need to be collected

for investigation of ova, cysts, parasites, and leukocytosis. Proper infection control techniques should be employed when collecting the stool specimen.

Every effort should be made to help these clients to the commode with all due haste or to have a bedside commode available. Try to keep these clients hydrated by offering ginger ale, which will inhibit vomiting. If infected food is suspected to be the problem, it is better to let the older person vomit and then provide the ginger ale. If the offending agent is a virus, like rotovirus, that often produces outbreaks among institutionalized elderly, the same general rules of excellent nursing care and infection control apply. In this instance, the nurse practitioner is the true primary health care provider, for there is little that medicine can do for these individuals.

Chronic diarrhea (i.e., persisting for more than several weeks) should be investigated thoroughly, to allow proper management and early treatment. Stress may produce episodes of diarrhea in clients suffering from irritable bowel syndrome, ulcerative colitis, or Crohn's disease (Cooper, 1980). In these instances, the best treatment is to help the client have a positive outlook on life and to deal maturely with stress to avoid bowel flare-ups of the disease. Lactase deficiency, cancer of the colon, ulcerative colitis, malabsorption syndromes, GI surgery, radiation therapy, and, of course, laxative abuse also contribute to chronic diarrhea.

Antidiarrheal and, when appropriate, antimicrobial therapy, with careful attention to hydration status, skin integrity, acid–base balance, and reality orientation, are the management techniques physicians and nurses should provide on a collaborative basis to help older persons with chronic diarrhea.

Fecal Incontinence

Although constipation occurs more frequently in older persons, fecal incontinence may be equally problematic. Decreased neural control of the anal sphincter due to cerebrovascular accidents, Alzheimer's disease, and other organic brain syndromes, altered mental states from drugs, rectal prolapse, and hemorrhoids may be the precipitating cause. Therefore, nurse practitioners must assess the older person for the presence of these etiologic factors and construct their nursing care plans accordingly.

The practice (Bustin & Iber, 1983) of giving the fecally incontinent older person constipating drugs and then evacuating the bowel periodically by enema is to be deplored. The better, more humane way to help control evacuation in the fecally incontinent elderly is to institute an appropriate bowel training program to establish normal, predictable regularity of bowel movements.

The assessment of the problem should include a 3–4-day log of the foods ingested and the hours when bowel movements occur. The latter is very important in planning the bowel training program. Although it is thought that ideally the bowel movement should occur after breakfast, an older person may have established some other time as being appropriate for evacuation. By knowing the usual time of evacuation, the nursing staff can then assist the person to the toilet at the appropriate time to avoid "accidents." If the fecally incontinent person has more than one bowel movement daily, the determination as to whether or not this is normal for the individual must be established. An analysis of the diet log might turn up foods that produce an unnecessary laxative effect. Intake of these foods can then be controlled (not necessarily eliminated). Incontinent pads can be worn until the bowel training program can be effected. Care must be taken to maintain skin integrity. The reader is urged to review the procedures for a bowel training program, which should be a basic component of nursing for all older persons in need of such help.

Ischemia of the Intestines

The vasculature of the heart and brain are not the only vessels to be subject to ischemia and infarct. Although relatively rare, ischemia of the bowel can be debilitating and even life threatening. The condition can be precipitated by de-

hydration, congestive heart failure, the use of digitalis, and polycythemia (Brocklehurst, 1980).

Sometimes the older person will complain of severe cramping abdominal pain beginning 15–30 minutes after eating and lasting for several hours. The pain may become so debilitating that the older person will refuse to eat in order to avert further pain. The gerontological nurse practitioner must be alert for clients in pain postprandially, for they may be having *abdominal angina*. This angina is caused by arteriosclerosis and atherosclerosis of the vessels of the bowel which are aggravated by the digestive/absorptive processes. The nurse practitioner can help clients with abdominal angina by encouraging small, frequent feedings and by making clients comfortable in a quiet environment for 30–60 minutes after eating.

The ischemic vasculature of the bowel may lead to occlusion and infarction. If this occurs, a surgical emergency exists, as the older person will be desperately ill with signs and symptoms of an acute abdomen—sharp, colicky pain, abdominal rigidity with rebound tenderness, nausea, vomiting, and evidence of shock. There may be loose stools with red blood or clots. Too often, however, the actual condition of the client is not appreciated: a "stomachache," from injudicious eating or constipation, or diverticulosis may be blamed. Laxatives are given, when the need is to save the abdominal vasculature from further ischemia and infarct. The gerontological nurse practitioner must keep ischemia in mind and be able to assess the abdomen, paying particular attention to a bruit over the superior mesenteric artery; the appropriate information can then be given to the physician and immediate steps taken to relieve the problem.

Cancer of the Colon and Rectum

Second only to lung cancer, colon cancer is responsible for approximately 140,000 deaths per year in the United States, more than 94% of victims being past the age of 50, and affecting men and women equally (American Cancer Society, 1986). Prevention and early detection, promoted by health providers, can help lower the incidence of this devastating disease.

Preventive measures to reduce the risk of colon cancer include a high-fiber diet, reduction of red-meat intake, positive bowel habits, and avoidance of environmental pollutants. Early detection of colorectal carcinoma includes digital rectal examination. Although it used to be said that most colorectal tumors were within reach of the examining finger, recent studies show that colon cancers are higher up in the colon than the examining finger and some sigmoidoscopes can reach (American Cancer Society, 1986).

The gerontological nurse practitioner should do a thorough rectal examination on all institutionalized elderly on admission and every 6 months thereafter. Included in the assessment must be an occult blood test of the stool, for this simple test can detect early asymptomatic cancers where the cure rate is high. The occult blood test takes advantage of the friability and bleeding tendency of colonic lesions (Vanneman, 1980). The nurse practitioner should remember that, for best results on the test, the client should be on a high-fiber, meat-free diet and should refrain from taking vitamin C and aspirin beginning 24 hours before the test and lasting until all slides are completed (Bolt, 1980). This will help decrease the incidence of false-positive tests and increase any bleeding from the cancer (Richardson, 1977). Older persons living at home can be instructed to collect their occult blood slides and turn them in to the nurse practitioner for reading.

If blood is present in the stools, and hemorrhoids or fissures are ruled out as the cause, the client should be referred to a physician for examination of the colon via a fiberoptic sigmoidoscope. Holt and Wherry (1979) found that the elderly tolerated this procedure better than when a rigid sigmoidoscope was used and found it valuable in finding lesions beyond the range of the rigid sigmoidoscope. If a lesion is found, it can be biopsied at this time.

Surgery, if warranted, may consist of colon resection with bowel anastamosis or the more extensive abdominoperineal resection with colostomy. The gerontological nurse practitioner should encourage self-care by these clients and not avoid such teaching in the erroneous belief that these persons are too old to learn. If at all possible, a family member should be included in the teaching. If these clients are being sent home or to a long-term care facility, nurses from the hospital, the community health agency, and long-term care facility should consult jointly with these individuals and their families about their continuity of care and health maintenance. No capable clients with a colostomy should ever be discharged unless they can care for themselves adequately and unless provisions for continuity of care have been made. Useful resources in continuity of care are the American Cancer Society's Ostomy Clubs and the United Ostomy Association, where volunteer ostomates help new ostomates adjust to their changed body images (American Cancer Society, 1981).

When older persons with colostomies are admitted to the nurse's care, it must not be taken for granted that they are able to care for themselves. The gerontological nurse practitioner needs to observe these individuals perform their self-care procedures to determine their adequacy, safety, and comfort. If problems are found, the nurse can readily correct them.

Colostomy care has changed over the years. Some ostomates have a regular daily bowel movement, precluding the necessity for irrigating the colostomy. The individual puts on a colostomy bag near the time of the regular evacuation and, after the evacuation, discards the bag and cleanses the skin. Other ostomates use a small amount of warm water inserted with a bulb syringe. This procedure stimulates peristalsis and the person readily evacuates. Still other ostomates need to utilize the traditional colostomy irrigation.

Clients with colorectal cancer may also have had chemotherapy and/or radiation therapy along with the surgery or they may have had these therapies in lieu of surgery. The gerontological nurse practitioner should recognize that the side effects of these therapies—skin reactions, nausea, vomiting, diarrhea, fatigue, hair loss, and infection—may cause severe emotional and physical stress for these individuals, so every effort must be made to help them conserve their energies and to reduce their discomfort. All the care-givers should confer on the care plan to ensure maximum assistance with whatever support and services are needed. Most of all, older persons with colorectal cancer need to be reassured that they are still live persons with needs and developmental tasks to pursue. The best nursing interventions here are listening and hugging (Edwards & Krouse, 1987).

BILIARY TRACT DISORDERS IN THE ELDERLY

Gallbladder Disorders

By far the most important problems of the biliary system confronting the elderly are gallstones and infections of the gallbladder. In fact, gallstones reportedly afflict one fourth of the population over 60, with a 3 : 1 female-to-male incidence of cholesterol gallstones (Redinger, 1980).

The American diet predisposes to stone formation because of its high cholesterol and low-fiber content. The lithogenic bile promotes the crystallization of the cholesterol, thus forming stones. If older persons are encouraged to eat high-fiber foods, the cholesterol content of the bile can be reduced and the levels of the beneficial bile salt chenodeoxycholate can be increased (Burkitt, 1982).

Cholecystitis in the elderly is often not appreciated by health care providers. Nausea, vomiting, and eructation may be attributed to problems other than gallbladder because pain perception may be diminished. If pain is present, it is colicky and perceived in the right upper quadrant, radiating to the back up under the right scapula. The temperature may or may not be elevated. In any event, the gerontological nurse

practitioner should carefully assess the older person and immediately report the findings to the physician. Surgery, often on an emergency basis, may be necessary. Although the uncompromised elderly can tolerate gallbladder surgery very well (Gaines, 1977), cholecystitis can be life threatening (mortality 10%), especially if jaundice from common duct obstruction is present (Bustin & Iber, 1983). The use of ursodeoxycholic acid, which is well tolerated by older persons, seems a promising nonsurgical treatment for gallstones (Bustin & Iber, 1983).

The gerontological nurse practitioner needs to reassure these acutely ill clients, making them comfortable in a low Fowler's position. Side rails on the bed should be in the ''up'' position. Nothing should be given by mouth except sips of tap water. Careful protection of the skin should be maintained, especially in transporting these clients from one location to another.

Pancreatic Disorders

The principal pancreatic disorder in the elderly as well as in younger persons remains diabetes mellitus (see Chap. 9). In spite of age-related changes in the pancreas, such as an increase in the fat content, making pancreatic cellular function less efficient, the pancreas is able to function adequately if the food intake is normally balanced (Fikry, 1968; Rosenberg, Friedland, Janowitz, & Dreiling, 1966). Unfortunately, the American diet is high in starches and lipids, and the diet of older persons tends to be even higher in carbohydrates; therefore, older persons may be at a disadvantage if meals presented to them are high in starches and fat or if the only style of cooking with which they are familiar contains large amounts of starches and fats. The pancreas of older persons may not be able to process this overload of food, thus causing acute indigestion. This may be equally true if the older person has overeaten in general, as the aging digestive system functions more slowly and cannot deal with large amounts of food at one time. It, therefore, behooves care-givers to see that the fat and starch contents in older persons' diets are restricted to the recommended average daily allowances and that the elderly themselves are taught how to prepare nourishing, balanced meals.

Acute pancreatitis may present in the elderly in the same way it does in younger persons or may be mistaken for other abdominal complaints, such as cholecystitis or ulcers. Pain, if perceived, is often excruciating and may quickly cause prostration. Nausea and vomiting accompanied by abdominal tenderness and rigidity also quickly debilitate older persons. Electrolyte imbalances, especially deficits in potassium, can quickly occur. Anxiety, hallucinations, and an acute confusional state may also accompany the acute onset of pancreatitis.

The gerontological nurse practitioner can be crucial in saving the life of the older person with acute pancreatitis. This is a medical emergency, so the nurse must endeavor to assess the client carefully and notify the physician immediately. The nurse should keep the client as comfortable as possible and be warmly supportive in order to reduce anxiety as medical attention is arranged.

The elderly, especially elderly women, are targets for carcinoma of the pancreas. The gerontological nurse practitioner should always be alert to the older person who complains of loss of appetite, weakness, and weight loss, or who develops a confusional state whose cause cannot be related to drug interactions or infections. When pain develops, it is usually described as "a red hot poker" going straight through the epigastrium to the back, causing the person to bend over for relief. The pain may increase at night. Common signs and symptoms of many other GI problems such as diarrhea may be present. Jaundice may appear early or late. The nurse practitioner should also suspect carcinoma of the pancreas when ecchymotic areas begin to appear over the flanks or around the umbilicus.

Carcinoma of the pancreas may also present initially with depression; therefore, investiga-tion of this carcinoma should be made in the depressed elderly, initially by the blood studies for elevations in the serum lipase, amylase, and alkaline phosphatase.

There is a 25% mortality for carcinoma of the head of the pancreas (Schein, 1979), so surgery may be waived. The nurse caring for these inoperable individuals is truly challenged to use nursing interventions to their fullest to protect, support, maintain, and comfort these clients. Careful attention to the skin is crucial in order to maintain its integrity, especially if pruritus from jaundice is present and if the client is too debilitated to move or eat well. Periodic mouth care must be given before and after oral feedings and several times a day if the client is receiving parenteral feedings. Active and passive range-of-motion exercises will maintain muscle tone and promote circulation. Every effort must be made to give these persons opportunities to express their feelings and be with their families. Control of pain should be a priority in nursing care, so an appropriate schedule of medications, relaxation therapies, and/or transcutaneous electrical stimulation should be designed with the health care team so activities can be planned for times that are most pain reduced or free.

Liver Disorders

As is true of other body organs, age causes the liver to decrease in weight, with little or no concomitant reduction in physiological effectiveness. What does constitute an important change is the age-related reduction in the microsomal-induced enzymes of the liver that are crucial to the detoxification and metabolism of drugs (Schuster, 1978). There may also be diminished albumin synthesis as well as reduced hepatic blood flow from a variety of causes, e.g., congestive heart failure and hepatocellular damage from alcoholism.

Viral hepatitis, with a mortality of 25%, is a serious threat to the older person (Berman & Kirsner, 1976). When being treated for another condition, older persons can be unwittingly infected with the virus via blood transfusions or contaminated dishes and medications. In institutional settings the elderly are particularly vulnerable to the disease if the staff fail to practice appropriate hygiene. The best therapy for viral hepatitis is prevention.

Drugs with high hepatotoxicity (e.g., the phenothiazines) can result in hepatocellular damage, causing the older person to become jaundiced. Any jaundice in the elderly should be reported to the physician immediately for appropriate medical diagnosis and management.

Cirrhosis of the liver, often in its end stages, is a reason for institutionalization of older persons. The gerontological nurse practitioner must remember that cirrhosis is not only a result of alcoholism, but may result from bile duct diseases (biliary cirrhosis) and from hepatitis (postnecrotic cirrhosis), as well as from unknown causes (idiopathic cirrhosis). The presenting pathological picture is similar to that for younger persons, so the reader is urged to review the current literature on this topic.

Bleeding can be an enormous problem in cirrhosis, so care must be taken to preserve the integrity of the skin whenever the skin is punctured, when the teeth are brushed, and in the course of any activity that can precipitate bleeding. Bleeding esophageal varices constitute a high priority emergency.

Jaundice may cause pruritus, so nonsoap baths, moisturizing lotions, and gentle massage are necessary. Fingernails and toenails will need to be kept short to prevent injury from scratching.

A flow sheet should be made listing all of the variables of observations and nursing care needed by these patients. In addition to bleeding, jaundice, pruritus, and skin integrity, the flow sheet should include vital signs, fluid and food intake (if on hyperalimentation, note condition of the insertion site), urine and stool output, behaviors, personality, rest, activity, level of consciousness, abdominal girth, condition of paracentesis site, presence of asterixis (hand flapping signifying developing encephalopathy), and anything else needing constant monitoring (Watson, 1981).

SUMMARY

Gerontological nurse practitioners, as advocates of the elderly, have the responsibility and the opportunity to teach the elderly bowel health and self-care for prevention of GI problems. Attention to older persons' body/mind/spirit in a number of socioenvironmental situations can assist in helping them to be as healthily involved in life as possible.

The nurse practitioner must be always alert and sensitive to pathological processes occurring in the aging GI system. Speedy intervention in the event of acute illness may be lifesaving. However, when no more can be done medically, the nurse practitioner can offer the support necessary to assist the terminally ill to die with dignity.

REFERENCES

American Cancer Society. (1981). *Facts on colorectal cancer* (revised, pamphlet). New York: American Cancer Society.

American Cancer Society. (1986). *1986 Cancer Facts and Figures*. New York: American Cancer Society.

Babka, J., & Castell, D. (1973). On the genesis of heartburn. *Digestive Diseases, 18*(5), 391–397.

Berman, P., & Kirsner, J. (1972, March). The aging gut. I: Diseases of the esophagus, small intestines, and appendix. *Geriatrics, 27,* 84–90.

Berman, P., & Kirsner, J. (1976). Gastrointestinal problems. In F. Steinberg (Ed.), *Cowdry's the care of the geriatric patient*. St. Louis: Mosby.

Bolt, R. (1980, December). Evaluation of screening tests for colorectal cancer. *Primary Care, 7,* 683–689.

Bond, J. (1982). Office-based management of diarrhea. *Geriatrics, 37*(2), 52–64.

Borda, I. T. (1987). Drug treatment of gastrointestinal disorders. In C. G. Swift (Ed.), *Clinical pharmacology in the elderly*. New York: Marcel Dekker.

Brandt, L. J. (1986). Managing GI disorders of aging: Noncardiac chest pain and rectal bleeding. *Geriatrics, 41*(7), 20–30.

Brocklehurst, J. C. (1977). How to define and treat constipation. *Geriatrics, 32*(6), 85–87.

Brocklehurst, J. C. (1980). Disorders of the lower bowel in old age. *Geriatrics, 35*(5), 47–54.

Brunner, L., & Suddarth, D. (1984). *Textbook of medical–surgical nursing* (5th ed.). Philadelphia: Lippincott.

Bulmash, J. M. (1981). Confronting the three most common medical problems of long-term illness. *Geriatrics, 36*(12), 79–85.

Burakoff, R. (1981). An updated look at diverticular disease. *Geriatrics, 36*(3), 83–91.

Burkitt, D. (1982). Dietary fiber: Is it really helpful? *Geriatrics, 37*(1), 119–126.

Bustin, M., & Iber, F. (1983). Management of common non-malignant G.I. problems in the elderly. *Geriatrics, 38*(3), 69–74.

Cooper, H. (1980). Irritable bowel syndrome: Diagnosis by exclusion. *Geriatrics, 35*(1), 43–46.

Edwards, J., & Krouse, S. (1987). Helping the emergency colostomy patient through reality shock. *Nursing 87, 17*(7), 63–64.

Fikry, M. (1968). Exocrine pancreatic functions in the aged. *Journal of the American Geriatrics Society, 16,* 463.

Gaines, R. (1977). Surgery for gallbladder disease in the elderly. *Geriatrics, 32*(6), 71–74.

Geboes, R., & Bossaert, H. (1977). Gastrointestinal disorders in old age. *Age and Aging, 6,* 197–200.

Geokas, M., & Haverback, B. (1969). The aging gastrointestinal tract. *American Journal of Surgery, 117*(6), 881–882.

Ham, R. J. (1987). *Incontinence and constipation: Issues in self-regard.* In G. Lesnoff-Caravaglia (Ed.), *Handbook of applied gerontology.* New York: Human Sciences Press.

Holt, R., & Wherry, D. (1979). Why flexible fiberoptic sigmoidoscopy is important in the geriatric patient. *Geriatrics, 34*(5), 85–88.

Jacobson, W., & Levy, A. (1977). Endoscopy of upper gastrointestinal tract is feasible and safe in elderly patients. *Geriatrics, 321*(1), 80–83.

Johns, M. (1980). Infections and tumors of the salivary glands: The best way to heal them. *Geriatrics, 35*(7), 79–81, 84–85.

Langer, A. (1976). Oral signs of aging and their clinical significance. *Geriatrics 31*(12), 63–69.

Lorand, A. (1912). *On the prevention and treatment of habitual constipation. Old age deferred.* Philadelphia: Davis.

Painter, N. (1976). Diverticular disease of the colon: A bane of the elderly. *Geriatrics, 31*(2), 89–94.

Pathy, M. S. J. (1985). *Principles and practice of geriatric medicine.* New York: Wiley.

Posner, G., & Rao, U. P. (1979). A diagnostic approach to occult blood in the stool. *Geriatrics, 34*(7), 52–58.

Ravdin, J., & Guerrant, R. (1983). Infectious diarrhea in the elderly. *Geriatrics, 38*(4), 95–101.

Redinger, R. (1980). Advances in the diagnosis and treatment of gallbladder disease in the elderly. *Geriatrics, 35*(4), 105–109.

Reynolds, J., Ouyang, A., & Cohen, S. (1982). Recent advances in Dx and Rx of esophageal disease. *Geriatrics, 37*(6), 91–93, 97, 101–104.

Richardson, J. (1977). Colorectal cancer: A mass screening and education program. *Geriatrics, 32*(2), 121–131.

Robbins, S. L., & Angell, M. (1971). *Basic pathology.* Philadelphia: Saunders.

Rosenberg, I. R., Friedland, N., Janowitz, H. D., & Dreiling, D. A. (1966). The effect of age and sex upon human pancreatic secretion of fluid and bicarbonate. *Gastroenterology, 50,* 191.

Rossman, I. (Ed.). (1986). *Clinical geriatrics* (3rd ed.). Philadelphia: Lippincott.

Schein, C. (1979). A selective approach to surgical problems in the aged. In I. Rossman (Ed.), *Clinical geriatrics* (2nd ed.). Philadelphia: Lippincott.

Schramm, V. (1980). A guide to diagnosing and treating facial pain and headache. *Geriatrics, 35*(8), 78–90.

Schuster, M. (1978). Disorders of the aging G.I. system. In W. Reichel (Ed.), *The geriatric patient.* New York: H. P. Publishing.

Smith, L. (1978). How to treat hemorrhoids: Five nonsurgical alternatives. *Geriatrics, 33*(10), 43–48.

Teutsch, E., & Hill, M. (1987). Sjögren's syndrome

adding moisture to your life. *American Journal of Nursing, 87*(3), 326–329.

Unger, J., & McGregor, D. (1976). When esophageal carcinoma is obscured by other factors. *Geriatrics, 31*(2), 53–58.

Vanneman, W. (1980). Toward the control of colon cancer. *Geriatrics, 35*(9), 51–63.

Watson, J. (1981). Cirrhosis and fibrosis. In Nurses Reference Library, *Diseases*. Horsham, PA: Intermed Communications.

GENITOURINARY CHANGES

7

Genitourinary disorders are relatively common in the elderly. As the male and female genitourinary systems are fundamentally different, it is not surprising that men and women are affected differently as those systems age and undergo progressive degeneration. On the other hand, the many common aspects of the urinary tracts in men and women are such that the older person will be prone to certain disorders simply as a result of aging, regardless of that person's sex. Despite the physiological and psychological changes that older persons normally undergo, however, the older person will often remain interested in and capable of sexual activity for an extended period of time. As in any other area of nursing, the older person with genitourinary problems must be managed as a unique individual.

AGING OF THE FEMALE REPRODUCTIVE SYSTEM

Bleeding, pain, and vaginal discharge are the most common gynecologic complaints of the elderly female client. High on the list of such complaints from women over 65 are those referable to the bladder and urinary tract. Generally speaking, most gynecologic problems in the elderly are related to postmenopausal bleeding, genital prolapse, infection, or alterations of normal urinary bladder function. These are due in part to decreased hormonal secretions and in part to weakening of the structures that support the urinary bladder, often as a result of damage to the pelvic floor that was suffered during labor and delivery, many years previously. In this age group, detection of a mass in the breast, abdomen, or genital tract must be considered highly suspicious of a malignant disease, particularly when accompanied by vaginal bleeding.

Correction of gynecologic disorders in the elderly client often involves surgery. Although the client might be reluctant to undergo elective surgery, she might submit to it if there is a reasonable chance of survival for a respectable period of time afterwards. Undoubtedly, the elderly client's physician will also find cardiovascular, renal, and/or pulmonary abnormalities, but such problems need not automatically contraindicate needed surgery, provided that reasonable surgical judgment is exercised and modern principles of preoperative and postoperative care are implemented. The important consideration in recommending surgical correction to the elderly client is not simply the opportunity to live longer, but rather the opportunity for her to live her remaining years more comfortably, usefully, and happily. Age itself should not be considered a contraindication for surgery. The chances for success improve, of course, when the condition is recognized and treated early in its course of development. The value of prevention by periodic examinations cannot be overemphasized.

Uterine Prolapse

Uterine prolapse (the abnormal protrusion of the uterus through the pelvic floor) is a common problem in elderly women. Although the associated mortality is not significant, uterine prolapse does cause considerable discomfort, disability, and suffering. Normally, the pelvic floor supports and contains the pelvic viscera and withstands increased intra-abdominal pressure during straining, lifting, or coughing. The disorder occurs most frequently in postmenopausal, multiparous, Caucasian women as a gradually progressive, delayed result of childbirth trauma, congenital anomaly, musculofascial weakness, pelvic tumor, sacral nerve disorder, or diabetic neuropathy.

The degree of uterine prolapse is related to the extent of separation or alteration of the supporting structures. In *slight intravaginal (incomplete) prolapse,* the uterus extends partially into the vagina; in *moderate prolapse,* the uterus descends to the extent that the cervix can be seen at the inferior entrance to the vagina; and in *complete prolapse* the entire cervix and uterus protrude, and the vagina is inverted.

Anterior and posterior vaginal relaxation, as well as perineal incompetency, often accompany uterine prolapse. A large *cystocele* (herniation of the urinary bladder into the vagina) is more common than *rectocele* (rectovaginal hernia) in prolapse, because the bladder is more easily carried downward (Symmonds, 1980).

For unknown reasons, the cervix often becomes elongated in prolapse. Prior to menopause, the prolapsed uterus hypertrophies and becomes engorged and flabby. After menopause, the uterus atrophies. In complete prolapse, the vaginal mucosa thickens and cornifies, resembling the skin.

Assessment Parameters

Signs and symptoms of uterine prolapse include urinary frequency, dysuria, and voiding difficulty. Most clients with uterine prolapse have a history of at least one traumatic delivery. A sense of heaviness in the lower back, pelvis, or inguinal regions can be the result of traction on the uterus or cervical ligaments by the inadequately supported uterus. After menopause, there can be excessive vaginal mucus and bleeding, due to trophic ulceration and infection of the prolapsed uterus. Urinary tract infection is common with prolapse because of compression or herniation of the bladder by the displaced uterus and cervix.

Uterine prolapse can cause significant ureteral obstruction, leading to renal failure. Early diagnosis and correction are required to prevent hypertension, severe postobstructive atrophy, and permanent renal insufficiency. Ureteral obstruction can also be present when renal function is normal, as assessed by blood urea nitrogen (BUN) and serum creatinine values; therefore, an intravenous pyelogram (IVP) should be considered an integral part of the investigation of patients with uterine prolapse (Churchill, Afridi, Dow, & McManamon, 1980).

Partial ureteral obstruction also can occur, leading to urinary stasis and hydronephrosis. Urinary frequency, urgency, and overflow voiding are common, but incontinence is rare. Constipation and painful defecation can occur with prolapse because of pressure or rectocele. Hemorrhoids can result from straining due to constipation.

Regardless of the mechanism of obstruction, correction of uterine prolapse results in correction of the ureteral obstruction. Delay in the correction of obstructive uropathy secondary to uterine prolapse can result in severe postobstructive renal atrophy and significant renal failure and/or hypertension (Churchill et al., 1980).

Pelvic examination in the supine or standing position (first with the patient bearing down and then straining) will demonstrate downward displacement of a prolapsing uterus; a firm mobile mass will be palpable in the lower vagina. A rectal–vaginal examination might reveal a rectocele (Symmonds, 1980).

Medical and Surgical Management

General treatment measures include bed rest, and a well-fitted pessary might give relief if surgery is contraindicated. *Pessaries* (varied forms of vaginal appliances) are generally used to support the uterus, cervical stump, or pelvic floor hernia. They can be effective in reducing vaginal relaxation and increasing the tautness of pelvic-floor structures. Pessaries are especially useful in the poor-risk patient who might refuse surgery for uterine prolapse or other gynecologic hernias, and they can be used as preoperative aids in the healing of cervical stasis ulceration or for the correction of urinary stress incontinence. Pessaries are contraindicated in cases of acute genital tract infection and adherent retroposition of the uterus.

Acetic acid douches, medicated tampons, or chemotherapy (for ulceration) might be prescribed. Estrogen in suppository or vaginal cream form are useful for the elderly client. Prolonged cyclic estrogen therapy for postmenopausal women often conserves the strength and tone of the pelvic floor.

Prolapse of the uterus remains unchanged, or ultimately progresses, unless corrected surgically. For the postmenopausal woman who is sexually active, vaginal hysterectomy and repair are usually recommended (Ellenbogen, Agramat, & Grunstein, 1981). In elderly clients, colpocleisis (closure of the vagina by suturing) or colpectomy (surgical excision of the vagina) might be performed (Symmonds, 1980). Preoperative instances of urinary tract infection, diabetes mellitus, or cardiovascular complications should be controlled by proper treatment.

In the aged woman, vaginal hysterectomy might help restore activity and relieve disability, but the client's medical status must first be determined. The client should be evaluated for hypertension, heart disease, diabetes mellitus, chronic lung disease, and anemia. Routine laboratory tests include a complete blood count (CBC), renal function tests, and an electrocardiogram (ECG). A diagnostic curettage is also performed, to rule out uterine malignancy (Ellenbogen et al., 1981).

Nursing Care Management

Client education is an important nursing function. The client with uterine prolapse who needs a pessary should be instructed in its use and care. Several types of pessaries are available, with the choice dependent upon the patient's condition. Fitting is very important, since a pessary that is too large can cause irritation and ulceration, and one that is too small might fail to remain in place. Bee-cell and inflatable pessaries should be removed nightly for cleansing and preservation of the vaginal mucosa. Firm pessaries should be removed every 4–6 weeks; a pessary of slightly different size and shape can be substituted. Frequent low-pressure acetic acid douches or acidic vaginal creams are helpful when pessaries are worn (Symmonds, 1980).

For the client who has had a hysterectomy, colpocleisis, or colpectomy, postoperative care includes the maintenance of fluid intake and early ambulation. Antibiotics are given at the first sign of infection. Common postoperative complications include fever, urinary tract infection, retention of urine, and stump abscess.

Fibroid Tumors

Fibroid tumors are benign masses of muscle and connective tissue. Often called simply *fibroids,* they are the most common type of gynecologic tumors. The true incidence of fibroids is not known, but it is estimated that 20–50% of women over 35 years of age have had or will have them. Fibroids are rarely seen before menarche or after menopause, and it appears that estrogen is an important factor in their growth. Genetic factors may also be involved in their development.

Assessment Parameters

The vast majority of small fibroids are asymptomatic, grow very slowly, and need only be monitored. If they are not causing problems, they are best left alone. On the other hand, large fibroids can exert pressure on the bladder or rectum and cause pressure symptoms such as urinary frequency, constipation, and abdominal fullness. If the client is approaching menopause and can tolerate the discomfort, a wait-and-see attitude might be taken; the discomfort will usually diminish as the tumor stops growing in the absence of estrogen. The risk of fibroids becoming malignant is less than 0.3%; although the operative mortality for a hysterectomy is also low, it is more than three times higher (1%).

Medical and Surgical Management

When a woman over 40 has a fibroid that is larger than a grapefruit, growing rapidly and causing pain, pressure, or bleeding, a vaginal or abdominal hysterectomy is often performed. Usually, the surgeon will perform a *total abdominal hysterectomy* (surgical removal of the cervix and uterus). An *oophorectomy* (removal of an ovary) is usually not performed, however; the risk of ovarian cancer in women over 40 is approximately 1%, but there is a significant chance that the ovaries will continue to function for many years after menopause.

Uterine Cancer

More than 90% of uterine cancer involves carcinoma of the endometrial lining of the uterus. Generally speaking, this cancer is an adenocarcinoma that metastasizes late, usually to the cervix, fallopian tubes, and other peritoneal structures. Systemic spread to the lungs and brain takes place via the circulation and lymphatic systems. It is primarily a disease of older women, occurring most frequently after menopause. Women who no longer ovulate or who have estrogen-producing ovarian tumors exhibit the highest incidence of uterine cancer; it occurs spontaneously in 1 of every 1000 postmenopausal women. It has been suggested that the use of oral contraceptives has increased the incidence of endometrial cancer, although the in-

creased incidence may also be due to the fact that women are living increasingly longer. There is a general consensus, however, that hormones are implicated as well.

Endometrial cancer is more prevalent than cervical cancer in the older adult female. An average of 37,000 new cases of uterine cancer are reported annually; of these, approximately 35,000 (95%) are eventually fatal. White women of higher than average socioeconomic status who are more than 30% overweight, who have had low fertility or have not borne children, and who have diabetes and high blood pressure are particularly at risk for uterine cancer (Sloane, 1980). Obesity is the principal culprit; the diabetes and hypertension are there by association rather than as direct contributors. In this case, the primary source of estrogen is the adrenal glands. Estrone produced in the adrenals is converted to estrogen in fat, muscle, liver, kidneys, and adrenal glands, and because this conversion is proportional to body weight, heavier women have higher circulating levels of estrogen. The increased estrogen levels stimulate endometrial growth and are believed to lead initially to endometrial hyperplasia and ultimately to endometrial carcinoma.

Assessment Parameters

The major initial symptom of uterine cancer is abnormal but painless vaginal bleeding. Such bleeding irregularities include *polymenorrhea* (cyclic bleeding that occurs at intervals shorter than 21 days), *hypermenorrhea* (heavy bleeding at the time of menstruation), and *metrorrhagia* (bleeding that is independent of the menstrual period). The discharge might at first be watery and blood-streaked, but it gradually becomes bloodier. Pain and weight loss do not appear until the cancer is well advanced. Sloane (1980) reports that 20–50% of the time, vaginal bleeding that occurs 6 months after the cessation of menstruation is an indication that the client has a cancer someplace in the reproductive organs. Because vaginal bleeding is such an early sign of the disease, and endometrial cancer tends to be such a slow-growing tumor, the chances of a cure are very good if medical care is sought promptly.

Ovarian enlargement in the postmenopausal woman must be treated as a malignancy, until proven otherwise, because of the high incidence of malignancy in that age group. Approximately 40% of cases of ovarian enlargement result in ovarian cancer.

In advanced stages, the tumor can extend directly into the myometrium and cervix and into the bladder, rectum, or other pelvic structures. Using the staging of endometrial cancer given in Table 7–1, 75% of cases are in stage I, 14% in stage II, 9% in stage III, and 3% in stage IV (Rosenshein and Rotmensch, 1982).

Diagnosis of uterine cancer requires endometrial, cervical, and endocervical biopsies, suction curettage, or dilation and curettage (D & C). An endometrial biopsy yields an accurate diagnosis in 75–90% of cases. Other diagnostic procedures include a complete physical examination, chest x-rays, IVP, sonography, computed tomography (CT), laparoscopy, cytological studies, ECG, and barium enema studies.

Medical and Surgical Management

Treatment of endometrial cancer depends upon the extent of the disease, but surgery combined with radiation therapy is the normal procedure, regardless of the stage, and is associated with the highest cure and lowest recurrence rates. For stage I endometrial carcinomas, the primary mode of therapy is total abdominal hysterectomy and *bilateral salpingo-oophorectomy* (removal of the fallopian tubes and ovaries)—alternatively referred to as *panhysterosalpingo-oophorectomy*—in conjunction with radiation therapy. In stage II, when the tumor is not well differentiated, intracavity or external radiation will be employed 6 weeks prior to the surgery. In stages III and IV, when the cancer has metastasized to the vagina, pelvis, and lungs, a combination of radiation, surgery, and chemotherapy often is used (Rubin, 1987b). In some cases of advanced endometrial cancer, it might be necessary to perform a *pelvic exenteration* (radical hysterectomy, pelvic node dissection, cystectomy, vaginectomy, and rectal resection). The chemotherapy might consist of intravenous doses of doxorubicin, massive doses of progesterone, or a combination of vincristine, actinomycin D, and cyclophosphamid.

Nursing Care Management

Care of the surgery patient. Prior to such surgery as will be required in cases of uterine cancer, it is very important that the nurse prepare the client psychologically as well as physically. The uterus is commonly considered the source of femininity, and women facing a hysterectomy

TABLE 7–1. STAGES OF ENDOMETRIAL CANCER

Stage	Description
I	The cancer is confined to the corpus of the uterus
Ia	Uterine cavity is not longer than 8 cm
Ib	Uterine cavity is longer than 8 cm
G1	Adenomatous carcinoma is highly differentiated
G2	Adenomatous carcinoma is differentiated, with partly solid areas
G3	Carcinoma is predominantly solid or entirely undifferentiated
II	The carcinoma involves the uterine corpus and the cervix
III	The carcinoma extends beyond the uterus but not outside the true pelvis, i.e., it might involve the vaginal wall or parametrium, but not the bladder or rectum
IV	The carcinoma involves the bladder or rectum, or it extends beyond the true pelvis

typically fear a change in body image as a result of the operation. The gerontological nurse practitioner should encourage the client to express her fears and should offer support and understanding in attempting to dispel such fears. Often, the older client will also fear the surgical procedure itself, perhaps feeling that she might die during the operation or suffer some other grave consequence, e.g., a stroke. Uterine cancer at any age is a frightening prospect; the special counseling and psychological support that are necessary to enable these clients to cope with this dread disease are essential components of the required nursing care.

Preoperative counseling should address specific aspects of postoperative recovery and subsequent effects on sexual functioning. To avoid unnecessary apprehension postoperatively, the client should be prepared for the special equipment and procedures that might be needed, e.g., intravenous infusions, catheterization, and nasogastric intubation. The nurse practitioner should explain how and why it is frequently necessary to turn, cough, and breathe deeply after the surgery. The need for careful cleansing of the perineum also should be emphasized. The client anticipating a pelvic exenteration needs to understand that her vagina and rectum will be removed; in her case, ileal conduits and colostomy also must be explained.

If the hysterectomy patient is premenopausal, she should be prepared for the "surgical menopause" that will result from the operation. She should understand that she might experience hot flashes or other previously described menopausal symptoms that women sometimes have when their bodies are no longer producing estrogen. If sexual functioning will be possible (depending upon the extent of the surgery and the patient's general condition), that fact should be explained. Since vaginal dryness can be anticipated, the use of a lubricant might be suggested.

Preoperatively, the client requires bowel and skin preparation. Residue in the client's diet is decreased for 48–72 hours prior to surgery; the client is then provided a clear liquid diet and,

finally, nothing by mouth. Enemas are given to empty the bowel, and occasionally an antiseptic vaginal douche is ordered, to decrease the chance of infection. Antibiotics are administered orally and/or intravenously, as ordered, and the perineum is prepped (often more than once) with antibacterial soap. A nasogastric tube might be inserted if the physician anticipates abdominal distention postoperatively.

Postoperative nursing goals include preventing infection, hemorrhage, respiratory complications, and pain, providing adequate nutrition, and promoting elimination. The nurse practitioner must remain particularly alert for hemorrhage. The hysterectomy client's vital signs should be assessed frequently, and dressings and/or perineal pads should be checked regularly for bleeding (particularly if the hysterectomy was performed vaginally). Any bleeding or foul-smelling drainage should be reported to the physician. Abdominal distention, severe pain, and breathing difficulties should also be noted and reported.

To prevent circulatory and respiratory problems, the client is encouraged to turn, cough, and breathe deeply. On the second postoperative day, she is usually assisted out of bed. As the elderly female client is particularly at risk for thromboembolic disease, antiembolic stockings, range-of-motion exercises, and low-dose heparin therapy are used to prevent the formation of thrombi and emboli. The client's calves should be assessed for tenderness, redness, swelling, pain, or a significant difference in calf measurements. Thromboembolic disease is also indicated by a positive Homan's sign (pain in the calf and popliteal area when the foot is dorsiflexed, passively).

The client's back and sacral areas should be massaged frequently, both for her comfort and to prevent skin breakdown; back- and side-lying positions should be changed frequently. Pain medication should be given, as ordered. (It might be especially helpful when given before the client ambulates.)

To promote urinary drainage, a Foley

catheter will be used; when it is removed (after 3 or 4 days, usually) the client must be checked for residual urine. Residual amounts in excess of 100–200 ml indicate that the catheter should be replaced. Following its removal, the client should be encouraged to drink copious amounts of fluids to promote urinary drainage.

Feminine hygiene is promoted by having the client wear a perineal pad (a sterile pad is used when there is danger of infection) until all drainage ceases. The pads should be counted, and the amount, color, and odor of the drainage recorded. Each time the pad is changed, the perineal area should be carefully cleansed with an antiseptic solution.

Following pelvic exenteration surgery, the client should be prepared to care for the stoma and skin surrounding the stoma. If soap is considered too drying, warm water and saline can be used for cleansing the stomal area. The perineal incision must be carefully watched, and the physician must be notified immediately of any bright red, foul-smelling, or purulent drainage.

Care of the radiation-therapy patient. The nurse practitioner should know if the client is to receive external, internal, or both modes of radiation therapy. Usually, internal radiation therapy is performed first when both types are needed. The radioactive source might be inserted in the operating room (*preloaded*) or subsequently, at the bedside (*afterloaded*). If the source is preloaded, the client will return to her room "hot," and safety precautions must be begun immediately. The gerontological nurse practitioner should explain that the procedure will be performed under general anesthesia, and the implant will be inserted by a physician. A hospital stay of 2 to 3 days is usually required. In preparation, the client should be given a bowel prep and a providone–iodine vaginal douche. A clear liquid diet will be prescribed, and a Foley catheter inserted.

If the radiation source is to be afterloaded, a representative from the radiation department will perform the implantation in the client's room. Safety precautions (involving time, distance, and shielding considerations) must be instituted as soon as the radiation source has been implanted. A sign that specifies all required safety precautions should be posted on the door to inform everyone of the radiation hazard. It is important that all health care providers organize their time spent in the client's room, to minimize their exposure to radiation. Because the client must remain still during the time that the implant is in place, items that the client might need should be located within her reach.

If the client is to receive external radiation therapy, she should be informed of the duration of treatment. Usually, treatment will be given 5 days a week for 6 weeks. The region to be irradiated will be marked on the surface of the skin. The client should be cautioned not to wash away these markings, as it is very important that the radiation be directed to the same region each day. To reduce the incidence of skin infection and breakdown, the treated area should be kept dry, and the client should avoid wearing clothing that would rub against the target area, exposing that region to heat, or using irritating skin creams.

Because diarrhea is a possible side effect of pelvic radiation, the client's diet should be high in protein, high in carbohydrates, and low in residue (to reduce bulk while providing the necessary calories). Diphenoxylate with atropine might be given for diarrhea.

Cervical Cancer

In the elderly female, atrophic changes usually cause the cervix to become flush with the vaginal vault, and endocervical polyps occasionally occur, which leads to vaginal spotting. The incidence of squamous-cell carcinoma peaks in the fifth decade of life, but it can occur at any age, as can adenocarcinoma of the cervix; therefore, annual Papanicolaou (Pap) smears are recommended for women of all ages. Any abnormal lesion should be sent for biopsy, as early detection and appropriate treatment of such lesions afford an excellent prognosis.

The incidence of cervical cancer is higher in low-income groups, and it is higher among Puerto Rican and black women than among whites. The disease is rare among virgins and lesbians, and it is well accepted that there is a direct relationship between frequency of sexual intercourse and cancer of the cervix (Sloane, 1980). About 95% of cervical cancer is squamous-cell carcinoma, and the remaining 5% is adenocarcinoma. About 2200 women die of cervical cancer in the United States each year. The overall survival rate is approximately 50%, and there are about 5000 new cases per year (Dickenson, 1980). Theoretically, annual cytological screening could eliminate further mortality due to cervical cancer, because it may take 10 years or longer for the disease to reach its invasive, life-threatening form.

Assessment Parameters

Cervical cancer first occurs as a mild abnormality of atypical cells that progress through a series of stages to malignant tumor formation or proliferation of anaplastic cells. In the early stages, the evolution is sometimes reversed or halted for an indefinite period. Even when an area of abnormality is not treated, it does not inevitably become cancerous. The Pap test, however, can detect cell abnormalities early, when they are preclinical and preinvasive and the progression to cancer can be stopped most readily.

Initially, cervical cancer is characterized by the presence of *dysplasia* (disorderly cellular arrangements) in the upper layers of the epithelium of the cervix. The nuclei are enlarged and stain darkly. Depending upon the number of atypical cells, dysplasia is categorized as slight, moderate, or severe, but even in severe dysplasia the abnormalities do not exist throughout the entire thickness of the epithelium. Many cases of dysplasia regress, and the epithelium sometimes returns to normal, but the possibility of regression decreases as the number of abnormal cells increases.

Medical and Surgical Management

Common treatments for dysplasia of the cervix include cautery, conization, cryosurgery, and laser treatment, but continued observation, i.e., no treatment, is also an option. A biopsy of the lesion may be performed via colposcopy. If the biopsy reveals severe dysplasia, conization (cone biopsy) is usually performed. Conization requires hospitalization and general anesthesia. Using a colposcope, however, the physician can perform electrocautery, cryosurgery, or laser-beam treatment in the office, painlessly, without using anesthesia.

Unless detected and treated early, cervical cancer can progress to *cancer in situ* (cancer in place). In carcinoma in situ, the entire thickness of the epithelial cell layer is involved. This next stage is still considered preinvasive or noninvasive, however, because the abnormality has not reached connective tissue or stroma underlying the epithelium. Once diagnosed, carcinoma in situ is usually treated by hysterectomy to remove the cervix.

The stages of invasive cervical cancer, which extends beyond the epithelium, are listed in Table 7–2. Invasive cancer is most commonly treated by radiation therapy, either externally (using supervoltage x-rays or cobalt) or internally (by means of radium implants, inserted into the cervical canal). Unless cancer of the cervix is treated in an early stage it might ultimately invade the vagina, pelvic wall, bladder, rectum, and lymph nodes. In some cases a radical hysterectomy is performed to remove the uterus, the upper part of the vagina and adjacent tissues, and the lymph nodes. In late stages of the disease, or if radiation fails, an even more extensive operation might be performed to remove the bladder and rectum.

Nursing Care Management

Regular Pap testing can detect cervical cancer long before symptoms of cancer appear. Preinvasive cervical cancer produces no symptoms, whereas early invasive cervical cancer usually causes abnormal bleeding; the menstrual flow

TABLE 7–2. STAGES OF INVASIVE CERVICAL CANCER

Stage	Description
I	The cancer is strictly limited to the cervix
II	Spreading extends beyond the cervix to the upper two thirds of the vagina, but not to the lateral pelvic walls
III	The cancer has spread to the lateral pelvic wall and the lower third of the vagina
IV	The urinary bladder and/or the rectum are involved, or the cancer has metastasized beyond the true pelvis

might be either irregular or excessive. An initial, persistent, watery discharge is followed by a dark discharge as the sloughing of necrotic tissue increases, and this discharge increases with douching, intercourse, or defecation. In advanced stages, as the cancer spreads to the lymph nodes, vagina, bladder, rectum, and uterus, the client might experience pelvic pain, vaginal leakage of urine and feces (from fistula formation), weight loss, anemia, anorexia, or malaise.

Nursing problems include emotional stress, bleeding, pain, and vaginal discharge. Each individual deals with the diagnosis of cancer in a unique way. It is important for the gerontological nurse practitioner to understand how the client views herself and what her relationship is with her family. In addition to psychological support, nursing care must include preoperative and postoperative nursing care and comprehensive patient education.

Vaginal bleeding might be severe, necessitating that blood pressure and pulse rate be monitored frequently and close attention be paid to hemoglobin and hematocrit levels, to prevent the occurrence of anemia. Blood loss can be estimated accurately by tabulating the number of perineal pads used during each 24-hour period (a saturated perineal pad holds approximately 60 ml of blood).

In assessing the client's pain, the nurse practitioner should determine its site, frequency, duration, and cause. Pain might be due not to the cancer but rather be a result of other problem(s), e.g., a full bladder requiring catheterization, constipation requiring laxatives, or immobiliza-

tion problems that can be avoided by frequent position changes. If the pain is due to cancer, the client should be given analgesics in dosages and at intervals that will enable her to continue daily activities free of pain.

Vaginal drainage is often profuse, has an offensive odor, and irritates the skin. Offensive odors can be reduced by using air fresheners and air cleaning devices. Skin irritation can be prevented by cleansing the perineal area frequently with soap and water and allowing it to dry thoroughly.

Care of the surgery patient. Following a positive cervical smear, the client should be prepared for further testing. If the client is to have a cervical biopsy, she should be advised that she might experience pressure or minor cramps, but there will be little if any pain, as the cervix has relatively few nerve endings. Following the procedure she might have some spotting, and she should abstain from sexual intercourse for 1 or 2 days.

Prior to cryosurgery the client should be informed that the procedure will take approximately 15 minutes and that she might experience abdominal cramps, sweating, or headache, but that there will be little pain at the operative site. Following the procedure she can expect to have a heavy, watery, yellowish discharge for about 2 weeks; she should not douche, use tampons, or engage in sexual intercourse until the discharge has ceased. The client who has had either a biopsy or cryosurgery should be impressed with the necessity for follow-up care within 3–4 months. She should also be taught the signs and symptoms of infection and told to report their occurrence immediately.

Care of the radiation-therapy client. Tumors of the cervix may be treated with radiation therapy (internally and/or externally) or hysterectomy. Radiation therapy is used to deter tumor growth and metastatic invasion of the pelvic cavity. Tumors of the cervix are particularly amenable to radiation treatment because they are well confined and readily accessible; the radioactive source can be inserted into the uterus via the vagina and dilated cervix, using a colpostat or Ernst applicator. Radiation therapy might include the use of external radiation, particularly as an adjunct to surgery for cancer of the uterine fundus. If an intracavitary implant is used, the radiation is directed at the cervix from the uterus or vaginal vault.

Before radiation therapy is begun, the physician and nurse practitioner should explain to the client the type and extent of the treatment. Usually, the length of treatment for cervical cancer is 2–3 days. During this time the client must lie on her back, to ensure that the implant is maintained in the proper position. The nurse practitioner should help her be as comfortable as possible while ensuring that the radioactive source does not become dislodged. A Foley catheter is inserted, but an enema might be given before the catheterization, to empty the bowel. The client is maintained NPO the night before surgery and is given liquid or low-residue diet following the implantation, to prevent gastrointestinal distention, bowel movements, or flatus. A fracture pan should be used if a bowel movement does occur.

For her comfort, the client can be allowed to turn slightly from side to side, and the head of the bed might be elevated slightly. The nurse practitioner should assist the client with her daily bath and rub her back frequently to relieve minor muscle aches and help prevent skin breakdown. Tranquilizers might help the client relax and remain still. Analgesics and antiemetics can be used to reduce pain and relieve nausea. Deep

breathing and arm-and-leg exercises should be encouraged, to help prevent respiratory and circulatory complications. To eliminate offensive odors, a room deodorizer should be used, and perineal pads should be changed frequently.

All required safety precautions must be scrupulously adhered to from the time that the radioactive source is implanted. Nursing care must be carefully planned so that the client will not feel hurried or isolated; usually this will include more than the primary nurse. Pregnant nurses should never be assigned the care of clients receiving radiation therapy. Visitors are usually not permitted, and a sign that lists all required precautions should be hung on the door of the client's room. If the implant should become dislodged, the radiation department should be called immediately, and only long-handled forceps should be used to pick up the radiation source.

Following removal of an implant, the catheter should be removed, and an enema may be given to empty the bowel. A low-pressure douche may be given also to remove necrotic tissue and soothe irritated mucosa. Some clients experience nausea, vomiting, or diarrhea, which are treated symptomatically. Fluids should be increased to prevent dehydration and cystitis. Soothing ointments can be used to relieve irritated tissue or pruritus. The client should be advised to avoid persons with infections, because radiation therapy usually results in a reduced white blood count. She should also be advised that a slight amount of vaginal bleeding can be expected for 1–3 months, and sexual relations can be resumed in 7–10 days.

Ovarian Cancer

Ovarian cancer, second only to endometrial cancer in frequency among gynecologic cancers, is responsible for more deaths than cervical and endometrial cancer combined. Furthermore, age-adjusted death rates for ovarian cancer have risen 4% over the last 30 years. After cancers of the breast, colon, and lung, ovarian cancer ranks as the most common cause of cancer deaths among American women (Rosenshein and Rotmensch, 1982). The exact cause of ovarian cancer is not known, but risk factors appear to include low parity (including nulliparity) and infertility.

Ovarian tumors spread rapidly intraperitoneally by local extension, surface seeding, the circulation, and lymphatics. Common sites of involvement include the diaphragm, omentum, peritoneal surfaces, and bowel.

Assessment Parameters

In early stages of the disease (Table 7–3) the client might complain of vague abdominal discomfort such as abdominal distention, dyspepsia, or pain. As the tumor increases in size, it can cause urinary frequency, constipation, pelvic pressure, and weight loss. In advanced stages, ovarian cancer might cause ascites, postmenopausal bleeding, pain, or symptoms related to the sites of metastases.

The highest incidence of ovarian cancer occurs in women between the ages of 55 and 65. Although only 1 case of ovarian cancer in 10,000 asymptomatic women will be detected, routine pelvic examination remains the most reliable means of detecting early disease. An ovary that is palpable 3–5 years after menopause should raise the suspicion of early ovarian cancer. Any pelvic mass that appears after menopause should also be considered a carcinoma unless and until proven otherwise.

Diagnosis of ovarian cancer requires a complete client history, histological studies, and surgical exploration. A complete physical examination (including a Pap smear) is followed by ultrasound studies of the abdomen to determine tumor size. IVP is used to determine renal function and possible urinary tract abnormalities, and a barium enema is used to determine obstruction and tumor size. Chest x-rays are useful for determining the sites of distant metastases or pleural effusion. Mammography can be used to rule out primary breast cancer, and lymphangiography can show lymph node involvement. Other tests

TABLE 7–3. STAGES OF OVARIAN CANCER

Stage	Description
I	Tumor growth is limited to the ovaries
Ia	Growth is limited to one ovary, and ascites (if present) is neither excessive nor pathological
	(1) The tumor is not on the external surface of the ovary, and the ovarian capsule is intact
	(2) The tumor is present on the external surface of the ovary, and/or the ovarian capsule is ruptured
Ib	Growth is limited to both ovaries, and ascites (if present) is neither excessive nor pathological
	(1) The tumor is not on the external surface of the ovary, and the capsule is intact
	(2) The tumor is present on the external surface of the ovary, and/or the ovarian capsule is ruptured
Ic	The tumor is in either stage Ia or Ib, but ascites or positive peritoneal washings are present
II	Tumor growth involves one or both ovaries, and there is extension and/or metastases to the pelvis
IIa	The extension/metastases are to the uterus and/or the fallopian tubes
IIb	The extension/metastases are to other pelvic tissues
IIc	The tumor is in either stage IIa or IIb, but ascites or positive peritoneal washings are present
III	Tumor growth involves either one or both ovaries, there are intraperitoneal metastases outside of the pelvis, and/or there are positive retroperitoneal nodes. The tumor is limited to the true pelvis, and malignant extension to the small bowel or omentum has been proved, histologically
IV	Tumor growth involves either one or both ovaries, and there are distant metastases. Stage IV includes metastases to the liver parenchyma. In case of pleural effusion, positive cytology is required for stage IV designation
Unexplored cases of tumors thought to be ovarian carcinomas form a special category, i.e., they are not designated as being in one of the listed stages	

used in the diagnosis of ovarian cancer include CBC, blood chemistry, ECG, liver function testing, liver scans, and aspiration of ascites fluid for cytological studies.

Medical and Surgical Management

Treatment of ovarian cancer usually requires the use of immunotherapy, chemotherapy, or radiotherapy (alone or in combination) in addition to surgery. Immunotherapy is somewhat controversial and consists of intravenous or intraperitoneal injection of *bacillus Calmette–Guerin* (BCG) vaccine or *Corynebacterium porvulum*. Chemotherapy extends the length of survival time for most clients, but it is largely used for palliative therapy in the more advanced cases. Instillation of a radioisotope, e.g., 32P, is occasionally useful if the peritoneal washings are positive. Often, surgery is followed by deep x-ray therapy, but the role of postoperative x-ray therapy is poorly defined. Surgical removal of the tumor and the ovary, as well as any other involved tissue, often includes total abdominal hysterectomy, bilateral salpingo-oophorectomy, omentectomy, appendectomy, lymph node dissection, tissue biopsies, and peritoneal washings.

Nursing Care Management

Nursing interventions include preoperative client education, postoperative care, and psychological support for the client and her family. In the preoperative period, the client should be prepared, both physically and emotionally, for the many tests that she must undergo. The nurse practitioner should explain the procedures (what will be done, and why), the expected course of treatment following diagnosis, and the surgical and postoperative procedures that will be implemented.

Following surgery, the nurse practitioner should monitor the vital signs frequently, check the dressing for bleeding or excessive drainage, and ensure patency of the catheter, in maintaining good catheter care. An abdominal support should be applied, and the client should be checked for abdominal distention. As with most postsurgical clients, she should be reminded to cough and breathe deeply, and an antiembolic hose should be applied. She should be repositioned frequently and encouraged to ambulate as soon after surgery as possible.

The client should be monitored for side effects of radiation and chemotherapy, and supportive care should be given, as necessary. If the client is receiving immunotherapy, flulike symptoms might occur for 12–24 hours following the administration of the drug. Antiemetics and aspirin should be given, as needed, and the client should be kept warm and comfortable.

Because of the poor prognosis and response to treatment, supportive care is a major nursing responsibility. The usual progression of the disease to a terminal stage is complicated by nausea, vomiting, abdominal distention, ascites, bowel obstruction, anemia, and pleural effusion. Supportive, empathetic nursing care often must be augmented by other health care team members such as the chaplain and social workers.

Vulvar Cancer

Vulvar carcinoma occurs most frequently in women 60 years of age and older and is associated with diabetes, obesity, hypertension, leukoplakia, syphilis, or granulomatous disease.

Assessment Parameters

Symptoms of vulvar cancer include intense pruritus, bleeding, and a vulvar mass. Cancer of the vulva is one of the few malignant tumors of the genitourinary system that is painful (due either to exposed nerve endings or to sepsis), so that the client might also complain of pain. The client might be reluctant to seek help, however, feeling that vulvar itching is far too personal a matter to warrant consulting a physician.

The diagnosis is made by biopsy, and because the vulvae are so sensitive, a small amount of novocaine is injected, beforehand. To determine the extent of the tumor, a 1% solution of aqueous toluidine blue is applied to the vulvae and allowed to dry for a few minutes before applying a 1% acetic acid solution. The test is considered positive for cancer if the cells retain a dark blue stain.

Medical and Surgical Management

The prognosis following therapy for vulvar carcinoma is directly related to the size of the primary lesion and the extent of lymph node involvement. Treatment might include a *simple vulvectomy* or a radical vulvectomy combined with bilateral lymph node dissection. Radiation therapy is normally not used unless the client refuses surgery or is in such poor general condition that she could not tolerate surgery. Radiation therapy is usually ineffective for several reasons. Vulvar tissue does not tolerate irradiation very well because it is too moist and contains too much fat. Necrosis of the skin is apt to develop, and the healing process generally is very slow. In addition, irradiation is ineffective in controlling squamous-cell carcinoma, which is the usual type of vulvar cancer.

Tumors confined to the vulvae respond well to surgical treatment, and the prognosis can be good. Once the disease has spread beyond the vulvae, the prognosis worsens. If there is no lymph node involvement, small lesions can be treated with a simple vulvectomy (surgical removal of the vulvae, without pelvic node dissection), but long-term follow-up is necessary for the detection of recurrent or persistent disease. A radical vulvectomy involves the removal of superficial and deep inguinal lymph nodes, together with a complete removal of the vulvae and (at times) resection of the urethra, vagina, and bowel, which leaves an open wound for up to 3 months. Following the healing process, plastic surgery is performed to reconstruct the pelvic structures.

Nursing Care Management

Preoperative nursing care should include explanations of the physical and psychological changes that can be expected following surgery. The client must be well hydrated and adequately nourished, and she should be provided an understanding of the surgical procedure and the postoperative course.

Postoperatively, nursing care is directed toward preventing infection and promoting healing. A Foley catheter is inserted, to prevent bladder distention and infection (from urinary drainage). Intake and output should be recorded and standard catheter care provided. Fecal contamination is difficult to control and often the physician will order an antidiarrheal drug to reduce the discomfort and possibility of infection. The initial diet of clear liquids should be followed by a low-residue diet and stool softeners, to combat constipation. The perineal area should be cleansed as ordered; aseptic technique must be followed, to avoid fecal contamination.

A Penrose drain or Hemovac drain may be used for 3 or 4 days to provide drainage (the nurse should expect approximately 300 to 500 ml of drainage per day). The dressing should be changed frequently, as it is a medium for bacterial growth. Any bleeding, foul-smelling discharge or other sign of infection should be reported to the physician.

Healing takes place slowly in these clients, due to their age and the fact that only a thin layer of skin remains (with a minimal blood supply) when the fascia has been removed. Special attention should be given to reducing pressure at the operative site and promoting better healing through improved circulation. The client may be placed on an air or egg-crate mattress, and a cradle should be used to support top covers. A sitz bath may be given to increase circulation if the physician concurs (some believe that the sitz bath could be a source of fecal contamination). A heat lamp may be used to dry the perineum, and the client's position should be changed frequently, to avoid pressure sores. The client is usually assisted out of bed in 3 or 4 days.

Edema of the lower legs can be a problem if the lymph nodes have been removed from the groin. Thigh-high elastic hose should be used immediately following surgery, to promote circulation and prevent embolism. The head of the client's bed should be elevated, to promote ve-nous return, and early ambulation should be en-couraged. The client should be advised to wear the elastic hose after she returns home; chronic edema often results in these cases.

The disfigurement of the surgery and the length of time required for healing are often de-pressing for the woman who has had a vulvec-tomy. Postoperatively, the client might com-plain of vulval numbness, and the nurse practi-tioner should explain that eventually (when the nerve endings have healed) most of the numbness will disappear. The client should be advised that sexual intercourse may be resumed in 6–8 weeks following surgery, that the vagina is still intact, but that the clitoris might not be functional. Lubricants may be used if the vaginal wall is atrophied or if intercourse is uncomfort-able. Less deep intromission of the penis also might help reduce discomfort. The geron-tological nurse practitioner should encourage the client to express her feelings and should help her adjust to the changes she has experienced.

Vaginal Cancer

Carcinoma of the vagina is a rare type of tumor in the elderly patient. When it does occur, it is most likely to be a metastatic lesion or a direct extension of a cervical lesion. Diagnosis is made by biopsy of the lesion (Rubin, 1987a). The inci-dence of vaginal dysplasias is increased among clients who have demonstrated cervical and/or vulvar dysplasia. Therefore, such clients should be evaluated on an annual basis. If cytological studies are suspicious in the absence of gross vaginal lesions, colposcopy is the method usu-ally used to determine the source of the abnormal cells.

AGING OF THE MALE REPRODUCTIVE SYSTEM

Most reproductive system disorders experienced by older men are associated with the prostate gland, a fibromuscular, glandular organ that weighs 15–20 grams and is normally about the size of a chestnut or walnut in the adult male. Comprising five lobes (anterior, median, pos-terior, and two lateral lobes), the prostate gland is completely enclosed in a dense fibrous capsule that resembles an inverted cone. It completely surrounds the prostatic urethra, with its base lying at the neck of the bladder and its apex resting against the urogenital diaphragm. The posterior aspect lies against the anterior wall of the rectum, and the anterior portion is attached to the undersurface of the pubis by the pubopros-tatic ligaments. Ejaculatory ducts pass obliquely through the prostate and empty into the posterior urethra. Blood is supplied to the prostate pri-marily from branches of the inferior vesical ar-tery, which is a branch of the internal iliac artery.

The prostate gland has no essential function except to produce a fluid that acts as a vehicle and source of nutrition for spermatozoa. Normal prostatic fluid is rich in acid phosphatase, which is excreted through the ductal system. Elevation of the serum acid phosphatase level (especially the prostatic fraction) is usually indicative of prostatic carcinoma with local ductal obstruction or distant metastases.

Benign Prostatic Hyperplasia (BPH)

Some enlargement of the prostate gland is evi-dent in most men by the age of 50 years, and the majority of men will have palpable evidence of hyperplasia by age 60. *Benign prostatic hyper-plasia* (BPH), sometimes referred to simply as *hyperplasia,* causes progressive obstruction to the flow of urine and, in later stages, causes *hydronephrosis* (back pressure in the kidneys) that contributes to the establishment of urinary tract infection.

The exact cause of the disease is not known, but BPH and hormonal activity appear to be re-lated. The growth and subsequent maintenance of prostate size and function are regulated by androgens; therefore, hyperplasia cannot be at-tributed to androgens per se, as the disease oc-curs at a time when androgenic activity is de-creasing. An imbalance between androgens and estrogens might be a causative factor, however, and high levels of *dihydrotestosterone,* the principal prostatic intracellular androgen (which is more potent in promoting prostatic growth than testosterone), might also contribute to hyperplasia (Smith, 1978). The five separate glands (lobes) that collectively constitute the prostate can grow independently or simultaneously. The size and position of each lobe affect symptoms, detectability, and the associated pathology.

Assessment Parameters

Rectal examination might be capable of revealing prostatic enlargement, depending on the lobes that are affected and the degree of enlargement. The surface of the prostate is usually smooth, but in BPH it can be *fibromuscular* (firmer than usual) or *adenomatous* (unduly soft and boggy)

An elevated white blood cell (WBC) count is an indication of infection, and a low hemoglobin is an indication that the client should be evaluated for anemia. Urinalysis and urine cultures might show pyuria, hematuria, or urinary tract infection. BUN and creatinine levels, if elevated, would suggest impaired renal function. Some (few) men will experience renal pain when voiding, due to reflux; however, the hydronephrosis secondary to prostatic obstruction is usually painless, unless there is infection. Symptoms of BPH that are related to pressure on the urethra include urgency, frequency, and retention. In an advanced stage of the disease, symptoms of uremia include somnolence, vomiting, diarrhea, and weight loss.

Cystoscopy is used to indicate the degree of prostate lobe enlargement and any secondary changes of the bladder wall, e.g., diverticula or irritation. Transrectal sonography of the prostate will reveal the size of the prostate more accurately. IVP can be used to indicate calculi, tumors, and filling or emptying defects of the bladder.

Medical and Surgical Management

BPH is usually treated with either conservative therapy or surgery. If conservative therapy is the selected approach to treatment, the client might be advised to engage in sexual intercourse regularly, to reduce prostatic congestion. Other forms of treatment used to reduce congestion include hot sitz baths and a sequence of three or four prostatic massages, given at 14-day intervals, but no medical treatment for BPH has been completely satisfactory. Prostatitis should be treated by prostatic massage (once a week for 3 weeks), and the infection should be treated with trimethoprim, sulfamethorazole, and minocycline. If urinary infection develops, antibiotics or sulfonamides are used, depending on the type of bacteria that is identified, but if there is a great deal of residual urine, these drugs might not be effective.

The client should be advised to avoid taking excessive amounts of fluids over short periods of time, as rapid distention of the bladder can exacerbate symptoms and even cause acute retention. The client also should avoid alcohol, tranquilizers, anticholinergics, and antidepressants, as they can cause urinary retention. The surgical procedure that is selected for treating BPH depends on the client's general health status, the size of the gland, the degree of prostatic disease, and the preference of the surgeon. The surgical procedures most often used to correct prostatic disease include transurethral resection, suprapubic transvesical prostatectomy, retropubic prostatectomy, perineal prostatectomy, and cryosurgery.

Transurethral resection (TUR), most often used in the treatment of BPH, is also used as a palliative measure in metastatic disease. In the TUR procedure, a resectoscope (which has been passed through the urethra) is used to remove prostatic tissue by means of an electric wire loop. The mortality is low (approximately 1–2%) and the incidence of impotence or incontinence is also low.

Suprapubic transvesical prostatectomy is commonly used when the enlarged prostrate remains in the bladder. This procedure is performed by making a low abdominal incision into the urinary bladder. The surgeon removes the prostatic tissue by reaching into the bladder. The mortality is 1–3%, and the incidence of impotence or incontinence is also low. Retropubic prostatectomy allows direct visualization of the prostate gland. The surgeon's incision is made into the lower abdomen, below the urinary bladder (which disallows treatment of bladder pathologies, as the bladder is not entered). The mortality for this procedure is 1 to 2%, potency is maintained, and incontinence is rare.

Perineal prostatectomy is used most often when the client has cancer of the prostate or an enlarged prostate gland (in the case of an older patient). If cancer is present, all prostatic tissue and the pelvic lymph nodes are dissected. The incision is made through the perineum, resulting in a high incidence of impotence, incontinence, and rectal injury; approximately 1–3% of the clients who have this procedure will develop a rectourethral fistula that requires surgical repair.

In *cryosurgery,* an instrument is passed through the urethra to the tumor mass, which is destroyed by freezing. There is minimal blood loss or other complications. This procedure is limited to poor-risk clients.

Nursing Care Management

The gerontological nurse practitioner should fully assess the client's ability to understand the diagnostic procedures and surgical intervention. All prediagnostic procedures, food and fluid restrictions, bowel preparation procedures, and immediate recovery room care (including the need for drainage tubes and catheters) should then be explained, to prepare the client for surgery. The physician will discuss the possible complications of the surgery with the client, but the nurse practitioner should be prepared to address the client's feelings. He should be advised that resumption of normal sexual function following this surgery will take time. Healing usually will be complete after 2 months, but he may be required to take antibiotics until all signs of infection have disappeared. Following prostatectomy, the client might have a regular catheter or a three-way indwelling catheter connected to a constant closed-bladder irrigation

system that uses sterile normal saline or an antibacterial solution, to reduce clot blockage of the catheter. The solution should be infused at a rate sufficient to maintain returns that are clear to light pink in color; *hematuria* (blood in the urine) might last for a few days following surgery, and the client should be watched carefully for fluid overload, as fluids will be absorbed into the client's system. It might be necessary to irrigate the catheter, if it should fail to drain properly because of clots. The physician's orders will usually call for 80–100 ml of normal saline solution to be instilled gently into the bladder while strict aseptic technique is maintained. A piston-type syringe is recommended, as a ball-type syringe puts too much pressure on the bladder-wall mucosa. The physician should always be notified if the catheter inadvertently falls out. In calculating the client's intake and output, it is important to remember to subtract the volume of irrigating fluid from the total input in order to accurately assess output. The client also should be questioned concerning a full feeling over the bladder, and the nurse practitioner should palpate over the bladder for fullness, to detect bladder distention. Early ambulation and increased intake of fluids should be encouraged while the catheter is in place.

Painful bladder spasms, if experienced, could indicate distention or irritation caused by the catheter balloon. If the catheter cannot be removed, antispasmodic drugs might be helpful. However, these drugs can diminish bowel function, leading to constipation, and they should not be used in patients with glaucoma or severe cardiac disease. Constipation should be prevented, and the client should be advised to avoid straining at stool for at least 6 weeks following surgery, as straining might cause bleeding. Colace, prune juice, or other stool softeners are recommended.

The length of time before the catheter is removed depends on the type of surgery, the physician, and the problems experienced by the client, for example, bladder spasms, hematuria, and so on. Following TUR, for example, the catheter might be removed in 2 or 3 days, whereas a perineal prostatectomy might require that the catheter remain in place for as long as 12–14 days. After the catheter has been removed, the client should be informed that he might experience urgency, dribbling, or frequency, due to changes in the bladder. The client also should be informed that such symptoms are not unusual and normal voiding patterns will return in time. He should be taught to urinate at his first desire and to perform perineal exercises (contraction of the abdominal, gluteal, and perineal muscles, 12–30 times per hour). The client who has had a suprapubic prostatectomy will also have a suprapubic catheter inserted through the abdomen into the bladder, and a Penrose drainage tube will be inserted through the incision. The drain is usually covered with a dry sterile dressing or ostomy appliance. Strict aseptic techniques must be followed in changing dressings, in order to avoid wound infections. Drainage tubes are usually removed before suprapubic tubes.

Prostatic Cancer

Carcinoma of the prostate most frequently arises in the posterior lobe of the gland and might invade the prostate, seminal vessels, urethra, bladder, or rectum. It usually metastasizes by way of the veins, particularly through the vertebrae. It is by means of this mechanism that metastases occur in the pelvis, heads of the femurs, and lower lumbar spine. Other bones, including the skull, are occasionally involved, and infiltration of the bone marrow is particularly common. Spreading to the skin and viscera (e.g., lungs, liver) is also seen. Adenocarcinoma of the prostate is staged as is indicated in Table 7–4.

Assessment Parameters

The symptoms of prostatic cancer are similar to those described for BPH. The presenting symptoms in 75% of men who have prostatic malignancy are due to obstruction to urine flow, infection, or both. Posterior urethral invasion frequently results in symptoms of bladder neck obstruction. Bladder symptoms include hesitancy and straining to begin the stream, a less forceful stream, terminal dribbling, frequency and nocturia, symptoms of bladder infection, and urinary retention. Bone and neuritic pain are often experienced when the cancer has metastasized to bone. Clients with nerve compression might complain of lumbosacral pain that radiates into the hips or down the legs. A mass in the right upper abdominal quadrant might indicate metastasis to the liver. Anemia, loss of weight, and hematuria occur late in the course of the disease, after cancer has invaded the bladder or urethra. For this reason, a CBC should be obtained. It is not uncommon for the elderly client to remain in bed with weakness and bone pain, become progressively immobile, anorexic, cachectic, and finally succumb to an intercurrent episode of bronchopneumonia.

Other signs of prostatic cancer include an enlarged nodular liver and pathological bone fractures from metastases. Chest x-rays might show evidence of metastases to the hilar nodes,

TABLE 7–4. STAGES OF ADENOCARCINOMA OF THE PROSTATE

Stage	Description
I	The tumor is found incidentally in prostatic tissue that has been removed because of BPH. The rectal examination is normal
II	A localized nodule is confined within the prostate gland. The serum acid phosphatase level is normal. Treatment is radical prostatectomy
III	The cancer extends beyond the confines of the prostatic capsule. The serum acid phosphatase might be elevated. Surgical cure is unlikely
IV	The cancer has metastasized to distant locations

lungs, or ribs. X-ray films of the abdomen might reveal osteoblastic metastases from the prostatic tumor. Excretory urograms might reveal hydronephrosis from bladder neck or ureteral obstruction. Scanning techniques are very sensitive means of demonstrating metastases, and the serum alkaline phosphatase will be elevated if there is metastasis to bone. Cystoscopy will usually show only nonspecific changes due to obstruction.

The diagnosis of prostatic carcinoma is based on rectal examination and acid phosphatase studies; cancer is confirmed by prostatic biopsy. Only in very late stages will invasion of the bladder be seen, in which case biopsy will be necessary for diagnosis. Bone marrow aspirated from the iliac crest might show evidence of malignant spread and is often more important diagnostically.

Tumor invasion of the prostatic capsule might not influence the prognosis significantly; tumor spread beyond the capsule is associated with a considerably higher death rate, however. Staging of the prostatic tumor as well as overall general health of the patient will also affect the prognosis. The 5-year survival rate is 70% when the tumor is localized. If the tumor has metastasized, the survival rate is less than 35%.

Medical and Surgical Management

The therapeutic management of adenocarcinoma of the prostate is determined by the stage of the disease, the age of the client, and the nature of the symptoms. If palpation reveals an indurated nodule in the prostate of a healthy man of less than 70 years of age, and if there is no evidence of metastasis to the bone, a radical prostatectomy is usually considered.

Radiation therapy might be employed preoperatively or postoperatively, depending upon the stage of the disease. Radiation is used preoperatively to reduce the size of the tumor or cure the cancer. Radiation also may be used as a palliative measure in metastatic disease, but radiation of the pelvic lymph nodes has not been shown to increase survival statistics significantly. Potency will be maintained in approximately 60% of the clients who were potent before radiation therapy was begun.

The prostatectomy may be accomplished by the perineal or retropubic routes. In a *radical prostatectomy* the entire prostate (including its capsule, the seminal vesicles, and a portion of the bladder neck) is removed. The *retropubic* approach enables the discovery of lymph node metastases and the dissection of affected lymph nodes. Urinary control is possible, postoperatively, but impotence can be expected. In the *perineal* approach to prostatectomy, often used in cancer of the prostate, an incision is made through the perineum. The procedure often results in impotence and rectal injury, but all the prostatic tissue can be removed, as well as pelvic nodes, if required.

In advanced prostatic cancer, particularly when it has metastasized to bone, three out of four clients will have markedly increased amounts of serum acid phosphatase. The administration of androgens usually increases the rate of growth of prostatic tumors and increases serum acid phosphatase levels. *Antiandrogen therapy,* which includes estrogen medication (Diethylstilbestrol), orchiectomy, medical adrenalectomy, and hypophysectomy, should be withheld until the client develops signs of metastases. Approximately 85% of prostatic cancers are androgen dependent; antiandrogen therapy can afford the client considerable comfort by decreasing the size of the tumor, lessening the degree of urinary obstruction, and decreasing bone pain. Usually, the client will gain weight and strength, and the anemia will tend to correct itself.

Estrogen therapy and orchiectomy slow the growth of these tumors and maintain normal levels of acid phosphatase in the blood. Determination of the serum acid phosphatase level is therefore an index of the extent of the tumor; it also indicates the degree of success that can be expected with antiandrogen therapy. After antiandrogen therapy, retrogressive changes can be marked; the gland becomes smaller and assumes a more normal consistency. Side effects of estrogen therapy include impotence and loss of sexual desire, tender gynecomastia, and edema of the ankles. The edema can be controlled by decreasing salt intake; the gynecomastia can be reduced by directing x-ray therapy to the areolae before estrogen therapy is begun. Clients receiving estrogen therapy should be watched closely for thromboembolic phenomena.

Orchiectomy (surgical removal of one or both testes) is similar in effect to the administration of estrogens in that bone pain is relieved. Cortisone may be given to perform a medical adrenalectomy and is normally used when the effectiveness of estrogen therapy begins to wane. Hypophysectomy is seldom used, and that only when all other methods of therapy have been exhausted. Chemotherapeutic agents such as fluorouracil and cyclophosphamide may be used when other palliative treatments begin to fail.

Follow-up care should include periodic rectal examination to detect local recurrence. Serum acid phosphatase levels should be determined, and chest x-rays, as well as x-ray films of the bones and lumbar spine, should be taken to search for metastatic deposits.

Nursing Care Management

The nurse should identify any physical or psychological problems that the client might have concerning the diagnosis and treatment of his disorder. In general, questions should be anticipated regarding the possibility of pain, type(s) of procedures to be performed, length of time involved, and expected outcomes. The client who has been diagnosed as having cancer will have many fears, worries, and uncertainties concerning his future. In providing the required emotional support, the gerontological nurse practitioner and client should explore the client's feelings regarding his future.

The prostatic cancer client will often be apprehensive concerning the use of radiation; he should be given a thorough explanation of the plan of therapy and the number of treatments he will receive. The use of skin markings should be explained, and the client should be advised not to use soap or ointments, to avoid removing the skin markings. The nurse should observe the client closely for skin erythema, rectal bleeding, fistula formation, diarrhea, cystitis, nausea and vomiting, dry skin, and alopecia. Plans to be worked through with the family and client include providing for adequate nutrition, hydration, and rest periods, and emphasizing the necessity for follow-up care and complete blood counts.

Occasionally, interstitial radiation therapy with implants (seeds) of radiation will be used. As many as 50 seeds may be introduced into the prostate gland at one time. The implants control tumor growth while causing only mild urinary, rectal, or sexual disturbances. The nurse practitioner should observe the client closely for hematuria, infection, and loss of the seeds postoperatively. If the seeds should become dislodged, they should be handled only with a Kelly clamp and be placed in a lead container.

Preoperative teaching should include instruction about postoperative procedures and the placement of tubes and dressings. Every aspect of care should be discussed, including anesthesia, medications, bowel preparations, food and fluid restrictions, recovery room care, catheterization, drainage tubes, waiting-room facilities for family members, and an approximate timeline for the procedures. Subsequent sexual functioning might also be discussed, but it is the physician's responsibility to inform the client of the expected outcomes of the surgical procedure. If a portion of the client's urethra is to be removed and the remainder of the urethra is to be anastamosed to the bladder neck, he should be made aware that he will be impotent and sterile and that there is the possibility of urinary incontinence postoperatively.

If the perineal approach to prostatectomy is taken, the client is given a bowel prep to prevent fecal contamination of the operative site. Cathartics, enemas, and neomycin are given 1 or 2 days before surgery. Only clear fluids are given on the day before surgery, and they will be continued well into the postoperative period, until the wound is healing well. The use of rectal thermometers or insertion of any type of rectal tube, postoperatively, should be avoided. Some physicians will order frequent sitz baths, to decrease the postoperative pain and inflammation. Perineal pads should be provided, to absorb urinary drainage, and they should be changed frequently, to keep the skin as dry as possible.

Following surgery, the client will have an indwelling urethral catheter in place. If he has had a suprapubic prostatectomy, a suprapubic tube will have been inserted through the abdominal wall into the bladder, and a Penrose drain will have been inserted through the incision. Following a perineal prostatectomy, the client will also have a drain inserted into the perineum. The skin surrounding the drain must be kept clean and dry; sterile dressings or ostomy bags may be placed over the drain.

Catheter care must be meticulous. Normally a three-way catheter that is continually irrigated with normal saline is used. The solution should flow continuously at a constant rate. The urethral catheter output should be monitored closely for clots or mucous plugs, which could block the catheter. In calculating the client's output, remember to subtract the volume of irrigant from the measured output. To detect urinary retention, palpate the client's bladder, and question him about a sensation of fullness. The urine will have a pink or red color for a few days, but then it should clear. Only a piston-type syringe should be used for catheter irrigation, which should be performed gently, using the prescribed type of solution. The catheter is usually removed within 2–3 weeks. Urethral catheters can cause bladder spasms, which may require treatment with anticholinergic drugs. While the catheter is in place, the client should be encouraged to drink large amounts of fluids. Early ambulation should also be urged, to avoid complications of immobilization.

The client receiving hormonal therapy should be observed for nausea and vomiting, gynecomastia, fluid retention, and thrombophlebitis. If the client is receiving chemotherapy, he can expect a loss of appetite, alopecia, and diarrhea.

The psychological implications of urinary incontinence, alopecia, sexual dysfunction, and the femininizing effects of drug therapies are often significant and frequently lead to depression and social withdrawal. The nurses can help the client resolve some of these problems by suggesting that the client wear a wig, and by teaching the client such sphincter-control exercises as squeezing his buttocks together for a few seconds and then relaxing. These exercises should be practiced approximately ten times per hour, to overcome incontinence.

AGING OF THE SEXUAL RESPONSE

Despite widespread beliefs to the contrary, there are no intrinsic biological limitations to the aging man's or woman's sexual capacity. Although elderly persons are often considered asexual, an interest in sex and sexual activity can and often does extend well into late life. Naturally, both men and women experience significant physiological changes as a result of the normal aging process, but if sexual partners are in reasonably good health, interested in sex, and sexually interesting, they can continue sexual activity indefinitely. The gerontological nurse practitioner can be of greater assistance to older clients if the nurse understands human sexuality, recognizes the physiological and psychological factors associated with aging, and intervenes in ways that are consistent with the individual client's concept of sexuality.

Physiological Factors

Physiological and psychological factors together determine and control a person's sexual identity and capacity for sexual activity throughout his or her lifetime. Unquestionably, sexual processes are as much a part of normal life as breathing, eating, and other natural physiological functions. Just as a person's respiratory, digestive, and other bodily mechanisms are affected by aging, however, a person's sexual mechanisms also undergo physiological changes as he or she grows older. These age-related changes can best be described, perhaps, in relation to what is known as the sexual response cycle.

Sexual Response Cycle

The act of sex (sexual intercourse) is a complex one, involving the mind and emotions as well as the body. Physiologically, the sex act involves the nervous system and hormonal activity as well as the genital organs. It is characterized by four phases: *excitement* (erotic-arousal), *intromission* (plateau), *orgasm* (climax), and *resolution* (recovery). Together, these four phases constitute the *sexual response cycle*. In different ways and to different degrees (and at different times, perhaps), male and female sexual partners both experience these four distinct phases. Physiologically, the human sexual response, in both sexes, is due primarily to *vasocongestion* (overfilled blood vessels) and *myotonia* (continued muscle contractions).

Sex hormones also play an active role in human responsiveness. Sex hormones, which are chemically steroids, are produced in the adrenal glands of both men and women—in the ovaries of females and in the testes of men. *Estrogen,* one of the most active female hormones, has a profound effect on the generative organs and breasts of women; the functions of *androgen,* the primary male hormone, are less well understood (Butler and Lewis, 1976).

Excitement. A person can become sexually aroused through thoughts and feelings as well as by the senses of sight, smell, and touch. As soon as a woman is aroused sexually (within seconds, usually) a mucoid-like substance appears on the surface of the vaginal mucosa (by transudation),

to lubricate the vagina for intercourse. Congestion of pelvic blood vessels causes several changes in the external genitalia; the clitoris becomes enlarged, and the labia minora flatten, separate from the vaginal orifice, and extend outward, effectively lengthening the vagina. At the same time, the uterus is raised, and the vaginal barrel increases in both length and diameter.

The woman's breasts also are affected in sexual excitement. The areolae become engorged with blood, erectile tissue in the nipples enlarges and extends them, and the network of veins in the breasts become accentuated. In some women, arousal is also heralded by a red "sex flush" across the chest, resembling a maculopapular rash.

Erotic arousal of the man is indicated primarily by the erection of the penis. The testes are drawn upward, closer to the perineum, as the scrotal sac contracts, and the man's nipples might become erect. An increased pulse rate and elevated blood pressure also accompany sexual arousal of the man.

Intromission. The intromission (plateau) phase of intercourse is marked by insertion of the penis into the vagina and by vigorous thrusts and pelvic gyrations. The highly vascular tissue comprising the external orifice of the vagina and the labia minora become increasingly congested and deeper in color. The Bartholin's glands secrete a small amount of a mucoid-like substance to lubricate the vestibule.

Although the clitoris is retracted upward, beneath the clitoral hood, traction on the labia as the penis is alternately thrust inward and withdrawn continues to stimulate the clitoris, indirectly. The uterus remains elevated, the areolae of the woman's breasts can become so engorged that the erect nipples become masked, and the sex flush can continue to spread from the chest to the neck, face, and even to the arms.

In the plateau phase, the man's penis continues to increase in diameter—particularly at the coronal ridge (the rim of the glans). The attendant increase in size of the elevated testes can be as much as 50% more than when unexcited. The Cowper's glands, too, secrete a mucoid-like substance to facilitate intromission.

Both partners experience hyperventilation and increased pulse rates (as high as 100–175 beats per minute). In women, blood pressures can be raised by 20–60 mm Hg systolic and by 10–20 mm Hg diastolic. Men similarly can experience blood pressure elevations of 20–80 mm Hg systolic, and 10–40 mm Hg diastolic.

Orgasm. The sex act culminates in orgasm, a climactic release of sexual tension accompanied by a feeling of intense pleasure. In the woman, orgasm (climax) is characterized by rapid contractions of the orgasmic platform (the extremely vascular tissue in the vicinity of the vaginal orifice), the rectal sphincter, and the uterus. Uterine contractions resemble those experienced in labor.

In the male, orgasm is characterized by contractions along the entire length of the urethra that result in *ejaculation* (sudden expulsion) of semen from the penis, in spurts. Contraction of the internal bladder sphincter prevents ejaculation of semen backward into the bladder. Men also experience rapid contractions of the rectal sphincter during orgasm.

Resolution. In recovery, following orgasm, vasocongestion diminishes rapidly from the orgasmic platform, and the clitoris returns to its normal position. More slowly, erection of the nipples recedes and vasocongestion of the breasts and labia subsides. The uterus descends to its usual position, and respiratory and cardiovascular rates return to normal.

The man loses his erection soon after ejaculation, although a complete return of the penis to its unexcited size takes place gradually, as vasocongestion subsides. The scrotal sac relaxes, and the testes descend to their usual location. Unlike the woman, who can respond sexually again, without delay, the man must undergo a refractory period before another sexual response cycle can be begun.

Female Physiological Changes That Accompany Aging

Older women experience little deterioration in their physical capacity for sexual activity as they age. More is known about the sexual changes affecting aging women than those of aging men because more is understood about the role of female hormones in sexuality than about the role of male hormones. Most sexual changes in females are directly related to decreased levels of estrogen following menopause rather than to "aging" itself.

Menopause. Defined as the cessation of menstruation, *menopause* (or *change of life,* as it is often called) marks the normal end of the transition from the reproductive to the nonreproductive stage of a woman's life. Usually starting between the ages of 45 and 50, the physiological process can continue for several years. Changes usually associated with menopause include decreased plasma levels of estrogen and progesterone (estrogen levels might fluctuate from normal to near zero), atrophy of the target organs of these sex hormones, increased plasma levels of follicle-stimulating hormone (FSH) and luteinizing hormone (LH), decreased numbers of primordial follicles in the ovaries, and reduced responsiveness of the follicles to gonadotropins.

Popular misconceptions concerning the effects of menopause include insanity, loss of physical (sexual) attractiveness (e.g., development of masculine characteristics), depression, and loss of sexual desire. In fact, however, only about 60% of women experience any physical or emotional symptoms in menopause, and most of these women have only minimal to moderate physical problems. Although it is a key sign of change in the basic hormonal mechanisms that mediate reproduction, cessation of menstruation does not ordinarily represent a clinical problem.

Common clinical symptoms of menopause

often can be attributed to variations in blood-vessel diameter caused by instabilities of the vasomotor system. The resulting changes that such fluctuations permit in blood-flow rates can cause hot flashes, headaches, neckaches, and profuse sweating. Other common symptoms include excessive fatigue and feelings of emotional instability. None of these symptoms are inevitable, however, and when they occur they usually can be greatly alleviated (if not entirely relieved) by hormone replacement. Life stresses can also precipitate or exacerbate menopausal symptoms, and psychological counseling in conjunction with estrogen therapy can be helpful under these circumstances. Even when left untreated, however, menopausal symptoms usually subside spontaneously.

Female changes in excitement. Following menopause, many women show signs of estrogen deficiency that can affect their sexual functioning. Lubrication of the vagina in preparation for intercourse is less spontaneous, and both the rate and volume of lubricating fluid are usually reduced. This may be due both to the loss of estrogen required for the production of secretions and to changes in the structure of the vaginal wall, through which the secretions ooze.

The reduced elasticity of vaginal tissue results in a reduced involuntary capability to increase the length and diameter of the vagina in response to sexual stimulation, although the vagina usually remains adequately large for intercourse. Oral estrogen replacement is the usual remedy. In extreme cases (if intercourse cannot be supported), dilation of the vagina might be attempted by the physician.

As some women age, they experience a marked decrease in general well-being and a resultant decrease in sexual interest that might be related to estrogen deprivation. Estrogen replacement can be helpful, although the hormone will not directly stimulate sexual arousal in women. Male hormones can facilitate sexual arousal, but they are not useful in treating wom-

en because of their potential for masculinizing effects (Butler & Lewis, 1976).

In general, aging sexual partners should try to spend more time in precoital stimulation, to offset the lengthened delays and reduced sexual responsiveness that accompany aging. Artificial lubricants can be used to offset the paucity of vaginal secretions, but such moisturizers should be nonallergenic, and they should have little, if any, lanolin content (Masters & Johnson, 1981).

Female changes in intromission. Without adequate lubrication, intercourse can feel scratchy, rough, or even painful. Thinning and atrophy of the vaginal wall can result in discomfort, *dyspareunia* (pain), or trauma. Sudden penile penetration and prolonged, vigorous coital thrusting should be avoided, as the aged vagina cannot as easily tolerate the thrusting penis, and cracking and bleeding, both during and after intercourse, can result.

The clitoris might become slightly smaller, late in a woman's life. The labia generally become less firm; the labia minora tend not to darken; and the covering of the clitoris and the fat pads in the pubic area usually lose fatty tissue, leaving the clitoris less well protected and more susceptible to irritation. Such changes with aging notwithstanding, the clitoris retains its responsiveness to sexual stimuli and continues to function without appreciable degradation as the focus of sexual sensation.

Female changes in orgasm. Women in good health who have experienced orgasms earlier in life can expect to continue to have orgasms, even well into their eighties. Although the onset of the orgasmic experience might be somewhat slowed, the duration shortened, and the intensity reduced, subjectively appreciated levels of sensual pleasure can continue to be derived.

Female changes in resolution. Following orgasm, vasocongestive effects recede rapidly. In postclimacteric women, the recovery phase might be shortened considerably.

Female Sexual Problems

Uterine spasms. Painful spastic contractions of the uterine muscles that do not release in the normal manner are sometimes (although infrequently) experienced during orgasm. If such spasms are experienced with any regularity, the apprehension of pain might understandably dissuade the older woman from sexual activity, at least to the point of orgasm. Relief from uterine spasms can usually be obtained with minimal levels of estrogen replacement (Masters & Johnson, 1981).

Vaginismus. Physiological alterations that produce dyspareunia often lead to the development of vaginismus, an involuntary constriction of the outer portion of the vaginal barrel, to guard against painful intercourse. Perhaps the most frequently missed diagnosis in the field of gynecology, vaginismus should be suspected when the aging female client has a history of painful coitus or prolonged continence from sexual intercourse. Vaginismus, when recognized, can usually be corrected by exercise to retrain the affected muscles (Masters & Johnson, 1981).

Vaginitis. The loss of estrogen that accompanies aging often causes the vaginal secretions to become less acidic, which can increase the possibility of vaginal infections and cause burning, itching, and discharge. This condition, referred to as atrophic ("senile") vaginitis, can lead to cystitis if allowed to progress untreated. Clients who suffer from atrophic vaginitis should have a complete examination (including a Pap test) to rule out the possibility of a tumor in the reproductive tract. Allergies and trichomonal and fungal infections (especially in diabetics) are other causes of itching; a prolapsed uterus can also produce a discharge. Clients should be instructed not to douche before the vaginal examination to avoid confusing the diagnosis.

Cystitis. As a result of aging, the walls of the vagina become thinner, the bladder and urethra consequently become less well protected, and these organs can become irritated during intercourse. Older women can develop what is sometimes called honeymoon cystitis, an inflammation of the bladder that results from the bruising and jostling of intercourse. Other than treatment of the bacterial infection, little can be done. When bacterial infection accompanies cystitis, the client can suffer an unrelenting, irresistible urge to urinate, accompanied by a burning sensation that must be treated medically. If left untreated, the client can experience an increasingly painful burning sensation during urination, frequent waking at night to urinate, and blood in the urine, occasionally.

Male Physiological Changes That Accompany Aging

Males are also subject to physiological changes as they age. From the mid 50s on, the aging man experiences a reduced intensity of sexual responsivity and changes in his sexual function that, even when not impaired, can have a significant impact on his female partner's experience of sex.

Male changes in excitement. It usually takes longer for the older man to obtain an erection, and full penile engorgement might not be achieved in every case. In the absence of more spontaneous response to sexual excitement, direct tactile stimulation involving participation of his partner might be required to achieve an erection. Elevation of the testicles, vasocongestion of the scrotal sac, and engorgement of the testes are diminished, if not absent altogether.

Male changes in intromission. Secretion of fluid to facilitate insertion of the penis is also reduced or absent. To the advantage of both partners, however, the older man often will be able to maintain ejaculatory control for a longer period of time, extending their enjoyment.

Male changes in orgasm. Ejaculation, when it comes, results in the expulsion of a smaller volume of seminal fluid, with less expulsive force than when younger. Although the older man usually maintains his interest in and continues to enjoy the sensual pleasure of intercourse, the previously automatic demand for ejaculation also might be reduced or absent. A man of 60 might be satisfied to ejaculate only once in every two or three occasions (Ludeman, 1981).

Male changes in resolution. Following orgasm, the penis rapidly returns to its normal flaccid state, as the period of detumescence becomes increasingly shorter. At least several hours are usually required before another erection can be achieved, as the refractory period becomes increasingly prolonged.

Psychological Factors

In addition to the previously described physiological changes, the psychological factors that accompany aging can have significant effects on the older person's sexuality. Men and women are affected differently, of course, but problems that affect one partner usually have at least an indirect effect on the other. Recognizing the important role that psychological factors play in determining a person's interest in sex and capacity for sexual activity, it is important to consider the types of events and circumstances that have significant potential for affecting people psychologically.

Female Psychological Factors

Physically, the woman's sexual ability might not be affected significantly by the normal physiological changes that accompany aging. Psychologically, however, the aging woman can be influenced greatly by several different factors. Her sexual attitudes will have been shaped primarily by experiences of childhood and early adulthood. Later, menopause will have added another dimension, and often the older woman will be faced with having to live the remainder of her life without a sexual partner.

Inhibitions. Older women grew up in times in which social conditions and societal attitudes were vastly different from those prevalent today.

Sexual matters were not discussed openly. Questions concerning sexual matters were not encouraged, and answers (when given) were not always correct. Typically, sex was considered a "wifely duty," to be tolerated but not enjoyed. Young women who enjoyed sex or sought it were considered "loose"; "nice" girls were not interested in sex, or they considered it distasteful.

In addition to the inhibitions that were ingrained by societal attitudes, parental pressures, and strict religious teachings, other factors might have hampered the free exercise of sexual activity. As most (if not all) of these women's premenopausal years were spent before the availability of reliable birth-control measures, the spontaneous enjoyment of sex was often thwarted by the fear of becoming pregnant. Promiscuous sexual activity also might have been inhibited somewhat more than at present by the (justified) fear of venereal diseases, for which effective treatments had not yet been found (Butler & Lewis, 1976).

Menopause. As previously discussed, the physiological changes associated with menopause sometimes are accompanied by emotional symptoms. Because menopause marks the end of a woman's childbearing years, it might be expected that in some cases the menopausal woman suffers a blow to her sexuality. She may consider herself less attractive, if not worthless—particularly in cultures in which the woman's primary role is to bear children. There is a positive side to menopause, however. Freedom from the fear of pregnancy and the lessening of earlier sexual inhibitions often lead postclimacteric women to a more relaxed enjoyment of sex and more satisfying sexual experiences.

Single life. Some of the most common and yet most significant emotional problems concerning the sexuality of aging women arise from the fact (or possibility) of being left alone, i.e., of being widowed, divorced, or separated. Because women tend to marry men who are older than they are (by 3 years, on average), and because women live longer than men (by 7 years, on average), the odds are that a wife will outlive her husband. With increasing age, older women increasingly outnumber men in their age groups, and societal attitudes are such that women have not yet obtained the degree of freedom that men enjoy to socialize with and/or marry younger members of the opposite sex (Butler & Lewis, 1976).

Male Psychological Factors

The principal emotional problem facing the older man is the fear of impotence. Although the cause of impotence can be organic, i.e., the consequence of a neurological, vascular, medicinal, hormonal, toxic, surgical, or traumatic problem, impotence is much more likely to be a psychological problem. In fact, the fear of impotence can itself cause impotence.

Described as the "barometer of man's feeling" (Butler & Lewis, 1976), the man's penis rapidly reflects the man's current state of mind. The nerves that control erection are extremely sensitive to emotions; anxiety, anger, and fear can result in a man losing an erection or failing to achieve one in the first place. Worse yet, the harder he tries to have an erection, the less likely he is to succeed.

Occasionally, at any age and for any one of several reasons, a man can experience episodes of impotence. If not of organic origin, the impotence might be attributable to fatigue (emotional as well as physical), depression, worry, illness, or excessive eating/drinking. In later life, problems with achieving and maintaining an erection can become chronic. The man who does not anticipate, or at least understand, the previously described physiological changes in his sexual performance (slowed arousal, decreased expulsive pressure, reduced volume of seminal fluid, and diminished ejaculatory demand) is likely to develop fears concerning his sexual capacity when such changes are first experienced. Furthermore, the man (regardless of age) who has on even one occasion seriously questioned

the effectiveness of his sexual performance is significantly at risk of moving into episodic (if not complete) impotence in the near future (Masters & Johnson, 1981).

To make matters worse, the man's sexual partner can both affect and be affected by his impotence. The wife who is unresponsive or disinterested or who merely acquiesces, perfunctorily, can be regarded as threatening, which can lead to impotence. The impatient or demanding partner will exacerbate the condition and can make a temporary impotence permanent. At the same time, the uninformed and unsuspecting wife is at risk of potentially serious psychological problems herself if, for example, she interprets her husband's impotence as a lack of interest in her or, worse yet, as an indication that he has transferred his sexual interests to another woman.

Attitudes toward the Sexuality of Older Persons

As previously discussed, men and women experience significant physiological changes in the aging process. Nevertheless, there is no evidence that these physiological changes by themselves limit the ability of the elderly to function sexually (Ludeman, 1981). There are, however, numerous misconceptions concerning the sexuality of older persons, with deeply established societal attitudes holding that the involvement of older persons in sexual activity is socially unacceptable, if not detrimental to their health. Masters and Johnson (1981) have attributed the increased withdrawal of many elderly persons from active expression of their sexuality to culturally enforced ignorance of geriatric sexuality—the widely accepted myth of "the asexual older person."

Ludeman (1981) cited earlier studies by Cameron and by La Torre and Kear that appeared to lend support to the asexual older person myth. Cameron (1970) had found that older people considered themselves (and similarly were considered by others) to fall below the general norm in several aspects of sexuality. These areas include desire for sex, skill in sexual performance, capacity for sex, frequency of sexual activity, frequency of attempts at sexual activity, and social opportunities to engage in sexual activity. La Torre and Kear (1971) had found that people generally considered coitus between aged partners less credible than masturbation, consistent with the earlier "disengagement theory" of Cumming and Henry (1961), which held it to be both normal and desirable that persons withdraw from societal activities in old age. Ludeman (1981), however, questioned the implication that sexual activity among the aged is considered unlikely or distasteful to young persons as well as old, including persons who work with the elderly. Instead, the possibility was raised that the respondents might have tended to answer in "socially acceptable" ways, i.e., in ways that were consistent with cultural myths supported and sanctioned by society rather than in accordance with personal beliefs.

Although sexual interest and activity are commonly supposed to decline over the course of middle and late adulthood, they typically persist well into late life. The pioneering research of Kinsey, Pomeroy, Martin, and Gebhard (1953) indicated that all measures of sexual activity decline with increasing age, for both men and women, although women typically reported lower levels of sexual activity than men (at any age), depending on the availability and preferences of a socially acceptable, functionally capable partner. Subsequent studies by other researchers generally supported these findings; however, a 6-year study of married couples conducted by George and Weiler (1981) indicated that sexual-activity patterns actually tend to remain more stable over middle and late life than had been suggested by previous studies. The observed stability of sexual activity across the study sample and the higher levels of sexual activity reported by younger age-cohort groups suggest that future groups of older persons might present different sexual-activity patterns than those of older persons today. The implication is

that, generally speaking, our current "understanding" of the sexuality of any age group might well be quite specific to the group of persons that are currently of that age.

Ludeman (1981) found that sexual interest and activity persist into old age, although the gap between continued interest and continued sexual activity widened with increasing age, even as the intensity (as opposed to the incidence) of interest in sex diminished. Strong sexual interest in persons over 70 was found to be exceptional. In persons over 75, a strong interest in sex was virtually nonexistent.

In the older woman, continued sexual activity depends primarily on her past enjoyment of sex and the present availability of a socially acceptable, capable, and willing partner. The woman's age is not considered to be a significant factor, per se, and the degree of pleasure derived from sex tends to remain essentially constant over the years. Among women, continued sexual activity and intact marriages are positively correlated. The older woman's interest in sex is based primarily on the satisfaction she experiences in the male/female relationship or in touching, as an expression of her sexuality. Sexual fantasies are commonly experienced by the older woman who is still interested in sex, and her sexuality might be channeled into nonsexual touching relationships with friends, children, or pets. Studies have indicated that masturbation is more frequent in women over 60 than in men of that age group, more prevalent among postmarital women than among married women, and less frequent than coitus in married women (Ludeman, 1981).

Increasingly, bisexual and/or homosexual relationships have been suggested as alternative forms of sexual expression for older unmarried women, because of the relative lack of available older men for heterosexual relationships. Generally speaking, today's older women have not accepted such nontraditional forms of sexual behavior, however, as their attitudes are typically more conservative than those of today's younger women. Although the current feminist and libertarian movements do provide women with opportunities (if not the stimuli) for homosexual behavior and/or bisexual identities, Ludeman (1981) found that even the older woman who is not involved in a sexual relationship overwhelmingly prefers not having sex at all to engaging in sex with another woman. As Ludeman points out, since it makes no sense to encourage behaviors that are inconsistent with a person's own system of beliefs, the growing advocacy for homosexuality among older women should be carefully examined for its relevancy to those persons it is intended to benefit.

In their study, George and Weiler (1981) found, as other researchers consistently have found, that men tend to report higher levels of sexual activity than women of the same age (since men in our culture typically are older than their wives). Cessation of sexual activity was attributed (by both men and women) mainly to the sexual attitudes or physical impairment of the male partner, as typically he is the one who initiates sexual activity in couples who are currently middle aged or older. In her research on sex and the elderly, Ludeman (1981) found that, in men, interest in sex and sexual activity is positively correlated with past sexual experiences, maleness, income, social class, health, and satisfaction with life, but that sexual activity declines with increasing age.

A Good Age (Comfort, 1976a), *The Joy of Sex* (Comfort, 1974), *Love, Sex and Aging* (Brecher, 1984), and *More Joy of Sex* (Comfort, 1976b) are reference sources that the gerontological nurse practitioner should read to assist in the understanding of sexuality of the aging client. The nurse practitioner should suggest these references to their clients who are experiencing difficulties in accepting the changes that occur during the aging process. These references will also help alleviate some of the concerns and taboos placed on sex during later years of life.

Sex and Health: A Practical Encyclopedia of Sexual Medicine (DeMoya & DeMoya, 1982) will provide the gerontological nurse practitioner with useful information regarding drugs

that are commonly prescribed for the older adult that are known to affect sexuality. The nurse practitioner must be aware of these drugs when assessing the client who is experiencing problems with sexuality.

AGING OF THE URINARY TRACT

Urinary tract disorders, which are very common in the elderly, are major causes of serious and distressing symptoms. They often require drug therapy, but only after an accurate diagnosis has been established. The diagnosis must be based on a complete history, consideration of current drug treatment, examination of the abdomen and nervous system, microscopy, and culture of the urine.

Traditionally, the urinary tract is divided into the upper tract and the lower tract. The upper tract consists of the kidneys and ureters, whereas the lower tract consists of the bladder and urethra. Most age-related problems affect the lower urinary tract and cause urinary disorders. Common problems include urinary tract infection, urinary calculi, and obstruction. Many older clients are also incontinent or have neurogenic bladders, which might necessitate chronic catheterization.

Many problems can be identified by taking a careful history and performing a complete physical examination. When taking a history, five urinary symptoms should be carefully noted:

1. *Nocturia.* Is the client awakened at night to void? How many times?
2. *Diurnal frequency.* Normal diurnal frequency is two to four times a day; eight to ten times a day is abnormal.
3. *Decrease in size and force of the urinary stream.* The decrease is usually progressive over several years.
4. *Urgency.* The urge to urinate can vary from acute distress to incontinence.
5. *Hematuria.* Blood in the urine always re-

quires investigation by intravenous pyelography and cystoscopy.

Other symptoms, e.g., dribbling or hesitancy, should also be investigated.

During the physical examination, the abdomen is palpated to identify a distended bladder. A rectal examination is performed to estimate sphincter tone: a lax sphincter implies impaired vesical innervation. In males, the size, contour, and consistency of the prostate can also be determined by rectal examination. The second voided urine specimen should be used for microscopic examination of the sediment, routine chemical tests, and culture for bacteria and colony count. The client should not be catheterized unless absolutely necessary. Bladder capacity (normally 350–450 ml) can be determined by inserting a catheter, measuring the residual contents, and then filling the bladder by gravity. To fill the bladder, water or normal saline is poured into a large syringe (attached to the catheter) until the client perceives the need to urinate. After the client has voided, the fluid is collected and its volume measured. This test also establishes the presence or absence of a urethral stricture. If a stricture is found, the client should be referred to a urologist. If the client has obvious acute retention, however, the physician may perform a suprapubic aspiration by passing a 20-gauge spinal needle into the bladder through the skin of the lower abdomen.

Urinary Tract Infection

Urinary tract infection (UTI) is common in older clients; it occurs in both the lower and upper portions of the urinary tract. UTI in the lower tract is often asymptomatic in the elderly client—especially if the client has an underlying disease (e.g., diabetes mellitus), has anatomic or physiological abnormalities of the genitourinary tract, or has been catheterized. Reasons for UTI in elderly people also include fallen bladders in women and enlargement of the prostate gland in men. Urine flow might be reduced, as older people tend not to drink enough fluids, and urine acidity tends to fall in old age, thus favoring bacterial growth.

Assessment Parameters

Symptoms of UTI include urgency, frequency, nocturia and dysuria, urinary retention, and ill-defined pain referrable to the lower back, perineum, pelvis, groin, abdomen, or flank. A change in the older client's state of alertness might also indicate UTI. Inflammation of the bladder also can cause hematuria and fever. Symptoms of upper-tract UTI (*pyelonephritis*) include fever, chills, and flank pain. Renal colic would suggest kidney stones or papillary necrosis. Upper urinary tract infection is more likely to occur in men who have diabetes mellitus, structural abnormalities, foreign bodies, or renal transplants, or in women who have had symptoms of UTI for more than 6 days (Yoshikawa & Guze, 1982).

Most urinary tract infections are caused by *Escherichia coli, Klebsiella, Pseudomonas, Proteus,* or *Serratia.* A clean-catch urine specimen is usually adequate for diagnosis. For a female with symptoms of UTI, a finding of more than 100,000 bacteria per milliliter in a clean-catch midstream urine specimen has an 80% probability of representing true bacteriuria; a second specimen yielding similar results increases the probability to 90%. In symptomatic men and women, a single urine specimen with more than 100,000 bacteria per milliliter is diagnostic for UTI (Yoshikawa & Guze, 1982). If for some reason a clean-catch urine specimen cannot be obtained, catheterization is recommended. A single catheterized urine specimen that contains more than 100,000 bacteria per milliliter is 95% accurate in diagnosing infection.

Management

Methods used to avoid UTI include urinary acidification and treatment with methenamine mandelate (Mandelamine) and long-term urinary antimicrobial therapy. If the client requires a Foley catheter on a long-term basis, closed-drainage sterile techniques must be employed for insertion, and the catheter should be changed when incrustations or cystals are present or if the catheter is not patent (Ruge, 1987). For incontinent clients, condom catheters (for men) or diaper pads might help prevent urinary tract infections, but they can produce local irritation that leads to decubiti (Finkelstein, 1982).

Treatment of UTI is usually first directed toward relieving symptoms, correcting the cause of obstruction (e.g., enlarged prostate), giving acidifying agents such as mandelic acid, and encouraging fluids, by mouth. Many older people will have UTIs that are confined to the bladder, but bladder infections are often troublesome, especially if the infection spreads to the kidneys. Urinary tract infections are usually treated with a sulfonamide.

A neurogenic bladder is the most common and most troublesome urinary disorder affecting elderly men. The presenting symptoms are nocturia, increased diurnal frequency, and urgency. Urgency is the most distressing symptom, as the patient can become incontinent before he can reach the toilet. Often he may have to carry a urinal for emergency use. Upon examination, the sphincter tone and prostate will be normal and the urine uninfected. Residual urine will be nil, but the bladder capacity will be less than 150 ml (possibly as little as 50 ml), as determined by simple cystometry. The disorder is almost always present in clients who have Parkinson's disease and in those who have had strokes. Clients may respond to oxybutynin (5 mg) three times daily, but caution should be exercised if the client has mild BPH, as oxybutynin can cause acute urinary retention.

Incontinence

Incontinence is a major nursing problem, especially if the client is bedridden or requires assistance to walk. Protective clothing such as stay-dry pants or disposable absorbent diapers, e.g., chux, can be used. External condom-type urine-collecting devices may be used for men and are preferred over indwelling catheters. The indwelling catheter can stimulate bladder contractions, resulting in involuntary voiding around the catheter. To ensure cleanliness and prevent odor, cleanse the client with mild soap and water when changing the stay-dry pants. The client's clothing also should be washed and changed frequently.

In the female client with urinary incontinence, exposure of the vulvar zone to constant moisture can lead to subsequent skin maceration and infection. In general, treatment should be gentle and consist mainly of cleanliness, nutritional supplementation, and soothing local applications. Many conditions respond well to careful local hygiene with either starch baths or a cool, dry, bland starch powder.

Vaginal or Vulvar Pruritus

Vaginal or vulvar pruritus is usually caused by candidiasis. In the older client, it is often associated with diabetes or antibiotic therapy. Vaginal pruritus is often accompanied by a watery or even bloody discharge, and the client usually complains of irritation. Treatment may consist of nystatin vaginal tablets (twice daily for 2 weeks), miconazole nitrate 2% cream (at bedtime for 1 week), or clotrimazole 1% cream or tablet (at bedtime for 7 days). Nearly immediate relief of vulvar irritation usually can be obtained by applying 0.01% cortisone cream, topically, with or without the nystatin.

Bladder Cancer

The majority of clients diagnosed as having bladder cancer are older individuals, and older persons are more likely to be affected by bladder cancer than by any other type of cancer. The incidence of bladder cancer in people 75–79 years of age is 155 cases per 100,000 persons. The average age at diagnosis is 68 years, and men are three times more likely than women to be affected by bladder cancer (Trump, 1982). Numerous carcinogens have been implicated as causes of bladder cancer, including aromatic amines, which are used in the rubber, leather, and dye industries. Cigarette smokers are particularly at risk, being twice as likely to incur bladder cancer as nonsmokers. Controversy surrounds the role that artificial sweeteners such as saccharin and cyclomates play in the development of bladder cancer. Part of the difficulty is that bladder cancer might not develop for 30–35 years following the heavy use of artificial sweeteners, and these substances were not widely used until the 1960s. It might be near the end of the century before it is known whether or not artificial sweeteners post a hazard. It is not clear whether viruses play any role in producing bladder cancer. On the other hand, the association of bladder cancer with urinary tract infection, urinary retention, and urethral strictures is well recognized (Prout, Garnick, & Canellos, 1982).

Three of four bladder cancer clients complain of painless hematuria. Dysuria or frequency is the next most common complaint (25% of clients). This triad of symptoms often suggests UTI; therefore, the client should be evaluated carefully, so as not to overlook an early bladder cancer (Trump, 1982). Hydronephrosis and subsequently pyelonephritis can occur if the tumor obstructs the ureteral orifice (Prout et al., 1982).

Most bladder tumors can be characterized as *noninvasive cancers* (bladder wall tumors) or *invasive cancers* (tumors that invade the muscle wall). Tumors seldom invade the surrounding pelvic organs or metastasize systemically. *Transitional cell carcinomas* (TCCs) comprise 90–95% of primary bladder tumors and primarily affect the elderly. TCC of the bladder is characterized by repeated occurrences at multiple distinct foci in the bladder, ureters, renal pelvis, and/or prostatic ducts. One client in four who initially presents with bladder cancer will have multiple separate tumors of the bladder. At least 30% of the clients who have a single cancerous tumor in the bladder will develop a new or recurrent tumor within 5 years of the original diagnosis. This feature of bladder cancer mandates vigorous follow-up of clients who have had bladder tumors, in order to detect and treat recurrences at the earliest possible time (Trump, 1982).

Immunology

Clients with bladder cancer have delayed hypersensitivity reactions to skin tests, and they become increasingly impaired in immunologic reactivity as the tumor size increases. It is for this reason that some physicians inject the thighs of the bladder-cancer client with BCG and then instill BCG (120 mg in 50 ml of normal saline) into the bladder (Prout et al., 1982). Removal of the tumor is accompanied by a return to the normal immunologic reactive state. From a prognostic standpoint, clients who do not regain reactivity are at greater risk for developing distant metastases (Morales, Edinger, and Bruce, 1976).

Assessment Parameters

In bladder cancer, the physical examination is generally negative, but in advanced disease a suprapubic mass might be felt. A rectal examination might reveal evidence of prostatic invasion or a palpable mass. A biopsy of the prostatic gland should always be considered. The diagnosis is nearly always confirmed by cystoscopy and biopsy of visualized lesions. It should be remembered, however, that it is difficult to visualize lesions with the naked eye; therefore, irritated or inflamed areas should also be examined for cancer. An IVP may be performed to identify a renal mass, stones, uretheral obstruction, or lesions of the collecting system or ureters.

The client's urine is examined for bacteria, to rule out inflammation masquerading as bladder cancer, and cytological studies are performed, to detect cancerous cells. At the present time, CT scans are not routinely indicated (Trump, 1982). Confirmation of metastasis requires positive bone and liver scans, lung tomograms, and evidence of elevated alkaline phosphatase levels.

Medical and Surgical Management

Low-grade noninvasive lesions can be managed by resection (via a cystoscope) and intravesical chemotherapy with thiotepa. The typical therapeutic dose is 60 mg, instilled in the bladder for approximately 1 hour at the time of surgery and then repeated at 1-month intervals for up to 1 year. Other agents that have been used include bleomycin, doxorubicin, and epodyl.

Lesions at or near the dome may be treated by *segmental resection* of the bladder, in which case a cuff of normal bladder is removed along with the lesion. The results of treatment depend upon selection and the degree of invasion; the larger the tumor and the deeper the invasion, the poorer the chance of survival. When the lesion has invaded the muscle, a cystectomy (with or without pelvic lymphectomy) is the procedure of choice.

The client who has a high-grade tumor that has infiltrated the bladder wall is a candidate for *cystectomy* (surgical removal of the bladder), if the client has a chance of survival. In females, the uterus and adnexa are also removed. In males, the surgeon also removes the seminal vesicles and prostate, which results in sexual impotence.

Removal of the bladder necessitates permanent urinary diversion. In the ileal conduit (Bricker's) procedure, the ureters are dissected from the bladder and transplanted into a 6–8-inch segment of the ileum that has been resected from the intestinal tract with its blood supply intact. The remaining intestinal tract is then anastomosed, and preoperative gastrointestinal function returns after it has healed. One end of the excised ileal loop is closed, to form a pouch, and the other end is brought out through the abdominal wall, to form a stoma. *Ureterosigmoidostomy,* a less preferred procedure, involves anastomosis of the ureters to the sigmoid colon, to direct the flow of urine into the colon.

Preoperative radiotherapy is important in reducing mortality and may be given safely if the volume and dose are modest (4000 to 5000 rads in 4 or 5 weeks). It is very important that the client understands the need for follow-up care, as 10% of low-risk malignancies ultimately will become life threatening. The 5-year survival rate following cystectomy is about 20%, but preoperative radiation can double it. The elderly client who is debilitated or who has severe cardiovascular disease is a poor surgical risk, however, and may be treated with radiation alone, which also provides a 5-year survival rate of 20%.

Nursing Care Management

If a partial cystectomy or segmental resection has been performed, the client should be reassured that a moderate bladder capacity (200–400 ml) will return, but it might take several months. For bladder training, postoperatively, the nurse practitioner should instruct the client to drink 2 liters of fluids daily, in large quantities (6–8 ounces at a time), but not for several hours before going out or retiring for the night.

The client who has had a segmental resection might experience burning upon urination, bladder spasms, and even some bleeding. These discomforts can be relieved by analgesics, antispasmodics, increased intake of fluids, and the application of heat over the bladder area. The urethral catheter is removed approximately 3 weeks postoperatively. The client will become aware of his decreased bladder capacity immediately, as he will need to void at least every 20 minutes. He must understand that tumors can develop and that fulguration might have to be repeated as often as every 3 months, for years.

Bladder instillation of the chemotherapeutic agent *thiotepa* might be required at weekly intervals for 4–6 weeks. The thiotepa is instilled via catheter by the urologist, and the client must try to retain it for up to 2 hours, changing positions every half hour (rotating between supine, prone, and left and right side lying positions). At the end of this time, instruct the client to void directly into the toilet, first informing him that dysuria or hematuria might be experienced. Fluids (up to 10 or 12 glasses per day) should be encouraged. Careful attention must be paid to the CBC, as thiotepa is extremely toxic and can cause profound anemia, leukopenia, and low platelet counts. Treatment with thiotepa must be suspended if the blood count becomes unstable.

Preoperative preparation for the cystectomy client must include psychological support.

In addition to the fear of cancer, the client is often apprehensive about the resulting change in body image and might feel dirty or less than whole. Clients need the time and opportunity to vent their feelings and learn how to cope with the changes facing them. They must be helped to maintain a positive outlook about the future and to accept the stoma.

Before cystectomy, the stoma site should be selected. The rectus muscle is the usual site, to avoid herniation and be readily visible to the patient. Usually, the stoma is located in the right side of the abdomen, below the waist. The site should be free of scars, skin folds, and bony prominences, and it should allow for comfortable standing, sitting, and reclining. The bowel is cleansed 3 or 4 days prior to surgery with cathartics, enemas, neomycin, and a clear liquid diet.

Following cystectomy, the client usually returns to the unit with catheters from the urethra and the cystostomy opening. The nurse practitioner must ensure patency of both catheters, to avoid stressing the sutures, as the client often has a bladder capacity of no more than 60 ml. If a catheter has not been inserted in the ileostomy to promote drainage, a plastic ileostomy bag will be placed over the opening. As the bowel normally secretes mucus, it might be necessary to irrigate the catheter, gently, every 2–4 hours. Any signs of urinary blockage (e.g., lower abdominal pain, distention, or decreased urinary output from the ileostomy) should be reported to the physician at once. Symptoms of peritonitis (e.g., fever or abdominal pain) likewise should be reported immediately, as there is a possibility of urine or fecal material leaking into the peritoneal cavity.

Approximately 5 or 6 days following surgery, self-care instruction should be begun. The client should be taught how to manage the stoma, including skin care and pouch changes. The stoma should be measured for a permanent appliance about 1 week after surgery, after most of the edema has subsided. The stoma size must be rechecked from time to time, however, as the stoma will continue to decrease in size for 6–8 weeks postoperatively. To select the correct size of pouch, the stoma should be measured and a $\frac{1}{8}$-inch margin added—most stoma manufacturers provide a card with various sized holes as a measurement aid. The pouch may be of either the reusable or disposable type and should have a pushbutton or twist-type valve at the bottom, thus facilitating drainage. The client should be instructed to empty the pouch when it is one third full or every 2–3 hours.

The skin surrounding the stoma should be inspected frequently and kept clean and dry. Following surgery, the stoma should be bright pink or red; some edema is usually present during the initial period. Any signs of infection or necrosis (gray or black coloration) should be reported immediately to the surgeon. The skin surrounding the stoma should be checked for signs of irritation caused by the leakage of urine, adhesive backing, or tape.

After the pouch has been removed, the skin should be washed with mild soap and water, rinsed well with clear water, and gently patted dry. Do not rub the skin. A gauze sponge or cotton ball soaked with a 1 : 3 vinegar–water solution may be placed over the stoma for a few minutes, to prevent the buildup of uric acid crystals. To collect the urine that might drain during the time that the pouch is being changed, a piece of gauze may be placed over the stoma. Coat the skin surrounding the stoma with a silicone skin protector, remove the gauze sponge, and then cover the stoma with the collection pouch. If the skin is irritated or breakdown occurs, an antacid precipitate may be applied to the skin just before the silicone skin protector is applied. Ensure that the adhesive area of the appliance is wrinkle-free, and gently press it into place. Tincture of benzoin may be used in place of the silicone skin protector, but it is irritating to some people. Karaya is not used for urinary appliances, as urine erodes the karaya, causing urinary leakage.

A pouch may be worn for 3–5 days, but after 5 days there is the potential for crystallization and foul odor. Reusable equipment should be washed with soap and water; if an odor develops, the appliance may be soaked in a half-strength vinegar–water solution or in full-strength white vinegar. One or two aspirin tablets also might be crushed and placed in the bag, to reduce the odor by acidifying the urine. Occasionally, alkaline urine will cause crusting of the stoma, which can lead to its occlusion. In this case, the physician might administer ascorbic acid, to acidify the urine, and the stoma may be bathed for 15 minutes, four times a day, with a half-strength vinegar–water solution placed in the pouch.

At discharge, arrangements should be made for follow-up home care. The client should be advised to avoid lifting heavy objects, as herniation of the stoma may result. If there is an "ostomy club" in the community, the client might be interested in talking with club members who have similar problems and can offer support.

AGING OF THE KIDNEY

Renal mass and function both decrease with age. Despite the decrease in renal function that accompanies aging, the normal volume and composition of body fluids are usually maintained. When disease or environmental stress places a greater demand on renal function, however, renal adjustments take place more slowly in the older individual.

Physiological Renal Changes

Kidney weight declines between maturity and old age by approximately 20–30%. The loss of renal mass is primarily cortical, the renal medulla being affected relatively little. The total number of glomeruli decreases with age, and the number of sclerotic glomeruli increases; as many as 30% of the glomeruli can be sclerosed in apparently healthy 80-year-old persons. Until the age of 40, a person normally has approximately 1 million glomeruli, but this number is decreased by roughly 300,000 (30%) by the seventh decade of life.

A loss of lobulation of the glomerular tuft, which is also associated with aging, decreases the effective filtering surface of the glomerulus. As a person grows older, diverticuli form in the distal tubules, with as many as three diverticuli per tubule present by age 90.

Age-related vascular abnormalities include sclerotic changes and increased tortuosity of the intralobular arteries. A thickening of glomerular and tubular basement membranes is probably due to ischemic atrophy that develops from vascular pathology. Renal plasma flow is approximately 600 ml/min in the young adult, but by 80 years of age the flow can be reduced by half. Factors that contribute to this decrease in renal plasma flow include age-related changes in the cardiac output and the previously described reduction in the renovascular bed (Rowe & Besdine, 1982).

The reduction in effective filtering surface of the glomerulus that occurs with aging results in a reduced glomerular filtration rate (GFR) and a corresponding reduction in creatinine clearance, which declines at a rate of approximately 1% per year between the ages of 40 and 80. Because muscle mass (from which creatinine is derived) decreases with age at roughly the same rate as the GFR, however, the rather drastic age-related loss of GFR is not reflected in an extremely elevated serum creatinine level. As a practical matter, then, serum creatinine concentrations in older persons must be interpreted very carefully when they are used to adjust the dosages of drugs that must be cleared by the kidneys.

Most drugs cannot be excreted as rapidly in late life, and because drugs tend to accumulate to toxic levels in the older person, antibiotics should be used with caution. Nephrotoxic antibiotics such as streptomycin, gentamicin, neomycin, and kanamycin must be used very cautiously. Tetracyclines accumulate in the body in the presence of altered renal function and they can cause further renal damage. Lincomycin and cleocin are considered highly likely to produce pseudomembranous colitis.

Fluid and Electrolyte Imbalances

Under normal circumstances, age has no significant effect on plasma concentrations of sodium or potassium, plasma volume, plasma pH, or the ability of the body to maintain normal extracellular fluid volume. However, the adaptive mechanisms required to maintain the normal volume of extracellular fluid are often impaired in the elderly client, and illness in old age is often complicated by the development of fluid and electrolyte imbalances that delay recovery and prolong hospitalization. These homeostatic perturbations are usually related to altered renal excretion of sodium and water.

Sodium Depletion

Renal response to an acute reduction in salt intake is relatively sluggish in the aged client who is capable of conserving sodium stores and achieving salt balance on a markedly restricted intake. Epstein and Hollenberg (1976) have reported that in older subjects the mean time required for reduction of urinary sodium after salt restriction is 30.9 hours, as compared to 17.6 hours for younger persons.

Other factors that can contribute to the depletion of extracellular fluid volume in the acutely ill elderly client include confusion, loss of the sense of thirst, and disorientation. This "salt-losing" tendency is aggravated by inadequate salt intake or impaired cardiac, renal, or mental function. Treatment of sodium depletion includes the prompt administration of sodium chloride. If the extracellular sodium depletion is mild, oral administration for several days of foods and fluids that are high in sodium content is usually sufficient. In more severe cases, marked by decreased blood pressure, tissue turgor, or orthostatic hypotension, the intravenous administration of isotonic saline is indicated (Coving & Walker, 1984).

Sodium Excess

Expansion of the extracellular fluid volume occurs primarily because of lowered GFRs in the senescent kidney when salt loads are abnormally high. Excessive salt loads are usually the result of the inappropriate administration of intravenous fluids, dietary indiscretions, or the administration of sodium-rich medications or dye (e.g., contrast agents used in IVP x-ray examinations). Volume expansion is treated by administering diuretics.

Hyperkalemia

Age-related decreases in the body's stores of renin and aldosterone place the elderly client at increased risk of developing hyperkalemia. Through its action on the distal tubules, aldosterone increases sodium reabsorption and facilitates the renal excretion of potassium. Because the GFR is often impaired in the older adult, serious elevations of plasma potassium can develop—especially if the client exhibits gastrointestinal bleeding, or if potassium is given intravenously.

The tendency toward hyperkalemia is further aggravated by an acidotic condition, as the senescent kidney responds sluggishly to acid loading. This slow response results in prolonged depression of pH and a concomitant elevation of potassium levels. Certain diuretics that impair renal potassium excretion (e.g., spironolactone or triamterene) should be administered to the elderly client with caution, and potassium should not be administered with such agents.

Management of hyperkalemia in the client with volume depletion or congestive heart failure includes the discontinuation of sources of dietary potassium or potassium-sparing diuretics. Severe hyperkalemia, which is indicated by ECG changes that include peaked T waves and broadened QRS complexes, requires prompt treatment with intravenous calcium salts (e.g., calcium chloride or calcium gluconate), which directly antagonize the effect of hyperkalemia on the myocardium and often normalize the ECG. Also indicated are sodium bicarbonate, glucose, and insulin (Toto, 1987b). Emergency treatment will have little effect on total body potassium; therefore, sodium–potassium exchange resin (Kayexalate) should be administered, orally or rectally, and diuretics such as furosemide or ethacrynic acid should be given (Rowe & Besdine, 1982).

Dehydration

In dehydration (hypernatremia), the capacity of the elderly individual to conserve water and concentrate urine is impaired. This can occur under conditions of water deprivation or when antidiuretic hormone (ADH) has been infused (Rowe, Shock, & DeFronzo, 1976). The cause of the aged kidney's decreased concentrating capability is not known, but it is probably related to the decline in GFR and an age-related decrease in renal response to ADH. Dehydration results when fluid intake is limited or when insensible losses are exaggerated, as with fever. Under such conditions, the serum sodium concentration rises, and the client shows evidence of impaired mental function.

Management of the client with severe hypertonic volume depletion should focus on restoration of volume as rapidly as possible by infusing isotonic saline intravenously until cardiovascular stability has been attained. In the presence of marked hypernatremia, isotonic fluids are actually "hypotonic," relative to the client's plasma, and the serum sodium level will begin to fall as fluid volume is expanded. Once the client's blood pressure and intravascular volume have been corrected, hypotonic fluid should be administered until the serum sodium concentration falls below 150 mEq/L.

The dehydrated client should be assessed for alterations in consciousness. The volume and concentration of extracellular fluid might be normalized as quickly as within 72 hours, but alterations of the older person's mental state might continue for as long as 2 weeks.

Water Intoxication

Water intoxication (hyponatremia) is a serious disorder of fluid and electrolyte imbalance that is frequently not well recognized in the elderly client. Common clinical findings that are nonspecific in hyponatremia include depression, confusion, lethargy, anorexia, and generalized weakness. When serum sodium concentration falls below 110 mEq/L, serious side effects can occur, e.g., seizures, stupor, or irreversible damage to the central nervous system (CNS). Hyponatremia can occur under stressful conditions such as surgery, fever, and acute viral illness.

Generally, there are two causes of hyponatremia in elderly clients. One of these causes is decreased renal capacity to excrete water, as a consequence of acute or chronic reduction in renal blood flow. This condition occurs in drug-induced hyponatremia, congestive heart failure, hypoalbuminemia associated with cirrhosis or nephrosis, and extracellular volume depletion. Clients with these conditions exhibit prerenal azotemia, in which BUN elevations are out of proportion to the elevations in serum creatinine.

Hyponatremia can also be caused by an oversecretion of ADH. In this case there are low serum sodium, evidence of good renal function (low BUN values), mild extracellular fluid expansion (normal to slightly full neck veins or trace edema), and evidence of inappropriate renal water retention, namely urine osmolality that is greater than maximally dilute and in many cases more dilute than serum. Excessive ADH secretion is often associated with pneumonia, meningitis, stroke, subdural hematoma, tuberculosis, and many other CNS and pulmonary disorders.

Treatment of water intoxication includes strict water restriction and avoidance of diuretics and agents that increase ADH, e.g., vasopressin, aspirin, acetaminophen, Haloperidol, narcotics, and barbiturates. In the client with reduced renal blood flow, therapy should be aimed at correcting the problem causing congestive heart failure, replenishing fluid volume, or, if the client is hypotensive, raising the blood pressure to normal.

In cases of excessive ADH secretion, fluid restriction alone usually results in a slow return of plasma osmolality to normal levels. In resistant cases, the oral administration of dimethyl chlorotetracycline, in dosages of 300 mg, two or three times per day, produces a diabetes insipidus state but usually corrects the hyponatremia in several days. Severe hyponatremia, often associated with seizures and CNS abnormalities, requires immediate correction. Hypertonic saline (500 ml of 3% sodium chloride), administered intravenously over a 12-hour period, usually increases the serum sodium to a safe level.

Renal Failure

Acute renal failure (ARF) occurs more frequently in older clients because its causes (hypotension due to blood loss, major surgery, sepsis, dyes used in angiography, and the use of antibiotics) are more common in the elderly. The older client's kidneys normally retain the capacity to recover from acute ischemic or toxic insults over the course of several weeks. In the usual case of acute tubular necrosis (ATN), 2–10 days of oliguria are followed by a diuretic phase that precedes recovery of function. The elderly, however, often have a nonoliguric stage in which the serum BUN and creatinine levels are abnormal for several days after a brief hypotensive period. Following this brief period of azotemia, renal function gradually returns. Because the clinical hallmark of ATN is the absence of a dramatic reduction in urine output, cases of nonoliguric ARF may go unrecognized. This can result in the client receiving an overdose of drugs, e.g., digitalis or aminoglycoside antibiotics (gentamicin), during the period of impaired renal function.

Elderly clients who suffer from ARF are managed in the same fashion as their younger counterparts. Dialysis (hemodialysis or peritoneal dialysis) is effective in the older client. Fluid and electrolyte balance must be monitored closely to avoid hypertension and cardiac failure; if fluid restriction is severe, the client's general condition or impaired CNS function can delay the recovery of renal function. In general, the administration of approximately 600 ml of fluid daily is adequate to maintain fluid and electrolyte balance. Maintenance of potassium balance is crucial; hyperkalemia must be avoided, if possible, or promptly treated, otherwise.

The major causes of death in cases of ARF are acute pulmonary edema due to fluid volume overload, hypertensive crisis, hyperkalemia, and infection. Infection can occur following unnecessary urinary catheterization. Serum levels of BUN, creatinine, and potassium are better guides to progress than is urinary output, although clients sometimes are unnecessarily catheterized on the basis of low urinary output. Infection from intravenous lines is also common. Intravenous lines should be carefully monitored and discontinued as soon as possible. The client's diet should be limited in protein, to prevent an increase in the BUN. Health-care providers also must realize the importance of monitoring and adjusting the administration of medications that are excreted via the kidneys—especially drugs such as hypnotics and tranquilizers (Hahn, 1987).

Chronic renal failure (CRF) is usually secondary to other age-related diseases such as BPH and cancer, which can lead to hydronephrosis, hypertension, atherosclerosis, multiple myeloma, diabetes, or perhaps to azotemia resulting from congestive heart failure. As previously noted, recognition of CRF in the elderly client might be delayed because the serum creatinine usually fails to rise to alarming levels (Coving and Walker, 1984).

Chronic dialysis (usually hemodialysis, but occasionally peritoneal dialysis) is the mainstay of treatment for the elderly uremic client; renal transplants are usually not considered for clients over 60 (Plawecki, Brewer, & Plawecki, 1987). Anemia associated with renal failure in the older client must be managed aggressively because of the coexisting cardiac disease. Dietary management of protein and salt is often not necessary, as most elderly clients normally ingest only 60–70 grams of protein and 4–5 grams of salt per day.

Pruritus is a major problem for clients in renal failure, especially if they also have xerosis (abnormal tissue dryness). Skin moisturizers and ultraviolet light treatments are usually effective. Antihistamines are rarely helpful because of the resulting sedation and the adverse nervous system effects that can be produced in the older person. Dosages and schedules of all medications, especially digoxin, must be carefully tailored to the individual client. Hypertension must be carefully controlled. Serum phosphate, calcium, and vitamin D levels must be closely monitored and controlled (Rowe & Besdine, 1982).

Diuretic-Induced Metabolic Disorders

The kidneys are the main route of elimination for most drugs. In a person of 65, the GFR is about 30% less than in a young adult, and tubular secretion also deteriorates. Impairment of renal function, combined with the decreased ability of the liver to detoxify toxic substances and the higher proportion of body weight that has been transformed to drug-storing fat, can cause even moderate dosages of drugs to accumulate quickly to toxic levels (Pagliaro & Pagliaro, 1983).

Diuretics, which are used to reduce blood pressure or edema by increasing urinary excretion of sodium and water, can cause metabolic complications resulting in significant morbidity and occasional mortality. Such complications include volume depletion, hyponatremia, hypokalemia, hyperkalemia, metabolic alkalosis, metabolic acidosis, hypercalcemia, carbohydrate intolerance, hyperlipidemia, and hyperuricemia. If recognized early, most of these disorders are easily managed.

Volume Depletion
Volume depletion (excessive reduction of extracellular fluid levels) is the most common complication of diuretic treatment, especially when furosemide or ethocrynic acid is used. Clients with normal renal function are more prone to develop diuretic-induced volume depletion than are those with renal insufficiency.

Mild volume depletion can cause tachycardia, orthostatic hypotension, and slightly re-

duced renal function (due to diminished renal perfusion). The elderly person might experience relatively less tachycardia, however, because of less responsive baroreflexes. In instances of mild volume depletion, the BUN is disproportionately elevated, compared with the serum creatinine, because there is a greater reduction in the renal clearance of urea than creatinine.

In instances of severe volume depletion, the client can experience life-threatening hypotension, coronary and cerebral insufficiency, or significant renal impairment. Treatment includes the immediate discontinuation of diuretic therapy, and fluid replacement might be necessary. Gradual diuresis may be accomplished by giving low doses initially, while monitoring the client closely. Alternatively, diuretic therapy may be given intermittently, e.g., on alternate days.

Hyponatremia
Hyponatremia (abnormally low blood levels of sodium) can occur during diuretic therapy for several reasons. First, excessive diuresis can cause significant extracellular volume depletion, which impairs urinary dilution. It also stimulates the release of vasopressin (ADH), which leads to further urinary concentration. Second, excessive water intake can cause hyponatremia, and third, profound diuretic-induced potassium depletion can cause sodium ions to migrate into the intracellular compartment. Elderly clients are more likely to develop hyponatremia from diuretics than are younger persons, probably because of the increased tendency for vasopressin release that accompanies aging. Furthermore, edematous disorders such as congestive heart failure, cirrhosis, and nephrotic syndrome, which are themselves characterized by water-excreting defects, exacerbate the effects of degraded nephron activity that accompany aging.

Symptoms of hyponatremia, including lethargy, convulsions, and coma, may occur when the sodium concentration is less than 120 mEq/L. When neurological symptoms are present, the electrolyte imbalance should be corrected immediately by the infusion of hypertonic saline. Treatment of asymptomatic diuretic-induced hyponatremia depends on the associated clinical features. When extracellular volume is depleted, the diuretic should be temporarily withdrawn and the fluid volume replaced.

Hypokalemia

Potassium excretion is enhanced by the administration of thiazide diuretics, which can lead to hypokalemia (blood deficiency of potassium). The gerontological nurse practitioner must be aware of the factors that can influence the extent of hypokalemia, e.g., dietary levels of potassium and sodium, metabolic alkalosis, and perhaps a secondary hyperaldosteronism. (Hyperaldosteronism is a clinical syndrome characterized by muscle weakness, polyuria, hypertension, hypokalemia, and the alkalosis associated with hypersecretion of the mineralocorticoid aldosterone by the adrenal cortex, due to stimuli external to the adrenal gland.) In the non-edematous client who is under little or no salt restrictions, only a mild degree of metabolic alkalosis or secondary hyperaldosteronism might develop. However, diuretic therapy can cause substantial potassium deficits in the edematous patient who has cardiac or hepatic disease. Edematous clients are frequently maintained on salt-restricted diets, and they tend to develop moderate-to-severe metabolic alkalosis and secondary hyperaldosteronism (Toto, 1987a).

Potassium deficits of less than 15% of the body's potassium stores (mild to moderate hypokalemia) usually do not give rise to significant symptoms of dysfunction. On the other hand, potassium depletions in excess of 20% are frequently associated with symptoms of muscle weakness and cramps, fatigue, polydipsia, polyuria, and palpations.

The asymptomatic, nonedematous client on diuretic therapy who has a serum potassium level of 3.3 mEq/L or greater and who is receiving potassium supplementation is at significant risk of potentially life-threatening hyperkalemia (abnormal elevation of blood potassium levels).

This is especially true of the elderly client who has impaired renal function. Therefore, a minimal deficit should be carefully monitored rather than treated. Clients who have significant hypokalemia, however, should be treated with potassium chloride; the high-potassium diet is an unreliable means of correcting potassium deficits.

Potassium-sparing diuretics, e.g., aldactone (spironolactone) and triamterene (Dyazide), should be avoided in clients who have renal insufficiency or who are receiving potassium supplementation. Potassium-sparing diuretics should also be avoided in the treatment of clients with diabetes mellitus, as diabetic clients appear to have a particularly strong tendency to develop hyperkalemia, even when they have normal renal function (Schwartz, 1987).

Metabolic Alkalosis

Diuretic therapy is a common cause of metabolic alkalosis (an abnormal physical state that is characterized by metabolic processes that tend to decrease hydrogen ion concentrations below normal or increase the loss of acid from the body excessively). Both thiazide and loop diuretics can generate metabolic alkalosis, since these substances promote renal excretion of sodium and potassium (almost exclusively in association with chloride), which causes hyperbicarbonatremia (abnormally high blood levels of bicarbonate ions). In addition, both types of substances stimulate renal excretion of hydrogen ions, thus further increasing the body's alkalinity. With the exception of clients with severe salt restrictions, thiazide diuretics usually induce only a relatively mild metabolic alkalosis. Loop diuretics, however, can induce severe hyperbicarbonatremia, even when the client does not have a strict salt restriction.

Symptoms of metabolic alkalosis include increased neuromuscular excitability, which can produce hyperactive reflexes, tetany, or generalized convulsions—especially if the client has hypocalcemia. The alkalemia can produce serious cardiac arrhythmias. The clinical signs and symptoms of coexistent hypokalemia may also be present.

Treatment of diuretic-induced metabolic alkalosis includes adequate replacement of chloride and potassium. Potassium chloride can be used to correct both deficiencies. If volume depletion is significant, sodium chloride may also be administered. Volume replacement in the cardiac client should be accomplished very cautiously, however, to avoid fluid overload, and the client's blood pressure and pulse rate must be monitored closely. Agents used for rapid correction of hyperbicarbonatremia include ammonium chloride (contraindicated for the client who has hepatic encephalopathy) and dilute hydrochloric acid. Response to treatment should be verified by the detection of significant amounts of chloride in the urine.

Metabolic Acidosis

Hyperchloremic metabolic acidosis (an abnormal physical state that is characterized by metabolic processes that tend to increase hydrogen ion concentrations above normal or increase the loss of base from the body) can develop during treatment with acetazolamide (Diamox), a weak diuretic that is often used as a urinary alkalinizing agent or as a means of lowering intraocular pressure in clients with glaucoma. Acidosis can also be induced by potassium-sparing diuretics, which can impair acidification in the renal nephons.

Hypercalcemia

Hypercalcemia (abnormally high blood levels of calcium) can result from chronic use of thiazide diuretics, e.g., Diuril, Anhydron, and dyazide. Persons with hypercalcemia (particularly those in whom serum calcium concentrations exceed 11.5 mg/dl) should be examined for an underlying primary hyperparathyroidism as an alternative cause of the hypercalcemia. Treatment includes withdrawal from the drug and replacement with furosemide, e.g., Lasix (Calloway, 1987).

Carbohydrate Intolerance

Thiazide diuretics, and to a lesser extent triamterene, furosemide, and ethacrynic acid, can cause carbohydrate intolerance. Thiazides depress and delay the peak insulin response to hyperglycemia, and they can cause increased glycogenolysis and reduced glycogensis. In addition, furosemide can have an anti-insulin effect.

Although diuretic-induced carbohydrate intolerance is usually mild, long-term effects can be significant. Therefore, during diuretic therapy the client's serum glucose concentration should be measured at regular intervals. Carbohydrate intolerance, if indicated, can be managed by correction of any potassium deficit, by administration of insulin or tolbutamide (Orinase), or by substitution of a nonthiazide diuretic.

Hyperlipidemia

Therapy involving the use of thiazide diuretics is associated with an increase in total serum cholesterol, low-density lipoprotein (LDL) cholesterol, and triglyercides—perhaps because of the effect that diuretics have on carbohydrate metabolism. Although such increases in serum lipids (hyperlipidemia) are usually mild, the client is at increased risk of atherosclerotic cardiovascular disease. This risk appears to decrease with age.

Hyperuricemia

Diuretic therapy involving the administration of thiazide, furosemide, ethacrynic acid, or spironolactone has been associated with increased levels of uric acid. Diuretic-induced *hyperuricemia* (abnormally high serum uric acid levels) is usually asymptomatic; in rare instances, however, gouty arthritis develops. The client who has hyperuricemia should have serum uric acid levels monitored frequently. If the level is greater than 10 mg/dl, hypouricemic agents, e.g., allopurinal, are usually prescribed.

SUMMARY

The aging woman is particularly prone to genitourinary problems. As a result of decreased hormonal activity and progressive weakening of the structures that support the urinary bladder (often as a result of damage to the pelvic floor suffered many years earlier during labor and delivery), the older woman often experiences postmenopausal vaginal bleeding, genital prolapse, urinary tract infection, or alterations of normal urinary functions. Detection of a mass in a client's breast, abdomen, or genital tract must always raise suspicion of cancer. Correction of gynecologic disorders in the older female often involves surgery, which should not be contraindicated solely on the basis of the client's age if it could afford her the opportunity of living her remaining years more comfortably, usefully, and happily. Preoperative teaching and discharge planning are a vital nursing function, and the gerontological nurse practitioner should be particularly responsive to the client's need for psychological support when faced with surgery perceived as disfiguring and a threat to one's body image and femininity.

The effects of reduced hormonal activity in the older man are not as well understood as they are for women. However, an imbalance between androgen and estrogen activity does appear to be related to the enlargement of the prostate gland and consequent obstruction to urine flow that eventually are experienced by most older men. By the age of 60, the majority of men will have palpable evidence of BPH. In the later stages, the resulting hydronephrosis can contribute to urinary tract infections. The only completely satisfactory form of treatment involves surgery; the attendant risk of impotence or incontinence varies with the procedure that is employed. The symptoms of prostatic cancer are similar to those of BPH, and adenocarcinoma of the prostate must be confirmed by prostatic biopsy. It is treated by radical prostatectomy and/or radiation therapy. Client education and psychological support are important facets of the nursing care required by the older male client.

Physiological and psychological factors together affect and control each person's sexual identity and capacity for sexual activity throughout his or her lifetime. Just as other body systems undergo physiological changes as a person ages, that person's sexual mechanisms also undergo age-related changes that affect his or her sexual functioning. Despite widely held myths to the contrary, however, there are no intrinsic biological limitations to the aging person's sexual capacity. Given reasonably good general health and interest in sex, sexual partners can and often do continue to enjoy sexual activity well into late life. In this particularly personal aspect of a person's life, gerontological nurse practitioners can be of greater assistance to the older client if they understand human sexuality, recognize the physiological and psychological factors associated with aging, and intervene in ways that are consistent with that individual's concept of sexuality.

Most age-related genitourinary problems affect the lower urinary tract (bladder and urethra) and cause disorders of urination. Urinary disorders affecting elderly men and women include UTI, urinary calculi, obstruction, incontinence, and neurogenic bladder. These are very common in the elderly and are major causes of serious and distressing symptoms. Urinary symptoms that should be assessed during physical examinations include nocturia, diurnal frequency, decreased size and force of the urinary stream, urgency, and hematuria. Although drug therapy is often required, an accurate diagnosis must be established first (based on a complete history, current drug treatments, examination of the abdomen and nervous system, microscopy, and urine cultures). Catheterization is often required, necessitating scrupulous nursing care to avoid causing or exacerbating UTI.

The adaptive mechanisms required to maintain the normal volume of extracellular fluid are often impaired in the elderly, and illness is often complicated by altered renal secretion of sodium and water, causing fluid and electrolyte imbalances that delay recovery and prolong hospitalization. Metabolic complications that can result in significant morbidity and occasional mortality include volume depletion, hyponatremia, hypokalemia, hyperkalemia, metabolic alkalosis, metabolic acidosis, hypercalcemia, carbohydrate intolerance, hyperlipidemia, and hyperuricemia. As most of these disorders are readily managed if recognized early, the gerontological nurse practitioner must be particularly vigilant to significant changes in the client's sensorium, vital signs, laboratory data, ECGs, skin turgor, and other signs of fluid and electroyte imbalance.

REFERENCES

Brecher, E. M., & Consumer Reports Books (Eds.). (1984). *Love, sex and aging.* Boston: Little, Brown.

Butler, R. N., & Lewis, M. I. (1976). *Sex after sixty.* New York: Harper & Row.

Calloway, C. (1987). When the problem involves magnesium, calcium, or phosphate. *RN, 50*(5), 30–35.

Cameron, P. (1970). The generation gap: Beliefs about sexuality and self-reported sexuality. *Development Psychology, 3,* 272.

Churchill, D. N., Afridi, S., Dow, D., & McManamon, P. (1980). Uterine prolapse and renal dysfunction. *Journal of Urology, 124,* 899.

Clinical Highlights (1985). Radioactive antibodies destroy cancer cells. *RN, 48*(1), 78.

Comfort, A. (1976a). *A good age.* New York: Crown.

Comfort, A. (1976b). *More joy of sex.* New York: Crown.

Comfort, A. (1974). *The joy of sex.* New York: Crown.

Coving, T. R., & Walker, J. I. (1984). *Current geriatric therapy.* Philadelphia: Saunders.

Cumming, E., & Henry, W. E. (1961). *Growing old: The process of disengagement.* New York: Basic Books.

DeMoya, A., & DeMoya, D. (1982). *Sex and health: A practical encyclopedia of sexual medicine.* Briarcliff Manor, NJ: Stein and Day.

Dickenson, R. J. (1980). Management of carcinoma of the cervix. *The Practitioner, 224,* 899.

Ellenbogen, A., Agramat, A., & Grunstein, S. (1981). The role of vaginal hysterectomy in the aged woman. *Journal of the American Geriatrics Society, 9,* 426.

Epstein, M., & Hollenberg, N. K. (1976). Age as a determinant of renal sodium conservation in normal men. *Journal of Laboratory Clinical Medicine, 87,* 411.

Finkelstein, M. S. (1982). Unusual features of infection in the aging. *Geriatrics, 37*(4), 65.

George, L. K., & Weiler, S. J. (1981). Sexuality in middle and late life: The effects of age, cohort, and gender. *Archives of General Psychiatry, 38*(8), 919.

Gault, P. L. (1982). Plan for a patchwork of problems when your patient is elderly. *Nursing 82, 12*(1), 50–54.

Hahn, K. (1987). The many signs of renal failure. *Nursing 87, 17*(8), 34–41.

Holden, L. S. (1983). Helping your patient through her hysterectomy. *RN, 46*(9), 42–46.

Kinsey, A. C., Pomeroy, W. E., Martin, C. E., & Gebhard, P. H. (1953). *Sexual behavior in the human female.* Philadelphia: Saunders.

La Torre, R. P., & Kear, K. (1977). Attitudes toward sex in the aged. *Archives of Sexual Behavior, 6,* 203.

Ludeman, K. (1981). The sexuality of the older person: Review of the literature. *The Gerontologist, 21*(2), 203.

Madias, N. E., & Zelman, S. J. (1982). What are the metabolic complications of diuretic treatment? *Geriatrics, 37*(2), 93.

Marron, K. R. (1982). Sexuality with aging. *Geriatrics, 37*(9), 135.

Masters, W., & Johnson, V. E. (1981). Sex and the aging process. *Journal of the American Geriatrics Society, 24,* 385.

Morales, A., Edinger, J. D., & Bruce, A. W. (1976). Intracavitary bacillus Calmette–Guerin in the treatment of superficial bladder tumors. *Journal of Urology, 116,* 180.

Neimark, P. G. (1979). *Female surgery.* Chicago: Budlong Press.

Pagliaro, L. A., & Pagliaro, A. M. (1983). *Pharmacologic aspects of aging.* St. Louis: Mosby.

Plawecki, H. M., Brewer, S., & Plawecki, J. A. (1987). Chronic renal failure. *Journal of Gerontological Nursing, 13*(12), 14–17.

Poe, W. D., & Holloway, D. A. (1980). *Drugs and the aged.* New York: McGraw-Hill.

Prout, G. R., Jr., Garnick, M. B., & Canellos, G. P. (1982). The bladder. In J. F. Holland and E. Frei, III (Eds.), *Cancer medicine* (2nd ed.). Philadelphia: Lea & Febiger.

Rosenshein, N. B., & Rotmensch, J. (1982). Combating postmenopausal gynecologic malignancy. *Geriatrics, 37*(5), 107.

Rowe, J. W., & Besdine, R. W. (1982). *Health and disease in old age.* Boston: Little, Brown.

Rowe, J. W., Shock, N. W., & Defronzo, R. (1976). The influence of age on urine concentrating ability in man. *Nephron, 17,* 279.

Rubin, D. (1987a). Gynecologic cancer: Cervical, vulvar, and vaginal malignancies. *RN, 50*(5), 56–63.

Rubin, D. (1987b). Gynecologic cancer: Uterine and ovarian malignancies. *RN, 50*(6), 52–57.

Ruge, C. A. (1987). Catheter-related UTIs. What's the best way to prevent them? *Nursing 87, 17*(12), 50–51.

Schwartz, M. W. (1987). Potassium imbalances. *American Journal of Nursing, 87*(10), 1292–1299.

Simonson, W. (1984). *Medications and the elderly: A guide for promoting proper use.* Rockville, MD: Aspen.

Sloane, E. (1980). *Biology of women.* New York: Wiley.

Smith, D. L. (1978). *General urology* (9th ed.). Los Altos, CA: Lange Medical Publications.

Symmonds, R. E. (1980). Relaxations of pelvic supports. In R. C. Benson (Ed.), *Current obstetric and gynecologic diagnosis and treatment* (3rd ed.). Los Altos, CA. Lange Medical Publications.

Toto, K. H. (1987a). When the patient has hypokalemia. *RN, 50*(3), 38–41.

Toto, K. H. (1987b). When the patient has hyperkalemia. *RN, 50*(4), 34–38.

Townsend, S. L., & Kurrle, G. R. (1980). Cancer of the cervix (stages 1B, 2A, and 2B): Treatment and results. *Australian and New Zealand Journal of Obstetrics and Gynecology, 20,* 224.

Trump, D. L. (1982). Update on diagnosis and management of bladder cancer. *Geriatrics, 37*(7), 87.

Yoshikawa, T. T., & Guze, L. B. (1982). UTI: Special problems in the elderly. *Geriatrics, 37*(3), 109.

What's New in Drugs (1985): Drug brings remission in prostate cancer. *RN, 48*(1), 82.

8

MUSCULOSKELETAL CHANGES

Musculoskeletal changes associated with the aging process affect the posture, function, and gait and may take on a variety of appearances. There is a general flexion and forward projection of the head and neck. The back becomes humped, the hips, wrists, and knees slightly flexed, the muscles of the arms and legs flabby and weak, and the overall height slightly reduced. The movement and gait become slower and appear clumsy and less than agile as the older person moves across the room. The steps are small and shuffling. The feet barely clear the floor.

The result of these visual changes are relative to complex life processes: birth, growth, maturity, hyperplasia, atrophy, and regression. The processes and their expected changes are as individual as life and time. The image of stooped shoulders, slow gait, and decreased ambulation should not be applied indiscriminately. The older adult who has maintained a philosophy of activity and a commitment to physical fitness is less likely to display this appearance.

AGING OF THE MUSCULOSKELETAL SYSTEM

In general, the skeletal system undergoes involutional bone loss or a reduction in the skeletal mass with aging. Because this loss of bone mass affects the bone strength, the older client is at greater risk for fractures. These lead to decreased mobilization, which, in turn, can contribute to and accelerate bone mass loss (Kart, Metress, & Metress, 1978; Aloia, 1981).

The decline in height and flexed posture of the elderly client is a result of a shortening of the vertebral column along with thinning of the discs and/or ankylosis of the ligaments (Grob, 1978). Kyphosis may be associated with progressive collapse of the vertebrae or there may be a shrinkage and sclerosis of tendons or calcification of ligaments with declining elasticity (Rockstein, 1975).

Movements and gait are affected by changes in muscle strength, endurance, and agility. The loss of muscle mass that occurs with aging can be attributed to a decrease in the number and size of muscle fibers. This is not as clearly defined as is bone mass of the skeletal system (Gutmann, 1977). Aging changes in muscles are not uniform among the aging population. Apparently, fibrous tissue replaces muscle tissue when muscle regeneration no longer occurs. This restricts the power of the muscle. In addition, movement, motor power, and locomotion are complex physiological functions that have interrelationships with the circulatory, endocrine, and nervous systems (Gutmann, 1977). Changes in these systems would directly affect

TABLE 8–1. SUMMARY OF MUSCULOSKELETAL AGING PROCESSES AND EFFECTS[a]

Process	Effect
Involutional bone loss (reduced skeletal mass)	Diminished weight bearing, at-risk for fractures (may be spontaneous)
Shortening of vertebral column, thinning of vertebral discs, calcification, ankylosis of ligaments, decreased elasticity	Posture changes, decline in height, flexed neck position, kyphosis with progressive collapse of vertebra
Fibrocartilaginous atrophy of muscles, decrease in size and number of muscle fibers, inter-relatedness of the circulatory, nervous, endocrine systems	Decrease or loss of muscle power, slowing of activity level, increase in time required to complete tasks
Cartilaginous ossification of joints (accelerated by obesity, and excessive use of joint)	Stiffness, pain, reduced mobility, ankylosis, foot joint effects: slow, small, shuffling steps, feet barely clear the floor

[a]Changes and effects are considered general rather than specific. Individual pathology, genetic makeup, and general life-style are factors that can affect the results.

physical activity and muscle reflex capabilities. The older person may adapt by taking longer to complete a psychomotor activity. Motor function of the body system also depends on nutrition, desire, activity level, and a healthy mental attitude about oneself. Essentially, the older individual must feel good about himself or herself to want to maintain musculoskeletal functioning at its potential.

Motor function also relies on joint functioning. Changes in joints can begin very early in the life cycle, i.e., ages 20–30 years. Joint pain and stiffness is expected in aging, and yet it is amazing how early the degenerative process can begin. Changes in joints can be accelerated by injury, obesity, and excessive use. The major change affected by time will be the joint cartilage. Pathological processes and joint stress seem to be the general culprits of decreased joint functioning (Tonna, 1977). Joint changes, with accompanying stiffness and pain, further limit activity levels of the older client. If problems with the feet are part of this process (e.g., hallux valgus, bunions, calluses, or hammer toes), ambulation becomes even more difficult. The nurse practitioners must *never* neglect the assessment of the older client's feet (joint movement, arches, skin, circulation, position, and function) and should refer the client to a podiatrist if necessary

(Shank & Conrad, 1977; Jahss, 1979). Table 8–1 summarizes the musculoskeletal aging processes and the expected effects.

DISORDERS OF THE MUSCULOSKELETAL SYSTEM

With the current and recent emphasis upon physical fitness, protecting the environment, and maintaining healthy nutrition, there is a need to collect and report data on the aging process. Research in the field of gerontology should provide answers that either substantiate current beliefs about the effects of aging or that may completely change what we believe about the body and aging. Presently, changes in the musculoskeletal system are thought to involve deterioration. The conditions presented in the remainder of this chapter are discussed relative to the aging or pathological process of the system.

Osteoporosis

Osteoporosis is a widely publicized and discussed problem of middle and old age involving demineralization of the bone and a decrease in bone mass; (Forbes & Fitzsimons, 1982, p. 44). Porosis, with the prefix osteo, is used to describe the bony, porous, cavernous, translucent appearance of the disease upon roentgenography.

According to Forbes and Fitzsimons (1981), osteoporosis occurs most frequently in postmenopausal women. This suggests that lack of estrogen, which is said to stimulate bone growth, is a causative factor. The etiology is also related to an excess of glucocorticoid affecting the protein matrix, such as occurs in Cushing's syndrome and aldosteronism (Price & Wilson, 1982, p. 707). Other possible causes of osteoporosis include immobilization after an injury or inactivity, inadequate calcium intake, lack of vitamin D, inadequate supply of protein, vitamins, and minerals, malabsorption syndrome, or conditions accelerating bone loss such as hyperthyroidism, hyperparathyroidism, or large doses of steroids (Forbes & Fitzsimons, 1981).

Assessment Parameters

What boundaries are included in assessment when a majority of clients have no major symptoms? The clinical picture is vague, elusive, and frustrating, with the salient problem being aches and pains. Associated physical findings may betray the location of aches and pains. The following parameters should be included in the nursing assessment:

1. Pain and its pattern are the primary foci of assessment. The client is asked to provide explicit data about location, quantity, quality, chronology, alleviating measures, aggravating activities, and associated symptoms. These are explored in relation to activity, rest, changes in sleep or daily routines, trauma, stresses, dietary patterns, and age-related physiological processes.

   Has the client experienced any trauma within the previous 1–3 months? Has the client changed activity patterns, like workouts at spas, health clubs, gyms or with home equipment? Has the client recently begun to jog or walk as an exercise routine? Was this recent jogging or walking activity a self-imposed life-style change or was it prescribed?

   Have there been any unusual stresses in the client's life? Death of a relative, mate, dear friend, or pet, a divorce, financial reversals, debts, problems, worries, difficulties with children or in-laws, or a loss or change of jobs for the client or significant other? Is the client concerned about his or her own death?

2. What is the age of the client? What has been the usual health pattern? During the client's life, from infancy to the present time, how was the general health?

3. A complete history is taken, including a complete menstrual, sexual activity, and child-bearing/childrearing history, menopausal history, birth control methods and/or drugs, hysterectomy, and any other significant gynecologic facts. A complete dietary assessment should be made using the basic four food groups and dietary requirements for age and build. A drug history is indicated, not only for present drug intake but for past drug usage as well. Over-the-counter drugs should be included in this history.

4. How does the client feel about himself or herself? Family? Living arrangements? Economics? Finances? The client's life-style should be explored with attention to habits, hobbies, recreation, social activities and changes. Does the client have any close relationships? What is the client's socioeconomic status? Does the client have sufficient income for a stable life-style, for emergencies, and for pleasures? Is housing adequate, comfortable, safe, free of major needed repairs, appropriately heated and cooled? Are there adequate provisions for storing and cooking food? Is there hot and cold running water? Are there neighbors who could respond in a crisis? How far away does the family live? Would the client call on the family if help were needed? How much help could be expected from the family, if requested?

5. How does the client get around? What type of

transportation does the client use? Is there access to the client's house of worship, a drugstore, a grocery store, a restaurant, a senior center, and other shopping facilities?

6. Family history should be explored, with the client representing the second generation, the client's parents the first generation, and the client's children the third generation. Is there any osteoporosis, arthritis, joint disease, or muscle problems in the family history? Could these have a relationship to client's current problem? Can hypertension, diabetes, mental problems, or other endocrine problems be related to the present problem? Is there a possibility of a genetic relationship to the problem? The nurse must be very knowledgeable of the genetic transmission process before pursuing this topic of inquiry.

7. The information obtained in the previous steps is reviewed, enabling the client to add, clarify, or verify data. The gerontological nurse practitioner must have sound, in-depth knowledge of the aging process. The nurse practitioner must also be alert for additional physical or psychological concerns and their relationship to the presenting problem.

Development of a subjective data base is extremely important prior to the collection of objective data. The nurse should be careful to obtain pertinent, complete data about the client's concerns, avoiding superfluous and irrelevant data that can, if necessary, be obtained at a later time. The same approach should be taken when collecting objective data.

Objective data can be gained by radiological studies, which in the presence of osteoporosis will show radiolucency of the bones on the roentgenograms. Tumors may be ruled out with bone scans, and a bone biopsy may be necessary to rule out a malignancy. Laboratory studies are most often normal for blood calcium, phosphorus, and phosphatase levels.

The physical examination includes evaluation of those movements and activities of the musculoskeletal system that the client is capable of performing under ordinary circumstances. Thus, a complete range-of-motion evaluation of all joints is made to include the degree of adduction, abduction, supination, extension, flexion, pronation, and hyperextension the client can accomplish. Any pain or discomfort should be further differentiated.

Pain in the joint is assessed in relationship to movement and increased movement, with the knowledge that a warm, erythematous, edematous joint may be indicative of arthritis, whereas pain without inflammation could represent arthralgia or be a precursor to arthritis. The nurse practitioner must consider tendonitis, which involves the periarticular process and may be localized to a single surface over or near a joint without involving the joint. This can be further differentiated upon active movement of the part within the proximal area. Arthritis involves the whole joint, and tenderness extends over the entire joint. Nonarticular discomfort can also result from muscle, bones, and nerves. Muscle pain (myalgia) is aggravated by direct palpation of the muscle group or inducing muscle contraction. Bone pain arises from the innervated periosteum. Nerve pain (neuralgia) presents a picture of symptoms that relate to specific nerves or roots. Sciatica is an example of a cause of lower back pain in the vicinity of the fourth and fifth lumbar area and first sacral area. Sensory loss, dysesthesia, and motor loss can also be related to nerve loss.

The posture is assessed with the client in an upright position, standing, walking, and sitting. Assess the attitude (body position) or balance of the head in relation to the shoulders, hips, and ankles. Lateral inspection involves observation of the cervical concavity of the neck, the dorsal convexity of the thorax, and the lumbar concavity of the lower back. The midspinal line should be straight with the shoulders level. The spine and paraspinal accessories are palpated for muscle tenderness, swelling, or spasm. Evaluate the gait as the client walks, noting the length of steps, the base (width) and swing or restriction of arm movements. Note any staggering, slapping, dragging, or shuffling of gait. Note the lift of the feet from the floor when walking. Complete the evaluation with the Romberg test.

Range of movement is further assessed to check major joints for mobility. During the assessment, the nurse must observe the client's safety at all times. Have the client bend forward from the waist to about 90 degrees from an erect position. Have the client open and close hands rapidly, supinate and pronate palms, extend arms forward, then abduct to side, touch shoulders, adduct arms to body, and then touch hands together over the head. The client should attempt a knee bend; this may be difficult or impossible for the older person.

With the client in a comfortable sitting position, evaluate flexion of feet. Have the client bend and raise the knees toward the chin. The client may need to use the hands to push against the chair while attempting this procedure. With your hands on the ischial tuberosities, evaluate the movement of the upper torso by having the client bend sideways, forward, and backward. While still sitting, have the client touch the chin to the chest, rotate the head laterally right and left, touch chin to shoulders, and hyperextend the neck and chin. Note and record any restriction, pain, or discomfort.

Assess the costo/vertebral angle by locating the lower border of the ribs at the junction of the spine. Percuss each angle with the ulnar side of the fist (blunt percussion), using the other hand to cushion the percussion.

The muscle strength is evaluated while the client remains seated. The nurse attempts to turn the head while the client attempts to resist. Shoulder resistance is evaluated in the same manner. The triceps and biceps are tested by having the client make a fist and push against the nurse's hand to further test upper extremity muscle strength. The lower extremity strength is tested in a similar manner and is probably best accomplished with the client in a supine position.

During the entire procedure, the nurse should note symmetry and comparison of left and right body parts. The nurse practitioner must also be aware of the fatigue factor and discontinue the examination should this or other disturbing symptoms occur. The examination can always be continued at a later date.

Finally, the general overall examination should include an integration of the musculoskeletal components. For example, the nurse practitioner must be aware of cerebral function, cranial nerve function, cerebellar function, and motor and sensory function. These areas are intricately interwoven; whether they will clarify the situation or merely mystify the nurse practitioner depends on his or her knowledge, skill, and patience to pursue all avenues of the musculoskeletal assessment with the older client.

Management

Most authorities agree that osteoporosis involves demineralization of the bones. There is also general agreement that reduced activity and a poor nutritional life-style promotes this progression. Thus, if the older person is kept active, maintains an adequate nutritional intake, strives to promote calcium retention, and maintains a safe and comfortable environment to prevent fractures, osteoporosis can be either slowed in its progression or prevented; the gerontological nurse practitioner and client can share in these goals.

There is a great deal of controversy regarding the treatment of osteoporosis. Estrogen therapy (which is the primary treatment) may slow the progression of bone loss because estrogen has an osteoblastic-stimulating characteristic. However, estrogen therapy (Gallager, Riggs, & Deluca, 1980) has been linked with increased hyperplasia of the breast and endometrial tissue, mandating that clients receiving estrogen also be given routine cytological and breast examinations. The risk of stroke and myocardial infarction may also be increased with estrogen therapy (Brunner & Suddarth, 1982). Adequate teaching and counseling of the client are essential. It is very important that the family history be explored for incidence of cancer and circulatory problems and that the client be followed very closely if estrogen therapy is initiated.

Calcium therapy may be instituted with or without vitamin D supplement (Draper & Scythes, 1981; Avioli, 1981). Numerous studies have shown that calcium therapy has a positive effect on bone loss. Another study strongly supported a calcium, fluoride, and estrogen combination (Riggs, Seeman, Hodgson, Taves, & Ofallon, 1982) for reduction of osteoporotic vertebral fractures. Still another study showed that a combination therapy of fluoride, calcium, and calciferol provided a significant ($p<0.05$) reduction in osteoporotic backache (Grove & Halver, 1981), using a 4-stage scale evaluation of pain, infirmity, and consumption of analgesics.

Gallager, Riggs, Elisman, Hamstra, Arnaud, and Deluca (1980) studied the effects of estrogen therapy on calcium absorption in 12 women with osteoporosis and 9 control subjects receiving a placebo for a 6-month treatment phase. Calcium absorption was unchanged with placebo treatment but was increased with estrogen treatment (0.53 ± 0.02 to 0.65 ± 0.04; $p<0.005$). The authors concluded that estrogen replacement increases calcium absorption in postmenopausal osteoporosis. Serum 1,25-(OH) 2D was unchanged with the placebo group but increased with the estrogen treated group (23.6 ± 2.7 to 33.2 ± 3.7 pg/ml; $p<0.005$).

Nordin, Horsman, Crilly, Marshal, and Simpson (1980) studied 95 postmenopausal women with spinal osteoporosis. They found that three of six treatments with calcium plus hormones, and 1 alpha-OHD3 appeared to be useful in modifying the problem. Vitamin D and 1 alpha-OHD3 as a treatment were considered useless or even harmful.

Much attention has been given to encouraging bone mass and stimulating new bone growth through various pharmacological and dietary activities. This later dietary treatment and/or prevention factor is directed toward foods that are high in calcium, protein, and vitamin D content. Calcium, phosphorous, and vitamin D are factors in bone growth. For the calcium to be absorbed, there must be more calcium than phosphorous in the food. Vitamin D regulates the absorption of calcium, which requires sunlight as the catalyst. Increased meat protein has been reported to reduce bone mass, leading to the conclusion that denser bone formation occurs in vegetarians (Forbes & Fitzsimons, 1981).

Foods such as processed cheese, milk, and dairy products provide excellent sources of calcium as well as protein. However, the older person with lactose intolerance could use broccoli, spinach, beans, nuts, and other dark green vegetables (Howard & Herbold, 1978). High-protein foods, such as meat, may be too costly for the elderly person to purchase regularly. The gerontological nurse practitioner can and should recommend other sources such as dry beans, peas, nuts, peanut butter, chicken, and fish. Tuna canned in oil is an excellent source of protein. However, fats and oils are usually not recommended for the older person. Fish is rich in vitamin D. Fortified foods such as cream, butter, eggs, and liver have a small amount of vitamin D, but these foods must also be evaluated for their cholesterol content. The exact dietary adult requirement of vitamin D is unknown, but a daily intake of 400 IU is recommended for the ages birth to 22 years (Howard & Herbold, 1978). Sunlight (ultraviolet light), a nonfood source, plays a major role in vitamin D absorption, converting 7-dehydrocholesterol to cholecalciferol. Is sunlight therefore an important therapeutic factor in osteoporosis? Older people may receive inadequate amounts of sunlight. Geography, climate, living conditions, and environmental pollution may diminish the exposure. Dark-skinned persons are less likely to receive a sufficient intake. The fortified foods must be considered. The multiple purposes of vitamin D include the metabolism of calcium and phosphorus, maintaining (in collaboration with parathyroid hormone and perhaps magnesium) the serum calcium levels, bone mineralization, and reabsorption of phosphate by the kidneys. The role of vitamin D is considered to be scientifically significant in the therapy of osteoporosis (Howard & Herbold, 1978). The nurse, as a teacher, counselor, and resource, becomes extremely important in dietary assessment and planning with older clients.

Activity is considered to be important in the management of osteoporosis, and yet there has been little research regarding its effects. Nursing has always considered activity and rest as therapeutic factors in health and sickness. The older person needs activity and rest (Ebersole & Hess, 1981), and yet often adopts the stereotyped role of being confined to a rocking chair. Prior to outlining an activity plan with the osteoporotic client, the nurse practitioner must have made a complete assessment of the client's musculoskeletal system. If the activity level has been less than desirable, the nurse practitioner must caution the client to proceed slowly, gradually increasing the level until it reaches the point of pain. Forcing the muscles and joints past this point can be just as damaging as a complete absence of activity.

Stretching, flexing, and walking may be a reasonable beginning, along with self-care activities. A safe stretching routine can be done in bed prior to arising. Housekeeping, gardening, and the like are forms of activity that are not usually considered by the older person as exercise. The nurse practitioner should make a full account of each activity with the client while planning an exercise routine (Ebersole & Hess, 1981). The client should be told that consistent follow-up is necessary with the nurse, the physician, and others in the health team. If the client is also taking cardiovascular drugs or other medications, it is extremely important that he or she have an individualized well-planned program of activity.

The National Council on Aging, the National Adult Physical Fitness Survey, and the Connecticut State Department on Aging are examples of agencies that have published facts, figures and/or physical guidelines for the older person. The "Life is Movement" publication of 1979 by Connecticut offers specific guidelines on posture, flexibility, exercise, warm-ups, and other selected material (listed in Forbes & Fitzsimons, 1981, pp. 233–240).

Fractures

In addition to experiencing a general weakening in the musculoskeletal system, the older person frequently suffers from a disturbed equilibrium; fractures are therefore not uncommon in the older person. The same physiological changes that contribute to the incidence of fractures lengthen the healing processes. This increases the risk of extended immobility, with its attendant hazards of pneumonia, decubiti, thrombus formation, urinary problems, fecal impactions, and contractures.

Assessment Parameters

The hip is reported to be the most common site of fracture, either intracapsular or extracapsular. These are also the differentiating characteristics of hip fractures. The assessment parameters are pain and external rotation of the affected leg with shortening. The greater trochanter may be palpated in the buttocks. The client must first be assessed for the first-line trauma, namely shock, blood loss, movement of toes, pulses (such as dorsal pedis), color, coolness, warmth, nails, and sensation. If the pain is severe, and it usually is, the client may lose consciousness. In this case, a neurological assessment is extremely important. The nurse practitioner should know that the most frequent cause of death after 75 years of age is hip fracture and the resulting complications. Osteoporosis may be the cause of the hip fracture, but accidents due to environmental hazards, errors in judgment or disabilities can also be responsible (Brunner & Suddarth, 1982, p. 288; Brocklehurst, Exton-Smith, Lempert-Barber, Hunt, & Palmer, 1978).

Basic assessment parameters of fractures should include:

1. *Pain:* Type, location, duration, radiation. Is pain sharp, piercing and relieved by rest and immobility?

2. *Function:* Is there loss of function? If yes, to what degree?
3. *Edema:* Is there edema localized to an area? Is there discoloration (evidence of trauma and hemorrhage)?
4. *Deformity:* Can definite deformity be seen? Can the deformity be palpated?
5. *Grating:* Crepetation? Is there a grating sensation felt on examination? *Warning:* Tissue damage can be provoked if the nurse practitioner does not proceed with care. Do not try to elicit this sign unless experienced.
6. *Mobility:* Is there "false motion" at fracture site? Is there abnormal mobility?
7. *Open fracture:* Is the bone visible through the skin?

Management

The first line of care is emergency care. This is directed toward the general condition: respiratory function, blood loss, shock. There is usually a heavy blood loss with a fracture of the femur and pelvis. The blood pressure must be maintained with intravenous fluids, plasma, and/or blood transfusions. Oxygen is needed for the tissues and an analgesic is needed for pain. The pain medication must be given with careful attention paid to the client's age and condition. Early treatment may involve splinting the extremity and possible application of traction. A constant assessment of pain is pertinent as treatment and care is carried forth. The nurse must then assess, evaluate, and care for other injuries. Trauma textbooks will provide the reader more definitive guidelines for emergency and continuing care for each area of the skeletal system.

The major objectives of managing the care are for the client to regain function of the involved part, regain and maintain appropriate position and alignment, and be returned to usual activities as soon as possible and at the least cost possible. Throughout the acute and recovery phases of the incident, nursing management is initiated to prevent complications such as fat embolism, thrombi, respiratory distress, mental

disturbances, fever, capillary occlusion (petechial), and urinary problems. The fat embolism syndrome results from an embolization of marrow or tissue fat or lipids within the pulmonary capillaries. The pulmonary capillary may leak, causing respiratory distress and central nervous system (CNS) dysfunction. This syndrome is likely to occur within 48 hours after injury.

Nursing management is aimed at promoting independence as soon as possible. A concentrated attempt should be made to prevent physical, psychological, or social dependence and to restore ambulation. Early in the restoration process, the client should be encouraged to move independently. If this is contraindicated during the first 2 or 3 days, the health team must plan to turn the client to a different position every 2 hours or more frequently if needed. Teaching the client the benefits of turning independently, deep breathing, and using side rails or trapeze will speed recovery. Appropriate positioning of the affected part should be considered when turning the client. Nursing management also includes consistent respiratory, circulatory, neurological, and integumentary assessment. Nurse practitioners should maintain current knowledge of theory related to musculoskeletal problems and proficiency in the skills assessment.

Nursing management is planned and implemented with the client and health team. Usually the plan of care moves gradually towards mobilization, for example, tilt-table, then upright, then wheelchair, then standing, and then ambulation. During these mobility activities, the nurse practitioner must continue to assess circulation, strength, respiration, and gastrointestinal and mental status. Often the older client may become discouraged and fear reinjury when ambulation is attempted, especially if the fracture is complex and the healing process is slow.

Active exercises should start as soon as possible after pain and soreness have subsided. These exercises are often planned in collaboration with the physician and physical therapist. Early activity, i.e., range-of-motion, stretching, and isometrics, is useful in prevention of contractures.

Urinary and bowel integrity is a primary concern of the older person and should be considered in regard to urinary infections and fecal impactions. There should be an earnest effort to avoid use of indwelling catheters. The color, volume, and odor of the output should be assessed daily. A liberal intake of fluid within the limits of cardiorenal function should be instituted as a preventive measure for urinary tract infections.

Dietary intake is likewise important in gastrointestinal functioning and to promote the healing process. Food intake should include adequate calories to sustain normal weight and activity in relation to height, weight, and body frame. If the client is obese, a reduction in calories may be indicated; if the client is underweight, additives or supplemental feedings are indicated.

Skin care is essential for the older person who has sustained a fracture. The immobility increases the risk of pressure sores. This, coupled with attendant decreases in circulation, muscle mass, subcutaneous fat pads, and sensitivity, mandates that careful attention be paid to skin care.

Once the client returns home, the same needs/problems and goals are continued. Before the client is discharged, the home environment should be assessed to ensure that safe and adequate care can be provided during the continuing recovery period. Additional client needs, e.g., homemakers service, Meals-on-Wheels, extended nursing services, and transportation to physical therapy or other services, may be discussed with the client and family. Referrals are best made during discharge planning so that a quality recovery can be maintained within a community and/or family support system. The older client left alone without a support system sometimes simply "gives up." Health care providers must ensure that the restorative level of health care is maintained for the older client. The major goal is to continue to encourage the client's independence in the postrecovery period.

Arthritis

Arthritis is defined as an inflammatory or degenerative change of a joint. It is generally considered to be a chronic disease, with its major symptoms being stiffness and pain in the musculoskeletal system. It affects mobility and can alter the entire life-style of the individual. There are more than 100 different types of arthritis, two of which are discussed in this section: rheumatoid (inflammatory) arthritis and osteoarthrosis (noninflammatory).

The causes of arthritis are unknown but a variety of theories have been proposed—by researchers, scientists, laymen, and quacks. Among suggested causes are nutritional, autoimmune response, bacterial, viral, metabolic, biochemical, and systemic disorders. Arthritis is a symptom, not a disease. It is an inflammatory process with associated manifestations.

Arthritis is painful. Its victims have difficulty describing the pain. Perhaps the best explanation is the constant dull ache experienced when very cold hands or feet are put in tepid water or held before a heater. The pain can be severe enough to rob the victim of clarity of thought. The client may become obsessed with pain. Every action exacerbates the pain. The client may accept the pain stoically, assume a posture of martyrdom, become angry with the world, or react in a number of other ways. The client is often willing to take any action, whether recommended or medically suspect, to obtain relief. The pain inhibits or prohibits the performance of simple activities of daily living. Walking, climbing stairs, moving a once functional part of the body, writing, grasping a fork, driving, working, sexual activity, and other common daily tasks may become too painful to continue.

Arthritis is reported as the major crippling disorder. In 1979, 31.6 million Americans had some form of arthritis. This included 16 million classified as osteoarthritis and 6.5 million as rheumatoid arthritis. The total economic impact was reported as $14.5 billion per year in medical cost, lost wages, and taxes. Approximately 1 million new persons are added to the statistics each year, with women affected more frequently than men (3:1) (Price & Wilson, 1981; Burnside, 1981; Phipps, Long, & Woods, 1979).

Rheumatoid Arthritis

Rheumatoid arthritis (RA) is a systemic chronic disorder involving the connective tissue. Inflammation of the joint is the predominant manifestation. The etiology is unknown. It follows a chronic, progressive course, resulting in deformities and disabilities. The disorder may occur between ages 20 and 60 years, with the peak incidence between the years of 35 and 45. At least one half of the 3.6 million RA victims are over 50 years of age. More women (3:1) than men are afflicted. In many instances medication and therapy are of little help in halting the progression of RA (Burnside, 1981; Kolodny & Kipper, 1976).

The disorder involves an inflammation of the synovial membrane, with gradual erosion of the cartilage and bone within the joint. The symmetrical involvement of the joints has an insidious onset, with pain both on motion and at rest. There is a general stiffness after inactivity, especially in the early morning on awakening. Rheumatoid arthritis is usually designated as polyarticular, with involvement of the small joints of the hands and feet. It is characterized by periods of exacerbation, with symptoms similar to those of influenza, cold, viral illness, or mononucleosis. If these symptoms last longer than 6 weeks and are accompanied by swelling of joints, shiny stretched skin over the joint, pain on movement, tenderness and stiffness lasting over 1 hour, RA must be considered (Burnside, 1981; Brunner & Suddarth, 1982). Pertinent differentiating signs and symptoms can be summarized as early morning stiffness, pain on motion with joint tenderness, heat and swelling in one or more joints, symmetrical joint swelling, signs and symptoms for 6 weeks or more, subcutaneous nodules, roentgenographic changes, a positive rheumatoid factor test, a poor mucin clot from the synovial fluid, histological changes in the synovium, and histological changes in the nodules.

Laboratory studies may reveal a hypochromic normocytic anemia. The RA factor is present in 60% of clients. A high titer is considered to be a bad prognostic sign. The synovial fluid is sterile with decreased viscosity. Radiological studies show soft tissue changes first, followed by narrowing of joint spaces and subchondral erosion.

Eventually flexor contractions can occur. Interphalangeal and metacarpophalangeal joint involvement leads to deviation of the phalanges, and hand function is impaired. Classic ulnar deviation can occur. Flexure contractions of the hips and knees result in further disability. Virtually all joints—hips, knees, wrists, fingers, elbows, toes, shoulders, and jaws—may become involved.

Osteoarthrosis

Osteoarthrosis is a noninflammatory deteriorating, abrasive insult of the joint cartilage. Degenerative joint disease (DJD) is the most common kind of arthritis. It *is* a disease of older people. The clinical picture of DJD shows an overweight, middle aged or older person with pain in the knees, hips, hands, neck, and lower back. The early manifestations show involvement of the stress- and weight-bearing joints. Later, pain occurs at rest and keeps the client awake at night. There is usually asymmetrical joint involvement, with painful small joint involvement of the hands. The distal joints may develop Heberden's nodules. Pain can be elicited with movement of the joints. Occasionally, crepitus can be heard with movement. Degenerative joint disease of the cervical spine may limit full flexion, extension, and rotation of the neck. There may be joint tenderness on direct palpation of the joint. Swelling and deformities may be present, especially of the knees. The laboratory studies are usually negative, with radiological studies as the only clear evidence of osteoarthrosis.

The etiology of osteoarthrosis is thought to be the breakdown of chondrocytes of the articular cartilage. It is said to be a wear-and-tear disorder attributable to age and initiated by biomechanical stresses. Although found in whites, blacks, men, and women, osteoarthritis most often affects women. The aching pain usually does not occur at rest; however, stiffness is present. Osteoarthritis is not as severe as RA, and activity can dissipate the stiffness. Limited motion and bony overgrowths (spurs) caused by DJD may irritate nerves and cause a numbness or tingling in that part.

Assessment Parameters

Assessment parameters for arthritis include a systematic evaluation of the client's needs, capabilities, and resources. As with any musculoskeletal problem, the most important data involve assessment of pain. The client's present dysfunction, specific strengths and needs/problems are evaluated to determine what the client can do for himself or herself. In addition to the musculoskeletal assessment presented in the first section of this chapter, other pertinent evaluation is necessary. How does the client perceive the dysfunction? How has the disability affected the client's life-style? Has the client accepted the diagnosis? Has the client accepted the required life-style adaptations? Is the client under treatment complying with the prescribed therapy?

The individual's own perception of the degree of dysfunction and his or her coping mechanisms, feelings of self-worth, and involvement in self-care reveal the client's understanding of the therapy and future expectations. This is essentially the most important aspect of learning about the client and establishes the basic groundwork for nursing goals, thus providing an idea of intervention for teaching, counseling and working with the client in a supportive, caring relationship.

How does the family perceive this event? Is the involvement what they wish? Do they perceive this as an interference in their own life-style? Is the client a burden? Does the client's condition create embarrassment or pity? Does the family profess this has not changed the way "we" feel or the love "we" have? Family roles *do* change when a member of the family develops RA. The changes in roles and feelings may have been so subtle that family members are unaware that any change has occurred. Can they express and work through these feelings as a "natural" part of change in their life-style? The gerontological nurse practitioner must support the client and family in an attempt to work through and understand feelings and emotions. If professional counseling is needed, this should be noted so that a referral can be initiated.

Objective physical data include a complete physical examination and laboratory and radiological studies. The assessment discussed in the section on osteoporosis is appropriate for the client with arthritis. Additional objective data needed include radiological studies of other organs to determine the extent of the involvement. The Latex Fixation Test is usually performed to further define a RA diagnosis. The nurse should be aware that x-rays and laboratory tests are costly. An older person may be living on a fixed income and have limited resources to pay for expensive testing. The nurse must also consider that false-positive tests may result when connective tissue disease is present, e.g., a serological test. In addition, the RA factor test may be inconclusive, e.g., negative, while the clinical picture is positive.

Nursing Care Management

The nursing care of clients with RA and DJD is directed towards the individual client's needs and problems. Relief of pain is the priority. No other care should be attempted until pain has been reduced. Then the complications of stiffness, decreased strength, loss of dexterity, loss of locomotor ability, and immobility may be addressed.

Consideration is first given to the pharmacological management. The physician and client must decide the appropriate drug therapy. In RA and DJD, analgesics and anti-inflammatory agents are used. Aspirin, indomethacin, ibuprofen, propoxyphene hydrochloride to supplement aspirin, meclofenamate sodium, fenoprofen calcium, mefanamic acid, naproxen, sulindac, tolmetin sodium, and diflunisal are examples of drug therapy. Some of the anti-inflammatory agents are very powerful and must be carefully monitored. Most anti-inflammatory agents cannot be used with aspirin, which is still the drug of choice by a majority of clients and physicians. When aspirin is the mainstay of the treatment, 12–20 tablets a day at regular intervals is considered a reasonable dosage. One or two new nonsteroidal anti-inflammatory agents are now available in once-daily dosages. The mechanism of physiological action and side effects of new products, such as piroxicam, have not been fully established as yet. Piroxicam may be an inhibitor of the biosynthesis of prostaglandins. Piroxicam is a highly protein-bound substance and might replace other protein-bound drugs. The side effects of this drug and other anti-inflammatory agents should be closely monitored. Clients receiving any of these pharmacological therapies must know and understand how these products act within the body, their possible side effects, and the importance of monitoring and follow-up.

Oral steroids should be avoided because of their potential toxicity. Intra-articular steroids (by injection) may provide the client relief for a hot, inflamed, painful joint. Drug therapy for arthritis is not a cure, however. In fact, the clients are often disappointed by the fact that the drugs give only partial relief.

If pain and deformities increase in severity, the client may require surgery for correction and pain relief. The advent of corrective surgery has allowed many clients to become partially independent in performing activities of daily living. Prior to surgery, clients may find that splints, braces, cervical collars, and other orthopedic aids provide rest and relief for the painful joints. Traction is also used by some clients when there

is cervical or lumbosacral involvement. Canes, crutches, and walkers can provide stability and relieve strain on weight-bearing joints. They also serve as safety aids. The client should discard these aids when they are no longer needed.

Through trial, and repeated efforts a combination of some of the above therapies, clients with arthritis do find general relief factors. It should be noted that some clients will use over-the-counter ointments and other means for relief. Rather than criticize the client, the team should work supportively with him or her, educating and building trust. Rather than chastising the client, the nurse can instruct him or her about the actual value of the product. This trust will go far in preventing clients from turning to expensive, often dangerous, advertised cures for arthritis. Clients are at risk and should know they can call on the team or the Arthritis Foundation for information on these cures. The nurse and other members of the health care team should consistently communicate with the client to provide information and support.

The palliative comfort measures of rest, activity, heat, and mild analgesics for pain are the basic modalities of a treatment program. The client should be counseled that the joints need both rest and activity. Routine, daily exercises must be to the point of pain but not beyond. They should be decreased if pain lasts 1 hour after the activity. Excessive exercise will increase the pain. Proper body alignment and good body mechanics also provide preventive relief, as does weight reduction if the client is obese. Gentle massage of the area(s) can be soothing, and some clients find a warm whirlpool bath gives much comfort and ease. Another form of activity the nurse may suggest is swimming, if the client has access to a pool. Many clients with arthritis purchase whirlpools or, if economically feasible, enroll in a health club or spa. Clients should be encouraged to plan all such exercise programs with the health team. If clients are unable to afford equipment or a health club membership, the nurse and the health team can help them plan an appropriate physical fitness program (see section on exercise in this chapter). Today, many senior centers do provide exercise equipment and classes for their participants.

Perhaps the primary goal of nursing care is to allow the client time to adjust to a different life-style and accept the fact that some previously enjoyable activities may no longer be possible. The nurse should help the client identify activities that do not induce pain and stiffness. Consistent supportive care by the nurse may be the most positive factor in the client's life. Clients soon learn their limitations and capabilities.

RA and osteoarthrosis differ in pathology and involvement of the disease. Thus, there are differences in treatment and therapy. Clients with RA may progress to extreme points of disability because of the devastating deformities. Osteoarthrosis does not usually result in such grotesque and debilitating deformities. RA may require a more intense drug therapy program, involving either aspirin, anti-inflammatory agents, gold or penicillamine, or immunopotentiating agents. Osteoarthrosis therapy may begin with lesser aspirin dosages, progressing to one of the anti-inflammatory agents if aspirin fails to provide relief. Generally, both disorders will have the goals of inhibiting the inflammatory process and its symptoms, preserving function, preventing deformities, and restoring function to the joint(s). The basic means of accomplishing these goals are rest and activity in equal parts and according to a regular program, heat (dry or moist) for soothing effect, analgesics such as salicylates for pain, and anti-inflammatory therapy on an individual basis.

It has been found recently that specific foods may trigger flare-ups in some clients with arthritis, with milk and milk products, cereal grains, shrimp, and sodium nitrate among the foods implicated. Eicosopentaenoic acid (EPA) has been shown to help alleviate arthritic problems. This fatty acid is found in fish such as tuna, rainbow trout, mackerel, sardines, and salmon. It seems to stimulate production of prostaglandins, which have anti-inflammatory effects (Cerrato, 1987). A well-balanced daily in-take suitable for the individual should be encouraged.

Other factors involved in the nursing care for clients with arthritis include working with the family, instructing clients in drug therapy and home safety factors and cautioning them about quack remedies and therapies, counseling clients and family regarding help available through community agencies and providing supportive care and a regular follow-up program.

Many elderly persons with arthritis will not see a physician, feeling that there are few real benefits to justify the expense. The nurse can be of great service in helping clients live with their arthritis rather than simply existing with it (Burnside, 1981; Brunner & Suddarth, 1982).

Paget's Disease

Paget's disease (osteitis deformans) is a metabolic disease of the bone involving excessive bone reabsorption. The etiology is vague but may involve developmental defects, chronic inflammation of the bone, or wear and tear of the skeletal system over a number of years. The disease seems to affect middle-aged and aged males. The skull, sacrum, pelvis, and long bones are most often involved. The pathology involves an increase in the size and a thickening of the skull. Kyphosis is usually present, as is bowing of the femur and tibia. There may be bone pain, and headaches and fracture may occur easily. Major complications can include paraplegia as a result of pressure on the spinal cord and deafness due to pressure on the optic nerve. The prognosis is poor, with a predisposition for the client to develop sarcoma of the bone. In extreme cases the cardiac output is increased, and failure results due to the highly vascular bone lesions acting as arteriovenous shunts in the affected bone.

Assessment Parameters
Assessment of the client is directed initially toward the bone pain, swelling, limitation of motion, weight loss, palpable tenderness, and increased temperature of skin over masses.

The client exhibits tenderness on pressure over the involved bone and an increase in the skin temperature. Skull measurements should be taken to establish a baseline for further evaluations. The bony skeleton is further assessed, with attention to areas about the spine, femur, and tibia for deformities and masses. The client's height is recorded, since a decrease in height indicates further progression of the disease. Neurological assessment should be directed specifically to hearing and visual acuity, muscle strength, vibratory and touch sensation, and reflexes. Roentgenograms of the skeletal frame can reveal porotic areas. These films may show evidence of sclerosis and bone repair. The laboratory studies show a markedly elevated serum alkaline phosphatase. The 24-hour urine analysis indicating hydroxyproline excretion reflects increased bone resorption. A bone scan is needed to locate the disease process and evaluate its progression or degree of activity.

Because Paget's disease may be related to developmental defects, the nurse should obtain a complete developmental history, from birth to the present. Were there any problems at birth? What were the usual measurements, e.g., head circumference, length, etc? When did client sit? Walk? Perform other motor skills? Does client remember any unusual problems during adolescence regarding skeletal integrity? Does the client have measurements at different stages of growth, e.g., height, weight, etc? Was the client ever injured in sports or otherwise? Does the client's occupation require constant use of the skeletal system?

Nursing Care Management

This disease requires extremely careful handling by the health team. This is especially true as the disease progresses and places the client at risk for fractures. Total care should focus on supportive measures and relief of symptoms.

Aspirin plus nonsteroidal anti-inflammatory agents may be used to treat pain and inflammation. Corticosteroids have been used but can result in calcium excretion and hypercalcemia.

Etidronate disodium may be prescribed as an oral medication to slow the rate of bone turnover (bone resorption and new bone accretion). The client must be told that nausea and diarrhea are major side effects of this drug. Other side effects relate to the drug dosage. Methramycin, a cytotoxic antibody, has been used in the therapy of Paget's disease, but the toxic and side effects may limit its use to severe bone pain and headaches. Basu, Smethurst, Gillett, Donaldson, Jordan, Williams, and Hicklin (1978) administered high doses of ascorbic acid to 16 clients, 8 of whom had decreased pain 5–7 days into the therapy. Three of these eight clients showed no pain. Calcitonin was administered subsequently, with noted improvements in most of the clients.

The nurse should caution the client about bathing in warm to hot water. The heat may increase the demand on the circulatory system, resulting in hypotension, dizziness, and fainting. Given the client's predisposing proneness to fractures, it is critical that the bath temperature be kept moderate.

The dietary requirements call for the client to limit calcium intake and increase fluid intake. The diet should be balanced with supplements or increased protein and minerals to help maintain the structure and function of the musculoskeletal system. If the client is obese, weight reduction may decrease the discomfort.

GENERAL HEALTH PARAMETERS OF THE MUSCULOSKELETAL SYSTEM

The general integrity of the musculoskeletal system is related to its physiological functions of protection of internal organs, body shape, mobility, stability, coordination, and balance. Maintenance of the machinery requires an appropriate level of activity, adequate rest of its parts, and adequate nourishment. As can be seen from the discussion of the preceding disorders, a balanced program of rest and activity is helpful. An essential factor in any program of activity and exercise, especially one for the older client, is safety. The following sections consider exercise, rest, nutrition, and safety with regard to the musculoskeletal system.

Exercise

Many older clients, with or without professional counseling and teaching, have "taken to the road" to walk, to jog, or to run. The media advocate and sell staying fit. Older individuals often appear on television to credit their physical fitness to some form of exercise: swimming, bicycling, dancing, and so on.

Today exercise is planned and sold by various groups and individuals. Health professionals must realize that exercise is part of today's society. Health professionals must also understand two very important facts before recommending an exercise program to any individual, especially the older client. First, nurses and other health professionals need in-depth knowledge of exercise physiology. This may require a college credit or continuing education course, preferably taught by an expert in this area. The course should include instruction on the anatomy, physiology, and functions of the skeletal, muscular, and joint systems. Range-of-motion, adduction, abduction, supination, pronation, hyperextension, rotation, flexion, stretching, and other terms must be well understood by the professional nurse. Heat release, warm-ups, and cooldowns are relative to understanding the physiological process of an exercise program. This depth of knowledge of exercise physiology must include an equal knowledge and integration of the neurological, circulatory, endocrine, nutritional, and elimination processes of the body. The nurse cannot recommend exercise to a client unless he or she possesses this knowledge.

The second important factor relative to exercise is the need to provide each client with an individualized program. This means that the health professional must know how to plan an exercise program and what it should include. By definition, exercise is prescribed or planned physical activity.

There is universal agreement that exercise is beneficial. It improves the circulation, restores vigor, helps remove wastes, supplies energy, and ensures joint mobility. Research has shown that exercise increases an older individual's physical abilities (Welford, 1977; Hellebrandt, 1979). Maximum oxygen uptake levels have been shown to be greater in an active person than in a sedentary person of the same age. Exercise programs were also found to improve maximum oxygen uptake (Shock, 1977).

Does physical fitness decline with age? Strandell (1976) believed that regular, appropriate exercise for the individual should help to maintain physical working capabilities. Most of those who study the effects of exercise agree that training in an exercise program does improve general fitness. None of the researchers actually stated that it stopped or slowed the aging process. Exercise cannot be a spontaneous or a random activity, however, it must be planned for the individual client. Physiological age, not chronological age, influences the individual's capabilities (Furlow, Oberman, & Eggert, 1980). Pathological processes may affect or moderate the prescribed program but should not be an excuse for having no program. Factors such as obesity and respiratory, cardiovascular, or balance problems may require that the health team (of which the client and family are members) include safety factors in the exercise program.

What is the positive effect of exercise for the older individual? The cardiovascular, respiratory, and neurological systems should show increased work capacities, thus ameliorating the problem of atherosclerosis (Furlow et al., 1980). Among the cardiorespiratory benefits of a regular exercise program are reduced heart rates at rest and during exercise. Regular exercise also increases cardiac output and circulation, blood flow to skeletal muscle, and ventilatory efficiency, as well as improving carbohydrate metabolism through cellular glucose uptake.

The first obligation in an exercise fitness program is determining baselines. These may differ in various locales but essentially are based on the client's tolerance level. How much exercise can the client accomplish before experiencing discomfort and pain? These factors are very important and can be obtained in a scheduled data-gathering health fitness assessment. Height, weight, resting pulse and blood pressure, exercise (such as stationary bicycling or treadmill), blood pressure and pulse, an ECG strip during the bicycle exercise, handgrip measure, measurement of percentage of body fat, and number of situps per minute are measures to obtain baselines. Also, a fasting laboratory chemistry should be secured prior to this data gathering. These baseline data, along with a complete health history and physical assessment would provide a parameter for designing the client's program. Subsequently, the health team should be involved in a total physical fitness program. This includes nurse, technician, physician, physical therapist, nutritionist, and others, as needed or as necessary. The form shown in Table 8–2 represents a sample of a prescription as just described.

The exercises should be demonstrated with a return demonstration if at all possible. The

---

TABLE 8–2. SAMPLE FITNESS PROGRAM PRESCRIPTION[a]

Exercise program for _____DATE _____

1. Warm-up exercises

    Check your pulse at the carotid
    a. Minutes of general body exercises
    b. Seconds, repeat times of flexibility exercises
    c. _____ (#number) _____ times of sit-ups
        _____ (#number) _____ times of push-ups
        for your muscular endurance exercises make sure you understand each of the exercise directions and what they are

2. General body exercises

    until heart rate reaches minimal threshold
    a. _____ is your heart rate target zone (MT)
    b. _____ (number of days) of week or _____ times a week
        Check carotid pulse (your heart rate) for 10 seconds, multiply by 6, to obtain your heart rate count
        Check your rate at the beginning of this program, after 1 minute of exercise, 3 minutes of exercise, 5 minutes of exercise until your heart rate reaches the target count set for you (see 2a above)

3. Cool-down activity

    a. _____ minutes of general body exercises
    b. _____ minutes of flexibility exercises

Nutritional plan

    Caloric Intake: _____ calories a day
Add _____ calories a day for each day of physical fitness activity

Call the health team or come to the clinic if you have questions or need information

Phone numbers are _____

[a]A sample prescription, would need adapting for each individual depending on need, tolerance level, or restrictions.
Ward's adapted prescription form, University of Texas at Arlington.

client should be given explicit instructions, i.e., demonstrations, printed copies of the different exercises, nutritional dietary description of caloric intake, which includes how to count and which food group selection matches the count, and how to count the pulse. The client should understand the limits of endurance, and how much exercise is enough for him or her. The minimal heart rate is computed several ways depending on who is doing the computations. A general rule of computation is to subtract the client's age from 220 to obtain the rate at which he or she should work up to but not beyond. This figure supposedly represents 60% of the maximum capability of the heart. Some health professionals assume a 70–80% percent maximum capability, however, the older client should know that a physical fitness program is a gift one gives to oneself. The results can bring the client an improved self-image and an improved independence; both factors are significant for the older individual. It is important that the client have follow-ups by phone and regular home or clinic visits.

Rest

Rest is that period of time during which the individual restores and energizes the power of concentration necessary for the well-being and for the performance of activities of daily life. Rest is not the opposite of fatigue, although fatigue may force the individual to rest. Rest is not necessarily sleep, although sleep is universally expected to result in rest. Much research has been published on the subject of sleep and the stages. The reader might be interested in pursuing the topic of sleep relative to the older individual (see Chap. 4). Rest does not mean inactivity, for the older person may be restoring and energizing by reading, playing checkers, spending time with his or her grandchildren, knitting, or enjoying a warm soaking bath or a whirlpool bath. The important factor is that physical activity such as walking, running, swimming, dancing, and so

on be interspersed with rest and relaxation. There is a time for both. Older clients may need teaching and counseling about the advantages of both rest and exercise and in pacing or planning activities with adequate rest. Counseling may be needed in directing the client to perform stretch and/or flexion exercises after a prolonged rest period such as a night of sleep.

Nutrition

The nutritional needs of the aging musculoskeletal system are related to maintenance of skeletal-muscle stability and energy. Whether loss of bone mass in the older client can be slowed or prevented by additions or changes in the nutritional intake is not conclusive. Data on dietary calcium intake have yielded conflicting conclusions. Older clients with osteoporosis usually have calcium deficiencies. Older clients do frequently reduce their dietary calcium intake. The relation of vitamin D to calcium absorption can also result in a calcium deficit. Ascorbic acid and protein (for connective tissue), trace minerals, fluoride, phosphate, and acid-ash have all been indicated in a healthy, adequate nutrition of the musculoskeletal system.

The older client should be cautioned to avoid fad or quack diets. There is little evidence that certain foods prevent, cause, or cure musculoskeletal problems. Clients should be counseled to maintain a balanced and varied diet. Attractive, nutritional food and fluids served in a pleasant environment with adequate time for eating should be a basic goal. Caloric intake should match the weight and activity level. Older clients should plan (with minimal help) their own food intake, their own time for eating, adding their own personal and cultural dietary preferences, including supplements if desired, eating out, and any other activity pertaining to their own nutrition. If diet therapy has been prescribed, then the client, nurse, and nutritionist should have joint counseling and teaching sessions to discuss why, with what, and how to implement the diet. The social worker may need to visit the client. Too often the older client is given a written diet and simply told to follow it. When the client fails to comply, health professionals rarely accept the fact that they did not do their job.

Safety

Safety should be a cornerstone in the life-style of the older client. Emphasis should be placed on prevention of injuries by practice of good body mechanics and environmental and home safety. The nurse's concern for the older client within the home environment is an important point in facilitating safety measures. Prevention of falls and injuries is paramount to maintenance of independence. The nurse must encourage use of handrails in the bathroom and on entrances and exits. Loose throw rugs, poor lighting, faulty electrical appliances, overloaded electrical circuits, and extension cords strung across the room are examples of hazards that invite danger and impair mobility. When these hazards are combined with arthritis or decreased visual acuity, the older person's chances for having an accident are increased. The older person should be counseled to avoid moving heavy objects or climbing on unstable surfaces. Clutter and poorly arranged rooms should be altered to provide a clear, smooth passage and walkway. Safety factors also include the wearing of appropriate clothing, i.e., shoes and robes, the use of walking devices such as canes, and the ensuring that heating and cooling equipment are appropriately installed and maintained. The older person should have a plan for crisis situations such as falling in the bathroom. Emergency phone numbers should be readily available; this also includes the number of a neighbor and a significant other. If economically feasible, the older client may use a beeper hook-up with an emergency or home visiting system of a hospital, provided the hospital has such a plan for the seniors in the community. Medications should be labeled and safely stored so that the older person does not accidently ingest a dangerous substance. Use of a walker, crutches, a cane, or a wheelchair al-

ways carries some degree of risk; the environmental home barriers may present safety hazards and limit the client's mobility. Clients using such appliances may have difficulty in moving up and down ramps or crossing streets as quickly as needed. The older client may stop using an appliance entirely if it inhibits mobility of daily living. Careful attention to a safe environment promotes a healthier independent life-style for the older person.

SUMMARY

Changes in the musculoskeletal system during aging can affect movement, motion, balance, stability, agility, endurance, coordination, and the general sense of well-being. These are the functions of the musculoskeletal system, and aging can affect these functions. The overall normal change in the musculoskeletal system is loss of bone mass. Osteoporosis reduces bone strength and increases the risk of fractures. Researchers have not found a preventive factor. Rheumatoid arthritis and osteoarthritis, two major types of arthritis, differ considerably in pathology and treatment. Research has brought new pharmacological products and surgical advances in joint reconstruction. Cure and prevention are still in the future, however, a balanced, individualized program of exercise, rest, and adequate nutrition is the mainstay of treatment for musculoskeletal problems.

The majority of older Americans are vigorous and independent whereas some 45% have a degree of limited ability. Arthritis affects 44% of those aged 65 and older (The Surgeon General's Report, 1979). The stereotype of a stooped, slow, clumsy, shuffling, and fragile old person is being questioned, as increased attention to physical fitness, healthy environment, and appropriate nutrition have increased the mobility and activity of the aged. While attitude toward the aged is slowly changing, American society is growing accustomed to and a little shocked in realizing that "you are as old as you feel." Old does begin to look better and better, the nearer and nearer it gets.

REFERENCES

Aloia, J. F. (1981). Exercise and skeletal health. *Journal of the American Geriatrics Society, 29,* (3), 104.

Avioli, L. V. (1981). Postmenopausal osteoporosis: Prevention versus care. *Federation Proceedings, 40,* 2418–2422.

Basu, T. K., Smethhurst, M., Gillett, M. B., Donaldson, D., Jordan, S. J., Williams, D. C., & Hicklin, J. A. (1978). Ascorbic acid therapy for relief of bone pain in Paget's disease. *Acta Vitaminologica et Enzymologica, 32,* 45–49.

Brocklehurst, J. C., Exton-Smith, A. N., Lempert-Barber, F. M., Hunt, L. P., & Palmer, M. K. (February, 1978). Fracture of the femur in old age: A two-center study of associated clinical factors and the cause of the fall. *Age and Aging, 7,* 2–15.

Brunner, L. S., & Suddarth, D. (1982). *The Lippincott manual of nursing practice* (3rd ed.). Philadelphia: Lippincott.

Burnside, I. W. (1981). *Nursing and the aged.* New York: McGraw-Hill.

Cerrato, P. D. (1987). What diet can do for your arthritic patient. *RN, 50*(9), 69–70.

Draper, H. H., & Scythes, C. A. (1981). Calcium, phosphorus, and osteoporosis. *Federation Proceedings, 40,* 2434–2438.

Ebersole, P., & Hess, P. (1981). *Toward healthy aging.* St. Louis: Mosby.

Eliopoulous, C. (1979). *Gerontological Nursing.* New York: Harper & Row.

Forbes, E. J., & Fitzsimons, V. M. (1981). *The older adult, a process for wellness.* St. Louis: Mosby.

Frankel, L. J., & Richard, B. B. (1980). *Be alive as you live.* New York: Lippincott and Crowell.

Furlow, R., Oberman, A., & Eggert, D. (1980). A step-by-step guide to exercise for the CAD patient. *Geriatrics, 35*(9), 41–43, 46–47.

Gallager, J. C., Riggs, B. L., Elisman, J., Hamstra, A., Arnaud, S. B., & Deluca, H. F. (1979). Intestinal calcium absorption and serum vitamin D metabolites in normal subjects and osteoporotic patients: Effects of age and dietary calcium. *Journal of Clinical Investigation, 64,* 729–736.

Gallager, J. C., Riggs, B. L., & Deluca, H. F. (1980). Effect of estrogen on calcium absorption and serum vitamin D metabolites in postmenopausal osteoporosis. *Journal of Clinical Endocrinology and Metabolism. 51,* 1359–1364.

Grob, D. (1978). Common disorders of muscles in the aged. In W. Reichel (Ed.), *Clinical aspects of aging.* Baltimore: Williams & Wilkins.

Grove, O., & Halver, B. (1981). Relief of osteoporotic backache with fluoride calcium and calciferol. *Acta Medica Scandinavica, 209,* 469–471.

Gutmann, E. (1977). Muscle. In C. E. Finch & L. Hayflick (Eds.), *Handbook of the biology of aging.* New York: Van Nostrand Reinhold.

Hellebrandt, F. A. (1979). Exercise for the long-term care aged—Benefits, deterrents, and hazards. *Long-Term Care and Health Services Administration Quarterly, 33*(1), 33–47.

Howard, R., & Herbold, N. (1978). *Nutrition in clinical care.* New York: McGraw-Hill.

Jahss, M. H. (1979). Geriatric aspects of the foot and ankle. In I. Rossman (Ed.), *Clinical geriatrics* (2nd ed.). Philadelphia: Lippincott.

Kart, C. S., Metress, E. S., & Metress, J. F. (1978). *Aging and health: Biologic and social perspectives.* Menlo Park, CA: Addison-Wesley.

Kolodny, A. L., & Kipper, A. R. (1976, November). Bone and joint diseases in the elderly. *Hospital Practice, 11,* 91–101.

Nordin, B. E., Horsman, A., Crilly, R. G., Marshal, D. H., & Simpson, M. (1980). Treatment of spinal osteoporosis in postmenopausal women. *British Medical Journal, 280,* 451–455.

Phipps, W., Long, B., & Woods, N. (1979). *Medical surgical nursing concepts and clinical practices.* St. Louis: Mosby.

Price, S., & Wilson, L. (1982). *Patho-physiology, clinical concepts of disease processes* (2nd ed.). New York: McGraw-Hill.

Riggs, B. L., Seeman, E., Hodgson, S. F., Taves, D. R., & Ofallon, W. M. (1982). Effect of the fluoride/calcium regimen on vertebral fracture occurrence in postmenopausal osteoporosis compared with conventional therapy. *New England Journal of Medicine, 306,* 446–450.

Rockstein, M. (1975). The biology of aging in humans—An overview. In R. Goldman & M. Rockstein (Eds.), *The physiology and pathology of human aging.* New York: Academic.

Shank, M. J., & Conrad, D. (1977). A survey of the

well-elderly: Their foot problems, practice and needs. *Journal of Gerontological Nursing, 3*(6), 10.

Shock, N. W. (1977). Systems integration. In C. E. Finch & L. Hayflick (Eds.), *Handbook of the biology of aging*. New York: Van Nostrand Reinhold.

Strandell, T. (1976). Cardiac output in old age. In F. I. Caird, J. L. C. Dale, & R. D. Kennedy (Eds.), *Cardiology in old age*. New York: Plenum.

The Surgeon General's Report on health promotion and disease prevention, healthy people. (1979). U. S. Department of Health, Education and Welfare.

Tonna, E. A. (1977). Aging of skeletal-dental systems and supporting tissues. In C. E. Finch & L. Hayflick (Eds.), *Handbook of the biology of aging*. New York: Van Nostrand Reinhold.

Welford, A. T. (1977). Motor performance. In J. Birren & K. W. Schaie (Eds.), *Handbook of the psychology of aging*. New York: Van Nostrand Reinhold.

9

ENDOCRINE CHANGES

The neuroendocrine regulatory system forms the basis for one of the hypotheses of the mechanism of aging: the completion of a genetic program of differentiation and development. Because very little is known about the biological nature of aging, the following discussion must be regarded with caution and at best viewed as hypothetical. The endocrine system involves key regulatory processes and clearly plays a critical role in human health. It is logical, therefore, that the endocrine system should play a key role in the changes that occur with aging. What are these changes which have come to be expected? Dilman (1981) offers the following: hyperinsulinemia; decreased tolerance of carbohydrates and insulin sensitivity; obesity; lipolysis and increased use of fatty acids; high blood levels of low-density-lipoproteins, triglycerides, and cholesterol; increased cortisol secretion; decreased output of androgen-like hormones (17-ketosteroids); decreased cellular immunity; increased secretion of total gonadotropins and total phenolsteroids; decreased output of estrogens; elevated blood pressure; diminished thyroid function; and production of a high titer of autoantibodies such as thyroglobulin antibodies.

Considering the numerous diseases and other pathology that affect the older person, endocrine problems cannot be viewed as distinct disorders. One must differentiate between changes that are normal concomitants of aging and changes that indicate the presence of an associated or underlying disease.

Primary alterations in most endocrine glands do not result from aging per se. The alterations in endocrine metabolism that do result from the aging process "seem to be secondary to changes in neural metabolism—and decreased target organ responsiveness—more than degenerative changes in the glands themselves" (O'Hara-Devereaux, Andrews & Scott, 1981). As reported by Davis and Davis (1983), primary endocrine problems in the older person have a relationship to the thyroid, parathyroid, and pancreatic glands. Those disorders are diabetes, hypothyroidism, and hyperthyroidism.

AGING OF THE ENDOCRINE SYSTEM

The aging pituitary and adrenal systems have been studied in experimental animals, but caution is needed in transposing animal models onto human systems. There is consensus that the physiology of the pituitary–adrenal–cortex–endocrine axis in the human does not change greatly with aging (Dilman, 1981; Davis & Davis, 1983; Wolfsen, 1982).

Adrenocortical disease is not common in older persons. In the rare instances when Addison's disease, Cushing's syndrome, or adrenal carcinoma occurs in the older client, the signs, medical treatment, and nursing care do not differ much from that in younger clients.

The syndromes of hyponatremia or hyperkalemia are common in older clients: the etiology is frequently iatrogenic, with diuretics and oral sulfonylurea agents usually implicated (Davis & Davis, 1983) (See Chapter 7).

In hypopituitarism and myxedema, the diminished metabolic heat production can result in hypothermia (Collins, 1983). Endogenous causes of accidental hypothermia can be labeled either impaired thermoregulation or impaired temperature discrimination. At least two empirical studies (Fox et al., 1973) which compared elderly and young subjects on thermoregulatory function tests found that older persons had impaired thermoregulatory capacity within the vasomotor control zone and were not able to adjust properly.

According to Exton-Smith (1981), the older client in a state of hypothermia has a gray coloring, puffy face, slow cerebration, and husky voice, with skin that is cold (even those parts normally covered) to the touch. The person may be confused. The heart rate is slow and respirations are slow and shallow. Oliguria is usually a symptom, and the blood sugar level is raised.

The older client should be covered with a light blanket and the body temperature permitted to rise slowly. Oxygen and intermittent positive pressure breathing treatment may be ordered by the physician. Central venous pressure should be monitored and warm, isotonic intravenous fluids administered. A wide-spectrum antibiotic is normally prescribed because older clients with hypothermia often have accompanying infection.

Nursing management includes monitoring of room temperature, administration of intravenous solutions, medications, and oxygen, monitoring of pulse, blood pressure, deep-body temperature, airway, and ECG measurements, and frequent turning, positioning, and skin care.

THYROID DYSFUNCTION

Anderson and Williams (1983) report that about 2% of older persons are affected with thyroid problems. Because the signs and symptoms of thyroid dysfunctions may be atypical, these problems may either be missed or misdiagnosed.

Hypothyroidism

Assessment Parameters
As in any age group, hypothyroidism in the older person is a gradual process. Complicating the diagnosis is the fact that the signs, symptoms, and conditions of hypothyroidism—a general slowness, weight gain, depression, constipation, strong reaction to cold environmental temperature, loss of hair, confusion, and hearing losses—also occur as normal concomitants of aging. Other signs for which the gerontological nurse practitioner should be vigilant are paresthesias—burning, tingling, numbness, muscular incoordination, and polyneuropathies. A slowed pulse may be a sign of hypothyroidism but may also be drug related or indicative of a number of other physical problems. The client with hypothyroidism may have a poor appetite and, as a result, may have nutritional deficits (Davis & Davis, 1983).

The older hypothyroid client may also be a diabetic. Approximately 2% of hypothyroid clients have been found to be diabetic. In recent years, older diabetics have been tested for thyroid function, which may be responsible for the coincidence of diabetes and hypothyroidism having been uncovered. Researchers have hypothesized that viral attacks may destroy a sufficient number of beta cells to create a condition of insulin dependence. The viral attack may confuse the body's defenses. The dead beta cells may be related to the body's response of treating its own insulin-producing cells as though they were dangerous. Research has uncovered an association between the insulin deficiency and islet-cell antibodies. Both problems—diabetes and thyroid deficiency—may be related to an abnormal autoimmune reaction (Melmed & Hershman, 1982).

Hyperthyroidism–Thyrotoxicosis

Assessment Parameters

As is true of hypothyroidism, the classical symptoms of hyperthyroidism are not always present. Signs in the older client may be atypical or share some similarities with the typical signs. Green (1981) found the most common presentations to be mental changes, arrhythmias, and heart failure. Rather than being anxious and overactive, these older clients were lethargic and apathetic.

Older persons who have been identified as thyrotoxic may display angina, heart failure, tachycardia, atrial fibrillation, and/or edema of the legs. The thyroid gland may or may not be enlarged. Eye signs, if present, are mild. These include a fixed stare and a widening of the palpebral fissures or the opening between the eyelids and lid lag. Blepharoptosis or drooping of the upper eyelid may also be present (Melmed & Hershman, 1982).

As with hypothyroidism, many older clients complain of constipation, weakness, and extreme fatigue. Some elderly clients with hyperthyroidism are also diabetic. Physiological studies that examine the relationship of thyroid hormones to the pathology of diabetes have shown that thyroid hormones, like the glucocorticoids, have an effect on hepatic carbohydrate metabolism. Glucose tolerance is decreased in the hyperthyroid client. This stems from an increase of carbohydrate absorption from the intestinal tract and an increase in glycogenolysis and gluconeogenesis in the liver (Davis & Davis, 1983).

Diabetes occurs in about 3% of persons who are diagnosed as hyperthyroid. If the diabetic client is losing weight, is unusually nervous, and complains of tachycardia, he or she should be assessed for a hyperthyroid condition. Generally, removal of the thyroid hyperfunction will result in a decreased requirement for insulin (Anderson & Williams, 1983).

Nursing Care Management

Nursing care interventions should focus on the diet, a self-medication system, an exercise and activity program, skin care, and management of depression.

Based on an assessment of the dietary habits of the client and family as well as general principles of good nutrition, a diet should be planned for the older person. The level of caloric intake should be prescribed by the physician. Adequate hydration and a certain amount of fruits and vegetables should be incorporated in the diet to prevent constipation. A stool softener or a laxative may be necessary if constipation persists and cannot be controlled by diet.

Because the client may be taking medication in addition to that prescribed for the thyroid imbalance, a medication history should be taken. It should include the client's medication-taking behavior, the effects and side effects of medications currently being taken, known drug allergies, patterns of medication use, specific beliefs about medicines, and the names of physicians and pharmacists with whom the client interacts.

If the client has a workable system of self-medication, the gerontological nurse practitioner may wish to periodically evaluate it for safety. If the client has difficulty in summarizing the medications taken each day, the gerontological nurse practitioner may jog the client's memory by asking about the timing of their administration in relation to other activities such as sleeping or eating. A chart or flow sheet may be useful to some clients. The chart provides a memory bank for the client and family and can be used by the gerontological nurse practitioner to assess patterns of taking medication.

Medication will be ordered by the physician for the thyrotoxic older client. It may be 3–6 months before the positive effects of the medication are felt. The nurse is responsible for noting when the medication has taken effect; this is particularly important because hypothyroidism may subsequently result if the medication continues to be taken.

Exercise is discussed in the section on diabetes. Activity may take the following forms: socialization, reading, gardening, reflection, television viewing, volunteering service and activities of daily living. The activity theory (Lemon, Bengston, & Peterson, 1972) provides a guide for the nurse to assist the older person in determining the levels of activity that may be appropriate for providing individualized satisfaction. Three types of activity are described in the theory: (1) informal activities, e.g., those of a social nature and involving relatives, friends, and neighbors; (2) formal activities, e.g., social interactions in voluntary organizations and the church; and (3) solitary activities, e.g., hobbies, hand work, and playing a musical instrument. Though there is physical decline in the aging person, many of these activities can be rewarding and need to be supported by the gerontological nurse practitioner.

Skin care of the thyroid client is important and should be included in the nursing plan. Principles of skin care for the thyroid client are similar to those discussed for the diabetic client.

Management of depression of the older thyroid client should not be overlooked by the nurse in planning care. Because depression is prevalent in the aged and a significant problem for the older thyroid client, Chapter 13 discusses the nursing interventions that assist the older depressed client.

OBESITY

Obesity is defined as weight that is 20% or more greater than the ideal weight for a given height, frame, and age, using weight and height charts established by the Metropolitan Insurance Company (MacBryde, 1964). *Overweight* was defined as being 10% over the ideal weight. The

Metropolitan charts were revised in February, 1983, at which time the preferred weight in all height categories was increased by 5–15% (Yen, 1983).

In a study of the elderly in Britain and America, 20–40% of elderly persons were found to be either obese or overweight (Runcie, 1978, p. 134). Of newly diagnosed diabetics above the age of 45, half were found to be obese (Runcie, 1978). It is believed that "successful and sustained weight loss will ameliorate or even reverse the disorder" (Runcie, 1978, p. 137). Nelson (1984, p. 19) is in agreement with this statement: "It is probably safe to say that most patients with NIDDM could quite literally cure their diabetes if they strictly adhered to their diets; as we all are aware, however, they generally do not."

Assessment Parameters

There is agreement on the special features of obesity in older persons (Yen, 1983; Runcie, 1978; Cozens, 1982; Bernstein, 1983). Obesity is generally a problem that the aged client has had for a number of years. As a result, he or she lacks a positive attitude, which, in turn, complicates health management. The obese client is at risk for additional health problems, namely diabetes mellitus, cardiovascular and hypertensive disease, and osteoarthritis of the weight-bearing joints. These conditions may be accompanied by additional physiological problems. Increased ventilatory failure, which results in chronic carbon dioxide narcosis, is not uncommon.

Nursing Care Management

Reduction in food intake is the therapy of choice but is often ineffective owing to noncompliance. Certain medications may help, but drug therapy for the older client carries a number of risks and is not preferred. If medication is used, the lowest possible dosage is recommended (Bernstein, 1983).

Amphetamines have been prescribed for

obesity. They have widespread effects resulting from catecholamine release and a number of particularly troublesome side effects, including nervous system irritability, cardiac arrhythmias, hypertension, acute glaucoma, and urine retention in the male. Contraindications include glaucoma and arteriosclerosis. Additionally, amphetamines are addictive, and the elderly have an increased susceptibility to drug toxicity (Lamy, 1984).

Albaneze (1980) claims that obesity is generally the result of eating a little extra each day and not exercising sufficiently to offset the additional extra calories. He advocates a balance between caloric intake and daily exercise with emphasis placed on exercise occurring on a daily basis in order to counteract the calories consumed that day.

If the client is bedridden or wheelchair-bound, weight reduction may be difficult or impossible. Although the diet must still be controlled, exercise may be limited. Some research shows that older persons can retain a healthful status while weighing more than they did when they were younger. There may even be some positive aspects to moderate obesity (Yen, 1983). For the obese diabetic client, however, weight reduction is preferred. To assist the diabetic client in adhering to the diet and exercise plan, the gerontological nurse practitioner could implement the following:

1. Assess the health care beliefs and patterns of the client and family
2. Clarify misperceptions and identify irrational beliefs
3. Provide reading materials that have been prepared specifically for the layperson and are clearly understandable
4. Develop an accepting and supportive environment conducive to learning
5. Teach the client about the power for change that exists within each person

Some specific suggestions the gerontological nurse practitioner could make are the following:

1. Record all the food eaten
2. Eat only while sitting at the table
3. Place the appropriate portions on the plate; avoid family-style meals
4. Reduce the amount and types of food kept stored in the home

DIABETES

Hyperglycemic Hyperosmolar Nonketotic Precoma and Coma

Onset of diabetes mellitus in an older person is insidious. Hyperosmolar nonketotic coma may be the first indication of the problem. Extreme hyperglycemia and dehydration are probably antecedents. These hidden alterations may occur in the older person whose diabetes is regulated or in the older person who has not been diagnosed as a diabetic. According to Williams (1978), the characteristics of hyperosmolar nonketotic coma are (1) plasma glucose level generally in excess of 1000 mg/dl, (2) serum osmolality frequently greater than 350 mOsm/L, (3) elevated serum sodium levels, and (4) absence of ketosis and acidosis due to lactic acid.

As is typical in diabetes, stress seems to be implicated in the development of hyperosmolar coma. The time period of development may extend for 12–14 days (Williams, 1978). Assessment of the older person, whether or not he or she has been diagnosed as diabetic, must be regular and frequent. Any change that could be perceived by the older person as a stressor should alert the gerontological nurse practitioner to increase vigilance in observation. Shock or dehydration are obvious problems. Glycosuria may be present. A change in cognitive functioning that is unrelated to other known factors in the client's situation may be a symptom.

Shuman (1984) believed that severe stress, infection, acute vascular and medical emergencies, and omissions of insulin are factors in hyperosmolar nonketotic coma as well as ketoacidosis and ketotic coma. Blood glucose levels must be tested immediately in the older comatose client. Depending on the severity of ketoacidosis, 10–20 units of regular insulin are initially administered intravenously or intramuscularly followed by 0.1 U/kg/hr for 4–6 hours. Blood glucose is checked every 2 hours.

Interdependent nursing actions involve administration of intravenous fluids and insulin. Continuous monitoring and accurate evaluation are mandatory. In the older client, the infusion rate for intravenous fluids is adjusted downward. Shuman (1984, p. 72) recommends 250–500 ml/hr less than normal. The physician may order central venous pressure monitoring and potassium supplements. Independent nursing management calls for measuring urinary output and observing for venous thrombosis and signs of embolism. Daily weight should be recorded. The skin and mouth must be inspected daily. The skin may be dry, thin, inflamed, cracked, or broken. The mouth is examined for signs of nutrient imbalance, such as stomatitis, glossitis, gingivitis, raw tongue, and soft, spongy bleeding gums (Beattie & Louis, 1983). Blood pressure should be taken regularly. When the client is able, fluids by mouth should be given in ample amounts and should be measured and recorded.

Assessment Parameters

A complete data base is desirable when assessing the health status of an individual. Although a comprehensive survey is beneficial, the older client may not wish to spend the time needed for a complete data base at one visit, in which case the information may be collected over several visits. At the initial visit, that data specific to the diabetic management must be collected.

The gerontological nurse practitioner should be sensitive to the knowledge that the diabetic problems are permanent for the client. Additionally, the diagnosis of diabetes for the older client will involve major changes in patterns of living and coping. This constitutes a situation of considerable stress. The nurse should keep in mind that health care actions will be implemented by the client or family members in the home setting.

Because older persons have normally been caring for themselves for many years, they may have accumulated considerable knowledge and experience regarding what is useful and helpful when health problems occur. These methods and techniques should be acknowledged and supported by the gerontological nurse practitioner. Older clients expressing interest should be supported in their desire to participate in all phases of the nursing process.

The initial assessment must include the following: income, coping mechanisms, level of understanding, readiness to learn, interest in self-care, exercise pattern, and diet patterns. Physical areas to be examined are weight, skin, eyes, mouth, hands and fingers, and legs and feet. Indications of urinary tract and vaginal infection should be elicited. The occurrence of headaches and dizziness should be determined.

During the continued assessment process, the data base is completed by gathering information in the following general categories: family demographic information, health history, review of systems, laboratory and other diagnostic values, and medications. In addition, health practices and patterns of functioning are important areas to be explored. During the interview, the client should be made aware of available and appropriate community resources.

Nursing Care Management

Diabetic Diet. Most older persons with diabetes can successfully maintain their health status if their diet is kept within the recommended guidelines. According to Fitzgerald (1978), when dealing with persons over 60 years of age who have difficulty in learning the principles of diet and nutrition, it may be more useful for the health care provider to recommend regular meals and overall caloric limitations than discuss what percentage of the diet should be allowed for proteins, carbohydrates, and fats.

Albaneze (1980) recommended that the daily diet of older persons contain 20% protein, 40% carbohydrates, and 40% fats. The revised guidelines of the American Diabetes Association for diabetics of all ages are 12% protein, 50–60% carbohydrates, and 20–30% fats (Nemchik, 1982). Research studies have found that animal fats are associated with cardiovascular disease; the American Diabetes Association exchange system has therefore divided meats into those of high, medium, and low fat content to assist planners and clients in more accurately determining the fat allowances (Nemchik, 1982). Podolsky and El-Beheri (1984), in discussing recent changes in the dietary management of diabetes, stated that atherosclerosis is now the most common complication of diabetes. The goal of the current methods is the prevention of atherosclerotic disease. Nelson (1984) maintained that, because of the possibility of atherogenesis and hypercholesterolemia, saturated fats should never exceed 10% of the total calories and cholesterol intake must be kept to under 300 mg daily.

Regarding carbohydrates, Podolsky and El-Beheri (1984) disclosed that, when the total caloric intake is controlled, diabetics can tolerate a high carbohydrate content. This would tend to support Fitzgerald's (1978) belief that discussing regular meals and overall caloric intake with the older person is more important than focusing on percentages of proteins, carbohydrates, and fats. Podolsky and El-Beheri (1984) present evidence linking the low-fat, high-starch diets in certain parts of the world with a low incidence of atherosclerosis. Diabetes was found to be negatively associated with starch consumption, that is, its rates were lowest in societies where the consumption of starch is highest, and vice versa (Podolsky & El-Beheri, 1984).

Though increased carbohydrate levels have been advocated for the diabetic, simple sugars must still be limited. Therefore, the increase in carbohydrates must come from complex carbohydrates or starches. These are digested more slowly than simple sugars, so that there is a less severe rise in postprandial blood glucose levels. Complex carbohydrates are found in rice, corn, potatoes, and white bread. The suggested breakdown within the carbohydrate category from the American Diabetes Association is 30–45%

starch and 5–15% sugars, primarily natural sugars which are found in fruit and milk (Crapo, 1981). Jenkins and colleagues (1981) cautioned that because there are significant differences in blood glucose and insulin levels due to different carbohydrates, prediction of physiological response must take into account all three categories (proteins, carbohydrates, and fats) and not only carbohydrate content. These researchers believed that classifying foods according to their effect on blood glucose would be more useful in terms of controlling by diet rather than the classification used now. Skyler, Beatty, and Goldbert (1984) emphasized use of the glycemic index approach and called for a full re-evaluation of the glycemic index of menus and specific foods.

In this appraisal of carbohydrates and dietary management of the older diabetic, Albaneze (1980) expressed support for fructose, which, unlike glucose, is metabolized by certain enzymes, is used almost solely by liver tissues, and is absorbed independently of insulin. His research has demonstrated that, unlike glucose utilization, which decreases conspicuously with age, fructose utilization is affected very little by a person's age. The inference drawn from these studies is that fructose-containing foods, such as fruits, some green vegetables, and honey are a better source of sugars for the older diabetic.

In their studies of complex carbohydrates, specifically starches, O'Dea, Nestel, and Antonoff (1980) found significant differences in blood glucose and insulin levels between the ground rices and the unground rices, with the ground rices showing increased levels. The implication of this seems to be that the physical form of the rice is more important than the fiber in determining postprandial glucose and insulin responses. Certain starches may, therefore, be more beneficial for the diabetic than others.

Though this knowledge may be useful to practitioners, Crapo (1981) advised that such studies as O'Dea and colleagues (1980) conducted have tested a single isolated food, and the results may differ greatly in a clinical setting. Further studies that involve different amounts and mixtures of starches are needed. Additionally, considering the incidence of chronic illness in older persons, it is possible that other agents are responsible for altering the metabolic effect. This should not discourage the gerontological nurse practitioner who gives care to older diabetics. New hypotheses should first be tested and conclusions drawn with great care. For example, the possibility exists that the need for oral hypoglycemia medication may be lower in the client who has a higher intake of complex carbohydrates.

Should high-fiber diets be recommended for older diabetics? Whole grains, bran and whole grain cereals, whole grain flours, most common garden vegetables, beans, and fresh fruit are good sources of fiber. Anderson and Chandler (1981) presented research findings that support the use of a high-fiber diet in adult diabetics. They indicated that they have used the high-carbohydrate, high-fiber diet (HCF) for a number of years and that motivated clients followed the diet and did not have untoward side effects. Nelson (1984) agreed with these findings.

Anderson and Chandler (1981) asked each client in their study to institute a regular exercise program. The insulin dosage for these clients was adjusted to achieve fasting plasma glucose values of approximately 150 mg/dl. Insulin requirements dropped so dramatically that 13 of the 16 clients no longer needed their insulin during the study. An additional bonus of the diet was a reduction in blood lipid concentrations.

These researchers maintain that their high-fiber diet can be started with outpatients. Clients must follow the diet carefully, however. If the plan is neglected, fasting serum tryglyceride values quickly escalate to abnormally high levels.

Because older persons tend to gain weight, this diet may be advantageous for the older obese client. Anderson and Chandler (1981) claimed that the high-fiber maintenance diet is very effective for obese diabetics. In support of this diet, the researchers relate that, other than increased flatulence, they have found no side effects. They do emphasize the need for motivation on the part of the client. Because

shopping and food preparation patterns may need to be changed, some clients will refuse to alter their diets, regardless of the benefits. Two of the benefits that were anticipated of the diet were a reduction in diabetic complications and atherosclerotic vascular disease.

The User's Guide to HCF Diets may be obtained from: HCF Diabetes Foundation, 1872 Blairmore Road, Lexington, KY 40502.

With the older client and family who are interested in self-care and learning, the teaching in general can focus on the exchange program or the point program, taking into consideration the client's individual situation. An important concept to remember when working with the older client and family to develop a diet plan is that the usual patterns of living—purchasing, preparing, and consuming of food—should change as little as possible.

Albeneze (1980) specified that, for older nonoverweight clients, the daily calories should generally total 1500 for females and 2100 for males. There is agreement in the literature that older clients who are not overweight must consume an adequate number of calories each day. Otherwise, the client with insufficient calories that day will not receive the necessary protein. To support the use of counting calories with no overdue focus on distribution of proteins and fats, Stucky (1982) noted that, when calories and carbohydrates are controlled, fats are self-regulated as a result. In general, however, each client's meal plan must be determined by checking and adjusting according to the needs observed, the diet prescription, and the patterns developed.

To assist clients with the diet, the gerontological nurse practitioner may recommend the use of one of two plans: the exchange list for meal planning or the point system. The exchange list has been supported by the American Diabetes Association since 1950. Six food groups comprise this program. Depending on the prescribed diet plan, the client may exchange foods within allowed groups. The American Diabetes Association or American Dietetic Association can provide the Exchange List for Meal Planning: American Diabetes Association, Inc., 2

Park Avenue, New York, NY 10016; and from: American Dietetic Association, 430 North Michigan Avenue, Chicago, IL 60611.

The point system comprises three nutrient groups and one calorie group. Within this system, the client selects foods that provide the prescribed number of calories and percentage of carbohydrates. As in the exchange system, proteins, fats, and carbohydrates are considered. Materials on the point system are available from: Kansas Wheat Commission, 1021 North Main Street, Hutchinson, KS 67501.

Within the assessment of the older diabetic person and family, the history and habits sections must be detailed and inclusive of diet and nutrition. The usual patterns of purchasing, preparing, and consuming of foods should be delineated; planning with the client and family is essential to keep changes minimal. The emphasis needs to be on ease and simplicity for the client and family. When the client and family are in agreement with the formulated objectives, there is an increased likelihood that they will cooperate and continue to maintain the methods to meet the objectives.

The elderly use many drugs, both prescribed and over-the-counter, and these may inhibit synthesis of food nutrients. However, adequate nutrition may be important in the proper distribution and use of necessary drugs.

According to Albaneze (1980), salicylates have a serious effect on carbohydrate metabolism. When given in large doses over a prolonged period, salicylates will reduce blood sugar levels.

Prolonged treatment of arthritic symptoms with corticosteroids may cause abnormal protein breakdown, with loss of nitrogen and certain electrolytes. Albaneze (1980) listed the following as some of the attendant problems: hyperglycemia, glycosuria, and steroid diabetes.

The effects of alcohol on the diet are well known: malabsorption of food nutrients, alteration in absorption of medications, and drug interactions. Especially notable for this discussion is the change in rate of metabolism possible when alcohol and tolbutamide are found to-

gether. As more alcohol is ingested the metabolic rate rises (Albaneze, 1980). Nelson (1984) warned that fat intake must be reduced if alcohol is to be consumed. If the client has been fasting, alcohol may cause hypoglycemia. Further, Diabinese has a definite Antabuse-like effect. Finally, consumption of alcohol may aggravate hypertriglyceridemia. Many older persons consume alcohol on a daily basis. A number of these same persons may be taking tolbutamide; therefore, caution is urged.

Exercise. Pacing is critical for the older person who is beginning an exercise program. Rhythm and regularity are important, so that exercise should be planned to occur at the same time each day. Exercise should be alternated with periods of rest.

An exercise program for the older client should be formally planned and evaluated. Considerations should include body temperature, blood pressure, presence of pain, and time interval from the previous meal.

The motion in the various joints should be assessed. The nurse can use the Evaluation of Range of Motion Chart (Kamenetz, 1976) at the time of initial assessment and to record progress. Exercises for the elderly have been developed by Kamenetz (1976). He presents ground rules and instructions along with illustrations to assist the client and the gerontological nurse practitioner.

Harris (1983) acknowledged that, although exercise probably does not extend life, some research indicates that exercise and motion can improve the quality of life and may delay or prevent some of the changes that occur with aging. He designated the following as desired client outcomes of proper physical exercise for the older person: maintenance and improvement of physical fitness, better joint flexibility, stronger muscles, increased mobility, and improved neuromuscular coordination and cardiovascular fitness. For the older client, exercise should be prescribed only after a thorough physical assessment has been completed. Even then, the prescribed movements should be those developed for the older person.

As a result of a planned and conscientiously followed exercise program, the older person can expect results in several areas. According to Harris (1983), the walking pattern can be improved and the loss of equilibrium reduced. He contended that partial improvements may be made in the musculoskeletal, respiratory, cardiovascular, and central nervous systems. Additionally, exercise can reduce fatigue, stimulate metabolism, help digestion, and assist with bowel elimination.

Harris (1983) held that there are psychological benefits to be gained from regular exercise, including an outlet for the tensions and worries of daily life and improvements in the client's overall sense of well-being and sleep patterns. He indicated that carefully designed exercise will also help channel aggressive feelings and provide emotional satisfaction.

Exercise for the older person must be approached with care. The criteria that must be considered include at least the following: age, sex, overall physical ability of the individual, and the kind of exercise and length of time needed to perform the specific exercise. For the older client, stretching while still in bed is a safe way to loosen up muscles and joints. Calisthenics can safely be performed if done slowly. For ambulatory clients, walking is a safe and effective exercise. Walking at a prescribed rate and distance is recommended as long as the individual does not encounter shortness of breath, chest pain, or significant increases in heart rate. According to Fuller (1982, p. 95) walking at a rate of 1–2 mph on level ground is ineffective; however, moderate endurance can be developed if a person walks at a rate of 3 mph on level ground continuously for 15–30 minutes, good endurance developed by increasing the rate to $3\frac{1}{2}$–4 mph, and excellent conditioning achieved by increasing the rate to 5 mph. Alternative forms of exercise include cycling, riding a stationary bicycle, and swimming (Ullrich, 1984).

Range-of-motion exercise should be a part of activities of daily living. For the client with a metabolic problem who is not able to walk on a daily basis, the range-of-motion exercises and

exercises for the elderly can be performed either alone, with the family, or as a member of a group. Group exercise lends itself to increased motivation and enjoyment.

There is an abundance of literature including studies on exercise and its benefits for persons of all ages. Cardiovascular specialists have reported the findings of numerous empirical studies on the positive aspects of exercise. These studies have included persons above 60 years of age. Two nurses, Holm and Kirchoff (1984), reviewed the literature on aging and exercise and reported on approximately 47 studies. They maintain that more information is needed on the relationship between exercise and the health of the elderly. In general, the studies indicated that exercise provides physiological and psychological benefits to older persons.

For the diabetic client, the knowledge that exercise alters the balance between glucagon and insulin is important. When the glucagon supply is increased, the glucose in the extracellular fluid is also increased. With exercise, there is an increased need for glucose in the muscles. The diabetic who exercises 30 minutes or more daily may show approximately a 30–40% decrease in the need for insulin. Utilization of glucose is increased 7–20 times during exercise. The diabetic who exercises will have a reduced need for insulin and, at the same time, an improved glucose tolerance. Exercise can lower the blood glucose level without insulin, and calories will be used, thus retarding complications, promoting weight loss, and contributing to well-being (Nelson, 1984; Felig, 1981).

General rules for the older diabetic regarding exercise are the following:

1. Exercise the same amount each day
2. Exercise at the same time each day
3. Exercise when blood glucose level is high, after a meal
4. If taking insulin, the abdomen is a good site if the insulin is injected prior to exercise

In discussing exercise as one aspect of the treatment of non-insulin dependent diabetes

(NIDDM), Nelson (1984) advised that exercise sessions should begin with 5–10 minutes of stretching. Following that, the exercise should consist of 20–30 minutes of "strenuous exercise at a level of intensity sufficient to maintain the pulse rate at 75% of the maximal heart-rate response." The maximum heart rate can be estimated by subtracting one's chronological age from 220. The cool-down period, like the warm-up, should include about 5–10 minutes of stretching. These sessions should be practiced a minimum of three times weekly to receive the fitness benefits.

Medications. Though there has been some controversy over the results of the University Group Diabetes Program (UGDP) study of hypoglycemia agents (Seltzer, 1972), oral medications are used by some physicians as the therapeutic adjunct to diet control for the older client. Other physicians use insulin with diet regardless of the age of the client.

The UGDP was undertaken in 1961 to study blood glucose levels and whether control of blood glucose levels would be a factor in preventing or delaying vascular disease in persons who require insulin. About 1027 patients comprised the sample group which was derived from 12 university-affiliated clinics.

The major conclusions of the UGDP research were as follows:

1. Diet and either tolbutamide or phenformin together are no more effective than diet alone in prolonging life
2. Diet and either tolbutamide or phenformin may be less effective than diet alone or diet and insulin, in regard to cardiovascular mortality

Due to a fair number of problems in the methodology of the UGDP study, the conclusions were questioned. Skillman (1984, p. 77), referring to a 1979 policy statement regarding the UGDP controversy, stated that sulfonylurea drugs are now considered "effective when used in concert with diet, exercise, and monitoring."

ORAL HYPOGLYCEMIA DRUGS. The oral hypoglycemia agents fall into two categories: sulfonylureas and biguanides.

Although the pharmacological action of the sulfonylureas is not entirely clear, research seems to indicate that these drugs stimulate the pancreatic islet cells to secrete insulin, resulting in a decrease in blood glucose. The oral hypoglycemic drugs are prescribed only for type II diabetics (persons with adult-onset diabetes). Within that category, the drugs are given only to those type II diabetics for whom dietary control alone has failed. If the diabetic has good control with dietary management, that person should not be taking an oral hypoglycemia drug. Clients and their families should be taught that the oral hypoglycemia agents can cause complications. Even though there has been much controversy over the UGDP study, clients should be alerted to the information regarding a possible increased incidence of cardiovascular problems and cardiovascular fatalities as a result of the use of oral hypoglycemia drugs.

The current position of the American Diabetes Association is that the UGDP study does not warrant government restrictions on the use of oral hypoglycemia agents. The association does support the finding that diet is the important factor in treating type II diabetes. Physicians believe that, when dietary management fails, insulin and diet are a safer combination than oral hypoglycemics and diet, particularly for the younger type II diabetic who may have many years to develop and live with complications that may result from oral hypoglycemics (Nemchik, 1982).

The four principal sulfonylureas used in the United States are tolbutamide, acetohexamide, chlorpropamide, and tolazamide. These drugs differ in their duration of action, metabolism, and excretion.

The oldest hypoglycemia agent is tolbutamide (Orinase). Its action lasts only about 8 hours, and it is rapidly excreted. Because it is absorbed in a rather short time, it may be given several times each day. The dosage is 0.5–3.0 grams (Vestal, 1984).

Chlorpropamide (Diabinese) is the longest acting sulfonylurea, having a duration of action of about 24 hours. It takes approximately 8 days for Diabinese to be excreted in the urine. In the older person, whose diet may be irregular in terms of time and inconsistent in type of nutrients, the long action of this drug may be a factor in a hypoglycemic reaction. Because the effects of accumulation may be insidious, the potential for problems should be noted. The dosage range for Diabinese is 0.1–0.5 grams (Vestal, 1984).

Acetohexamide (Dymelor) may cause hypoglycemia due to its cumulative effects. Because it assists in the elimination of uric acid, Dymelor may be advantageous for the diabetic patient who also has gout. Its duration of action is between 12 and 24 hours, and its dosage range is 0.25–1.25 grams (Vestal, 1984).

Tolazamide (Tolinase) is the newest of these four sulfonylureas. It acts about twice as long as Orinase and does not accumulate in the blood. The dosage is 0.1–0.75 grams (Vestal, 1984).

The side effects are similar for all four agents. The oral hypoglycemia drugs can produce jaundice, gastrointestinal and hematological disorders, skin reactions, hypoglycemia, and hypothyroidism (Vestal, 1984).

The patient who is taking the oral hypoglycemic medication needs to know what the medicine is, how it works in the body, and how long it remains in the body. The gerontological nurse practitioner needs to instruct clients in the relationship between the medication and their diet and eating patterns. Additionally, the client and family should know that exercise can make a difference both in the amount of medication and amount and type of food needed by the body.

The gerontological nurse practitioner should be aware of the interactions of hypoglycemia agents with other drugs. Increased blood glucose levels are caused by Dilantin, corticosteroids, estrogens, nicotinic acid, oral contraceptives, and the following diuretics—thiazides, chlorthalidone, ethacrynic acid, and furosemide. Medications that tend to lower blood glucose levels are salicylates, monoamine oxidase inhibitors, oral anticoagulants, phenylbutazone, phenyramidol, probenecid, sulfinpyrazone, and sulfonamides. Alcohol and Inderal can either raise or lower the blood glucose level depending on the amount taken and other unknown factors (Vestal, 1984).

The second category of oral hypoglycemia agents are the biguanides. These drugs—phenformin and metformin—are not available in the United States. The biguanides were associated with lactic acidosis, particularly in elderly clients, and were implicated in several deaths. Subsequently, the U.S. Food and Drug Administration banned the biguanides in the United States (Nemchik, 1982).

A second generation of sulfonylureas is now available. Glyburide (Micronase or Diabeta) is the first of these newer drugs. Its effects last from 12 to 24 hours. The second drug, glipizine (Glucotrol), has a duration of 10–18 hours. These agents may prove to be useful for clients who are not able to tolerate the other oral hypoglycemia agents. Among the advantages of these second-generation drugs are (1) they are 100–200 times more potent than the first-generation agents, (2) they have a higher rate of long-term success, (3) they may be given in lower doses, and (4) side effects and drug-induced toxicity may be decreased (Nelson, 1984; Nemchik, 1982; Skillman, 1984).

INSULIN THERAPY. The use of insulin with the older diabetic person is similar to its use in younger diabetics, and a standard medical–surgical nursing textbook may be consulted for a general overview of insulin therapy. There are a number of additional factors to consider in treating older diabetics, however: (1) visual impairment, (2) decreased manual dexterity, (3) decrease in overall energy and motivation, (4) altered tubule reabsorption, (5) decreased subcutaneous fat, (6) fixed income, (7) loss of what may previously have been considered good health, and (8) alterations in coping ability.

If the client's vision and manual skill are greatly diminished, a family member or other responsible adult will need to administer the insulin. Arthritic joints may constitute part of the problem. Practice time may need to be extended. If a family member is not available, the community health nurse may become the actual care provider. The nurse may either administer the insulin or prepare a 1-week supply of labeled insulin syringes and leave them in the refrigerator. If the latter is the case, specific instructions must be written out by the nurse, including the times and sites for administration. These instructions should be reviewed verbally at the time of each nurse visit. The nurse should proceed with the teaching at a slow pace and allow time for discussion and questions.

A decrease in overall energy and a possible decrease in motivation may be related. There is obviously a physiological rationale for the decrease in overall energy that accompanies aging, for aging certainly involves physical change and decline. The reduction in physical energy, resiliency, and strength also has a definite effect on behavior. In older age, the difficulties of physiological function and susceptibility to fatigue may require greater attention by the client and family. Another reason for a decrease in energy may be depression; however, hypoglycemia should also be suspected. On the other hand, the older client who has been diagnosed as diabetic may need to move into a new role, and it may be possible to motivate him or her by a new set of expectations and by a new set of approvals from a different group of persons—health care providers.

Problems in tubule reabsorption of glucose can create havoc with urine tests. With the aging diabetic, there may be glomerulosclerosis. In this condition, the capillary basement membrane thickens. Capillary openings reduce and can become occluded. As renal function becomes increasingly impaired, there is a decrease in glycosuria. This is due to a decrease in glomerular filtration, thus permitting a greater proportion of the filtered glucose to be resorbed.

The decrease in fatty tissue under the skin is a concern when injection sites are being planned and when the technique of injection is being taught. Instruction should include site rotation and the angle and depth of injection. The injection of insulin should be rotated among several areas of the body: upper arms, abdomen, and thigh. Within each of these areas, the section can be further divided into eight 1-inch squares. This provides 48 different subsections for injection which can be rotated systematically. The angle of the needle is important because the insulin should be injected into the subcutaneous area, which is beneath the fatty layer. The subcutaneous area can be located by pulling up the tissue to separate the subcutaneous portion from the muscle. The needle is then inserted at a 90-degree angle into the pinched tissue. There are difficulties associated with administration in both the thin and the obese elderly person: the former has little fat under the skin and must take care to avoid injecting the insulin into muscle; and the obese client will need a longer needle in order to assure reaching the subcutaneous area. In general, for the older person, fat deposits tend to disappear in the periphery of the body, whereas fat persists in the abdominal section (Anderson & Chandler, 1981).

Changes in the economy have made the fixed income a frightening concept. The client whose ability to purchase adequate and appropriate foods is limited by financial constraints may be assisted by Title VII nutrition programs. Food cooperatives, which encourage community, backyard and container gardens, and gleaning, may be a help. Other alternatives may be food stamps and Supplemental Security Income. Any treatment must be carefully evaluated in terms of cost and benefits. Letters from physicians to third-party payers are generally useful. The refiling of claims may result in a sufficient return to be worth the effort.

Though the older client who must begin insulin therapy may view the move negatively and as yet another burden on present coping mechanisms, the gerontological nurse practitioner can emphasize the positive benefits of predictability and control. The gerontological nurse practitioner can begin by supplying information about the effects and use of insulin therapy in the older person. Such information may need to be shared regularly: it is also helpful if crucial material is written down so that the client can keep it readily available. The gerontological nurse practitioner should next inquire about the client's present routine; planning with the client and supportive family members can then ensure that few changes are made in the daily routine. This will reduce the number of stressors introduced into the immediate environment. Both of these interventions are designed to lower anxiety.

The client should be informed that transitions, losses, and illnesses are stressors that need to be managed. The gerontological nurse practitioner can begin in the management of the client's stress by encouraging the client to undertake self-care efforts, verbally emphasizing the client's health rather than illness, and being present for the client. Though there are others, five approaches to the management of stress are presented here: relaxation techniques; meditation; imagery or visualization; exercise and yoga; and massage.

Specific relaxation techniques include progressive relaxation, biofeedback, autogenic training, and certain exercises. Progressive relaxation is a systematic method of tensing and relaxing sets of muscles to achieve a relaxed state. The gerontological nurse practitioner can either lead the individual or act as the leader of a group of persons, or the nurse can teach the individual or the group the method. Biofeedback uses instrumentation to give the client information about brain-wave activity. Knowledge of this activity gives the client a degree of control over internal functions of the body such as heart rate and dilation of blood vessels. Biofeedback is useful in achieving states of relaxation; the client can receive a measurement of his or her degree of relaxation. Autogenic training is a form of self-hypnosis that produces relaxation. Two basic exercises that the gerontological nurse practitioner

can use with older clients to induce a relaxed state are described as follows:

- Identify the stressor(s)
- Briefly discuss the stressful situation
- Discuss the benefits of relaxation
- Verbally list the steps of the exercise
    Sit in a comfortable chair with eyes closed
    Inhale deeply and hold breath for a short period of time while thinking "I am"
    Exhale slowly through pursed lips while thinking "relaxed"

The inhalation and exhalation while thinking "I am relaxed" is repeated five to ten times.

The second set of exercises is similar in all respects with the exception of the thinking portion. In this exercise, the client goes from head to toe thinking a phrase appropriate to the part of the body, such as "my left leg and foot are heavy and warm." Both of the above exercises can be performed twice daily. Each time should take about 10 minutes. The instructions should be written down if the nurse is teaching the client to do the exercises on a self-care basis. The nurse should assist the client in the initial learning sessions by being present, verbally giving instruction, praising the client for completing the exercise, and emphasizing the positive feeling of relaxation at the completion of the exercise. Additional relaxation training programs are available from Simonton, Matthews-Simonton, and Creighton (1979) and Jasmin and Trygstad (1979).

Meditation can take many forms. All forms are aimed at achieving the same effect: a particular level of concentration. The easiest type of meditation is the repetition of a single word or phrase over and over. The nurse should have the client become comfortable in a sitting or a lying position. The client can select the word or phrase for repetition. The word or phrase does not have to have any meaning. Practice of this exercise should allow the client to achieve higher levels of concentration, thus relieving stress and anxiety. This exercise can be performed whenever necessary (Benson & Proctor, 1984; Benson, 1980; Bolen, 1973).

Imagery is also known as visualization and imaging. Imagery is a means of altering emotions through creating mental images or pictures. Physical changes can occur as a result of changes in emotional states. There are variations in the process of imagery when used by different practitioners for differing purposes. Simonton, who worked with oncology clients, used visualization within relaxation techniques. He asked his clients to see their cancer, visualize positive effects of their therapies, think about and see the immune system destroying malignant cells, and picture themselves as well again. Therapists who espouse the Jungian theories name subcategories of visualization: directed daydreams, behaviorist desensitization, healing, guided effective imagery, and psychosynthesis. The gerontological nurse practitioner can use the process of imagery with older diabetic clients by first seeing that they are made comfortable and then having them complete one of the relaxation processes. Then the client should picture the stressor(s). Next the client needs to see the therapy(ies) working to remove the stressor(s). Lastly, the client should see the stressor(s) removed from the mind/body and feel free of the stressor(s) (Brown, 1984; Dychtwald, 1984; Horowitz, 1970; Samuels & Samuels, 1975).

Exercise and its benefits for the older client are discussed earlier in the chapter. The range-of-motion exercises and other exercises by Kamenetz can be used or another system may be selected. There are numerous books that describe exercises for the older person. Yoga is a training discipline that also has an extensive body of literature to support its beneficial use. Essentially, it consists of a series of physical movements that are meant to result in physical, mental, spiritual, and emotional balance for the individual (Cantu, 1980; Getchell, 1979).

Nurses have traditionally used one form of massage, the backrub, as a therapeutic intervention. The advantages of massage are primarily seen as a relaxation of muscular tension. Massage is directed at the holistic person and should produce positive feelings in terms of the total individual. As with the other relaxation therapies, there are a number of manuals, books, and procedures available on the correct techniques of massage (Downing, 1972; Yokay, 1973).

The older client who is undergoing a major change, such as a need for insulin therapy, experiences a higher level of stress than usual. Due to the additional stress, the older person is more vulnerable to the other health problems; the gerontological nurse practitioner should therefore counsel the individual to maintain proper rest and nutrition. Supportive counseling and teaching by the gerontological nurse practitioner should help the client in predicting and controlling problems of living through a period of major change.

Skin Care. In general, an older person's skin is not as resilient as is the skin of a younger person. The older person's skin is thinner, drier, and, thus, more fragile and subject to problems. Skin breakdown can be prevented through control of temperature change, frequent position change, protection of vulnerable areas over prominent bones and joints, gentle cleansing only as necessary, and replacement of decreased natural lubrication with a lotion.

Foot care is mandatory. The major concept employed is vigilance. Regular, daily efforts must be made to maintain skin integrity and prevent even the slightest trauma. The current literature emphasizes the importance of including foot care for the diabetic person as one of the activities of daily living.

The most critical nursing intervention is teaching. The client or family member must be taught how to assess the client's legs and feet, the management measures, and how to evaluate the results of home/self-care.

Graham (1984) recommended a twice-daily examination that should include the entire leg as well as the foot. The examination should focus on dryness, cracking, fissuring of interdigital spaces, and fissuring about the heels. The shoes should be inspected every morning and evening. Any cracks or worn areas that could result in irritated skin should be noted. Signs of temperature change in the leg, pain, difficulty in palpating the various pulses, and progressive intermittent claudication require medical attention. If the leg appears pale and cold, with a minimal amount of hair and with skin that is dry, the client must be taught about maintaining skin integrity to prevent infection. Additionally, the client must be taught care in movement and ambulation so as to prevent trauma. The gerontological nurse practitioner should check the type and size of stockings and shoes the client wears to determine suitability and proper fit.

Graham (1984) advised that socks and stockings should be snug but not tight over the foot and leg. Socks should be ''33% wool, 32% cotton, and 35% nylon'' (Graham, 1984, p. 44). This fabric combination will keep the feet dry and cool in normal to very high humidity and temperature ranges. ''For extremely cold conditions, a thicker sock of 65% orlon, 25% cotton, and 10% nylon proves most comfortable—and causes fewer wrinkles and less blister formation'' (Graham, 1984, p. 44).

Clients whose extremities exhibit signs and symptoms of sensitivity, aching, tenderness, edema, dry skin, and hardening and thickening of tissues will need support hose, evaluation of legs and feet, and exercise. Proper application of support hose should be taught to the client and family. Support hose should be put on before the client gets out of bed in the morning. If the client has the assistance of a family member, the legs should be elevated while the support hose is pulled on. The support hose should be evenly distributed over the leg and end just below the knee. The top should not be turned down; this could create a tourniquet effect.

Buerger–Allen exercises may be prescribed for the client. The basic reason for doing these exercises is to increase blood supply to the tissues. Buerger–Allen exercises are specifically designed to alternately fill and empty the blood vessels in the legs and feet. The client should be flat in bed. The legs should be elevated to a level above the heart for approximately 2 minutes. Following this, the legs should be placed in a dependent position until they regain a pink color. In the third movement of the exercises, the client should lie flat for about 5 minutes. The three movements in the set should be repeated five times. The set is generally prescribed three times a day.

Overall care of the feet includes daily washing in lukewarm water and complete drying. Lotion should be gently applied and rubbed in lightly, leaving no excess. Nails must be cut straight across and kept meticulously clean and filed. The use of a heating pad and hot water bottles must be discouraged. Instead, soft, warm socks should be recommended. Socks should be changed when damp. When ambulating, socks and shoes are essential. Referral to a podiatrist is essential for corns, callouses, ingrown toenails or fungal infections of the nails (Graham, 1984; Drury & Reynolds, 1982).

General monitoring of the legs calls for avoidance of crossing the legs while sitting and careful choice of supportive undergarments and hose. Garters and hose with tight elastic tops must be discarded. Scratches or cuts must be cleansed with water and a mild soap. A sterile Telfa or nonadherent dressing should be applied. Frequent checks should be made to observe for signs of inflammation and rate of healing.

Graham (1984, p. 44) asserted that shoes should be made of soft leather and provided these further guidelines:

1. The toe-box should be high enough to provide room for contraction deformities of the toes. Sufficient height in this part of the shoe will reduce the occurrence of dorsal excrescences

2. Sufficient width of the shoe will accommodate bunions at the first or fifth metatarsal phalangeal joint

3. A double-last shoe is recommended for the person with a narrow heel
4. The arch, counter, and shank of the shoe should be strong while providing flexibility in the barefoot
5. For everyday wear, the heel should be less than $1\frac{1}{2}$ inches in height
6. To break in new shoes, a shorter stride is recommended—this allows better distribution of weight
7. To prevent neurotrophic ulcers, several suggestions are made regarding a molded insole: (a) soft density Plastizate; and (b) medium density Ali-Plast or pelite polyethylene
8. If an insole is needed, an extra-depth shoe, which is commercially available, will allow sufficient space for the insole to be inserted

The importance of leg and foot care must continually be emphasized. If the client or family member is not confident in home/self-assessment, the gerontological nurse practitioner should encourage the client and/or family to seek periodic professional assessment.

The client should be taught that smoking causes vasoconstriction. The gerontological nurse practitioner should be prepared to assist the diabetic client who is motivated to stop smoking. The American Lung Association offers classes and written materials.

Urine Testing and Blood Glucose Monitoring. Urine testing is widely acknowledged to be the least effective method for determining glucose levels. When used along with the client's subjective feeling about his or her status and the trends indicated in his or her records, it can, however, be a fair test. Many persons continue to use urine testing because it is convenient, inexpensive, and not time consuming.

For the older diabetic adult, urine testing is even less dependable than with younger persons. With increasing age, the renal threshold for glucose increases. The renal threshold for non-diabetic persons younger than 50 years of age is 60–180 mg of sugar per deciliter of blood. Thus,

in the older adult, the level of blood glucose may be fairly high before it can be detected in the urine. The trend or pattern of the results of urine testing is of value for all clients, but it is particularly so for the older diabetic who is doing self-management. Once the physician has determined the appropriate testing method and the necessary number of times to test each day, the client is taught the major principles of urine testing, which include what urine testing is, why it is done, how it is done, and why different urine specimens might be needed.

Urine testing is an assistive device—it helps in judging whether the diabetic condition is under control and the level of that control. Urine tests, along with specifics about blood levels, can provide reasonable answers. Better answers are achieved when urine tests are performed correctly. The gerontological nurse practitioner who teaches the client how to perform the urine test must emphasize the need for accuracy.

There are generally two types of urine specimens: the A specimen and the B specimen. To support accuracy, the urine specimen should be a premeal specimen. The A specimen is the first voiding collected 1 hour to 30 minutes before a meal or before bedtime. The B specimen is the second emptying of the bladder 30 minutes or less before a meal or prior to bedtime. The A specimen may actually comprise postmeal and premeal glucose values. At times this may be what is wanted; at other times this value may not be appropriate. The B specimen, which is collected only 30 minutes before the meal, allows approximately 20 minutes for the passage of urine from the glomeruli to the kidney. Thus, the second-voided specimen may be a better indication of the level of control *at that time*. Some practitioners request that both A and B specimens be obtained and tested. Because postmeal specimens are primarily used for checking on intermittent glycosuria, the A sample or premeal and first emptying of the bladder is designated by some as representative of the continuous level of the blood glucose. If the B sample is positive, a third specimen may be useful.

The protocol for collecting the A or B specimen that the gerontological nurse practitioner would teach is outlined below:

1. The bladder should be emptied about 30 minutes to 1 hour prior to the meal. The urine of this sample is known as the A specimen and should be tested
2. If the second specimen is needed, the client may drink a glass of water to facilitate the second sample
3. The bladder is emptied again approximately 30 minutes or less before the meal. This sample is the B specimen
4. If the physician has ordered the B specimen to be tested, this sample is then tested (Peterson, 1979)

The results of urine testing must be documented in order to establish the trend or pattern. A simple chart with day, time, and results can be constructed as a model for the client and family. The chart would be evaluated at least once each week. The client who is controlled by diet or oral agents should be taught that a change in the pattern necessitates altering the food intake first; a change in the activity and exercise pattern would be a second choice. The insulin-dependent diabetic client, however, who finds a major change in pattern should be advised to call the physician for an alteration in the therapy.

Tes-tape, Clinistix, Diastix, or Keto-Diastix are urine testing tools commonly used by clients who do not require insulin. When teaching the client how to use the tape or stick, it is important to stress that timing is crucial in the removal of the tape or stick from the urine sample. A larger size Diastix is available for the older person with vision or dexterity decrements.

The tape or stick is usually prescribed for clients with adult-onset diabetes because these tools are easy, simple, and able to register the presence of the smallest amounts of sugar in the urine. For the older client, these tools may be problematic. In order to read the tape or stick, the client is required to discriminate between green and brown tones. If the older client has a vision problem, the tape or stick is valueless.

Clients and families need to know which medications interfere with test results. There are many drugs that can obstruct a true reading. Aspirin, ascorbic acid, levodopa, and methyldopa can give a decreased value or a false-negative reading on a Tes-tape. Levodopa, ascorbic acid, malidipic acid, cephalosporin, and probenecid can result in elevated or false-positive readings for the client who is taking insulin or using Clinitest (Lamy, 1984).

When teaching urine testing techniques, the nurse should emphasize to the client that it is important to continue using the same type of tape or stick. The reason for this is that a particular color in one tape or stick may be a sign of a positive reading, whereas the same colors in another system may indicate a negative reading.

The gerontological nurse practitioner should be aware that some older clients who are on a fixed income may not be able to purchase the urine testing tapes or sticks. These are nonprescription articles and there is no reimbursement policy to cover the costs. Because urine tests are not as reliable for older clients as they might be for a younger group, some older clients do not believe the expense of urine testing supplies is warranted.

The effects of a new stressor should always be considered. Stressful situations require more energy and glucose yields energy. Under stress, glucose must be mobilized from storage sites. If the supply of insulin that is present is inadequate, the glucose level will become elevated and glycosuria will become evident upon testing the urine. The gerontological nurse practitioner needs to teach the client and family of this process for at least two reasons. Knowledge of this physiological process can help the client and family with their self-diagnostic skills. Secondly, with this kind of knowledge, measures can be instituted to ameliorate or eliminate the stressor(s).

Home blood glucose monitoring (HBGM) is another method for evaluating diabetics (Christiansen & Sachse, 1980). However, most older diabetics would not be candidates for HBGM. Among the indications for using

HBGM that could apply to the older person are the following: The first indication deals with those persons whose renal threshold is unstable or abnormal. The second consideration is to use HGBM with clients having impairments in color vision. The last indication is with clients who have difficulty recognizing true hypoglycemia.

Inasmuch as older persons may have an elevated renal threshold, they fall into the first category shown above. Particularly with the older client, the renal threshold will be an individual concern. To establish the older person's threshold, HBGM could be useful at the time of diagnosis. HBGM may be an improvement over urine testing for older clients with impaired color vision. Older diabetics who have retinopathy may have sustained a loss of color vision due to the retinopathy itself and to photocoagulation, which may have been a treatment. Because clients may experience similar types of symptoms in actual hypoglycemia and a rapidly dropping blood glucose, HBGM may help in determining which problem they are having (Hughes, 1987).

Because the HBGM devices are scarce and expensive, the older client who is relatively stable should not be encouraged to use this approach. Other aging processes constitute problem areas in the use of this method. Some of these would be arthritic joints, a decrease in fine motor ability, and visual acuity. Decreased circulation to the brain may lead to forgetfulness and, in general, it may take an older person longer to learn new skills.

Monitoring on a regular basis might better be accomplished by using the pattern of the results obtained through urine testing and relating them to the results of the Hemoglobin Alc test. This test gives a mean blood sugar concentration and covers a period of approximately 4 months. In the older person who is fairly stable, the HbAlc need only be done every 4–6 months (Peterson, 1979).

For the client over 60 years of age, the urine glucose should be checked twice daily. The outcome desired is aglycosuria and a fasting plasma glucose level of less than 150 mg/dl. Nelson (1984) maintains that a glycosylated hemoglobin on these clients should be obtained every 3 months.

Complications of Diabetes

Of the numerous possible complications associated with diabetes, a few of the more prominent ones are discussed: large- and small-vessel disease, nephropathy, retinopathy, and neuropathy.

Diabetes mellitus in the older person may appear to be nonexistent during the initial onset. One reason for this seems to be the relationship of diabetes to obesity found in older persons. Rather than being faced with the problem of insufficient insulin, the obese older person is dealing with a resistance to proper insulin utilization. Prior to diagnosis, there may be a mildly hyperglycemic state with no observable polyuria or polydipsia.

For those persons whose onset of diabetes occurs later in life, complications such as retinopathy and nephropathy are not prevalent. For adults with long-standing diabetes, complications seem to be related to the duration of the diabetic condition and are probably the result of the combination of aging and diabetes.

Large-Vessel Disease. All vessels of the body can be affected by large-vessel disease but most frequently involved are the heart, brain, and the periphery—generally the feet. Small-vessel disease involves the kidneys and the eyes.

If the arteries to the heart are atherosclerotic, there is decreased blood supply or possibly obstruction. If the load on the heart is increased through exercise or other unusually demanding physical activity, angina or an actual occlusion may result (Williams & Porte, 1974).

Cerebral hemorrhage, thrombosis, or vascular accident can be the result of arteriosclerosis. With cerebral hemorrhage, brain tissue can be destroyed. Early symptoms may include anxiety, speech difficulties, dizziness, or numbness on one side of the body. In thrombosis, the symptoms for cerebral hemorrhage are evident if there is occlusion of a large vessel. If a smaller vessel is involved, there may be headache, dizziness, and possibly confusion (Williams & Porte, 1974). The diabetic person who suffers a stroke must be closely monitored by the gerontological nurse practitioner. Observation for skin changes, infection, and ulceration is of prime importance.

Small-Vessel Disease

KIDNEYS. There are two problems associated with the kidneys: infection and nephropathy.

The symptoms of infection in the bladder include frequency of urination, burning upon urination, and lower back pain. Urinary retention may result in infection. Medication will need to be started to prevent further infection to the kidney tissue. Because up to 50% of older persons may exhibit these symptoms but be reluctant to notify or discuss them with a family member or health care provider, it is prudent for the gerontological nurse practitioner to include these problem areas in the routine assessment of the older adult.

Nursing actions include observation for symptoms of urinary retention and urinary infection. Teaching the diabetic person and family members the techniques of bladder training and the signs of urinary infection may be indicated.

The glomeruli are microscopic blood vessels in the kidney that function to filter waste materials from the blood. Diabetic persons experience changes in the form of thickening and separation in the basement membrane material. When the glycoproteins that constitute the basement membrane receive more glucose and galactose than is necessary, thickening and separation occur. Observable symptoms may include infection, proteinuria, hypertension, and edema (Williams, 1978; Brennan, 1984).

Glomerulosclerosis, also known as Kimmelstiel–Wilson syndrome, is a nodular form of glomerulosclerosis. Within the syndrome, renal function is decreased and hypertension is present. Control of blood sugar and hypertension seems to be advantageous. Tubular nephrosis, a second type of nephropathy, is related to hyperglycemia. This condition is found in the prox-

imal tubules and may be reversible with control of blood glucose (Parte & Halter, 1981).

EYE. Eye disease secondary to diabetes mellitus may be divided into two categories: background or nonproliferative retinopathy and neovascularized or proliferative retinopathy. Nonproliferative retinopathy is characterized by blood vessel damage that remains within the retina. Problems include both superficial and deep hemorrhages, microaneurysms, cottonwool patches, macular edema, and hard exudates. Damage initially takes place in the walls of the retinal capillaries. The capillary walls balloon out, forming aneurysms. Because these walls of the aneurysms are thin, blood may be released through them (Parte & Halter, 1981).

In proliferative retinopathy, there may be retinal and vitreous hemorrhages, formation of new vessels and fibrous tissue, and subsequent retinal detachment or tearing. Loss of vision may be anticipated.

The following signs and symptoms of eye disease should be taught to all older persons, particularly the older diabetic client (Williams & Porte, 1974):

1. More than normal sensitivity to light
2. Appearance of flashing lights and/or floaters
3. Pain that persists
4. Halos or rainbows around lights
5. Redness to the eye
6. Any abrupt disturbance in vision
7. Loss of vision

Observations for these problems should be a part of the regular assessment and evaluation techniques of the gerontological nurse practitioner. With the diabetic client, these would become routine questions. Any symptomatology would require immediate eye examination by an ophthalmologist. For those diabetics whose condition has been long standing, the gerontological nurse practitioner should recommend at least an annual eye examination because a great percentage of these clients will have changes in the blood vessels of the eyes.

Neuropathy. Diabetic neuropathy may involve loss of sensation, aching, burning and pain in the lower extremities, and loss of autonomic function, with bladder paralysis, diarrhea, and sometimes muscular paralysis. There is an association between neuropathy and an increased blood glucose level. As the blood glucose level is decreased, the pain diminishes.

There are four subareas under diabetic neuropathy: distal symmetrical polyneuropathy, autonomic neuropathy, proximal motor neuropathy, and cranial mononeuropathy. Distal symmetrical polyneuropathy appears as tingling and numbness in the feet. When the blood glucose level is well controlled, symptoms are minimal. Autonomic neuropathy includes problems with bladder muscle control and intestinal tract function. Additional problems are impotence, diarrhea at night, postural hypotension, loss of the sweat response, gastric retention, and other gastrointestinal problems. In proximal motor neuropathy, nerves to the muscles are impaired. The area of the body is overly sensitive to touch or clothing; pain may be mild or severe. Cranial mononeuropathy refers to the neuropathy that involves the muscles around the eyes. Among the symptoms may be pain, drooping eyelids, and double vision. Generally, the neuropathy is the result of poor control of blood glucose level (Brennan, 1984; Jordan, 1982; Christman & Bennett, 1987).

Nursing care in the neuropathies involves at least the following: emphasizing to the client the importance of blood glucose control via diet, exercise, and medication if prescribed; and regular evaluation by the physician to include the eyes and the gastrointestinal, genitourinary, and cardiovascular systems. Discussing the decreased sensation in the lower extremities and the necessity of daily examination of legs and feet for external lesions is essential. The need for visual examination as well as palpation with the hands should be emphasized. Persons who have neuropathy in the hands and fingers will need to depend more on the visual examinations. The loss of tactile sense and two-point discrimination in the fingers may prevent adequate palpation (Rossman, 1986). Other diabetic persons with increasing loss of vision may be more dependent on examination with the hands and fingers. Both types of problems may require that the examination of the legs and feet be done by a family member or another person.

SUMMARY

Endocrine changes and aging seem to develop together. The major changes are seen as diabetes, hypothyroidism, and hyperthyroidism. With the growing number of older persons, the gerontological nurse practitioner should be aware of the increasing incidence of hypothermia. Because the signs for both hypothyroidism and hyperthyroidism are atypical, the gerontological nurse practitioner should include pertinent questions in the routine assessment of each older person. Obesity is a common problem that requires creative measures on the part of the nurse. The hidden aspects of hyperglycemic hyperosmolar nonketotic precoma and coma are important. Changes in the older person are continuous; therefore, assessment must be frequent and cover the major endocrine problems.

Though all aspects of care are important for the diabetic, the diet is of primary importance. Researchers agree that many diabetics can control or reverse their diabetic state by maintaining a proper diet. The traditional methods of determining the diet may be replaced by use of the glycemic index approach. Exercise is second in importance to dietary control and should be planned for every day. Variety and novelty in planning for exercise may encourage older clients.

Oral hypoglycemia drugs are prescribed by many physicians for older clients. Now that they are available in the United States, the second generation of sulfonylureas may be preferred by some physicians. Insulin must be used by a percentage of the elderly population. For these persons, the gerontological nurse practitioner must provide continuous teaching, caring, support, and coordination. Mechanisms for coping with stress should be taught by the gerontological nurse practitioner.

Daily care of the feet and legs is imperative. Equally important is daily inspection of shoes and knowledge of the proper types of socks and stockings to be worn. Urine testing assists the client in the control of the diabetic condition. The gerontological nurse practitioner should emphasize the importance of accuracy in urine testing. Clients should be taught the signs of complications and be made aware of the critical importance of continuous preventive actions within their self-care.

REFERENCES

Albaneze, A. A. (1980). *Nutrition for the elderly.* New York: Liss.

Anderson, J. W., & Chandler, C. (1981, Summer). High fiber diet benefits for diabetics. *The Diabetes Educator, 7,* 34–38.

Anderson, F., & Williams, B. (1983). *Practical management of the elderly.* (4th ed.). Oxford: Blackwell.

Beattie, B. L., & Louis, V. Y. (1983). Nutrition and health in the elderly. In W. Reichel (Ed.), *Clinical Aspects of Aging* (2nd ed.). Baltimore: Williams & Wilkins.

Benson, H. (1980). *The mind–body effect.* New York: Berkley.

Benson, H., & Proctor, W. (1984). *Beyond the relaxation response: How to harness the healing power of your personal beliefs.* New York: Time Books.

Bernstein, R. S. (1983). Evaluation and treatment of obesity. In E. B. Feldman (Ed.), *Nutrition in the middle and later years.* Boston: John Wright, PSG.

Bolen, J. (1973, July). Meditation and psychotherapy in the treatment of cancer. *Psychic,* 20.

Brennan, M. D. (1984). How to manage the five kinds of neuropathy you are most likely to see in patients over 40. *Transition, 2*(6), 63–74.

Brown, B. B. (1984). *New mind, new body.* New York: Irvington.

Cantu, R. C. (1980). *Toward fitness: Guided exercise for those with health problems.* New York: Human Sciences Press.

Christiansen, C., & Sachse, M. (1980). Home blood glucose monitoring: Benefits for the patient and educator. *The Diabetes Educator, 6*(3), 13–21.

Christman, C., & Bennett, J. (1987). Diabetes: New names, new test, new diet. *Nursing 87, 17*(1), 34–41.

Collins, K. J. (1983). *Hypothermia: The facts.* Oxford: Oxford University Press.

Cozens, R. E. (1982). Obesity in the aged: Not just a case of overeating. *Nursing Clinics of North America, 17*(2), 227–232.

Crapo, P. A. (1981, Fall). Complex carbohydrates in the diabetic diet. *The Diabetes Educator, 1*(3), 37–39.

Davis, P. J., & Davis, F. B. (1983). Endocrinology and aging. In W. Reichel (Ed.), *Clinical aspects of aging* (2nd ed.). Baltimore: Williams & Wilkins.

Dilman, V. M. (1981). *The law of deviation of homeostasis and diseases of aging.* Boston: John Wright, PSG.

Downing, G. (1972). *The massage book.* New York: Random House.

Drury, D. A., & Reynolds, B. J. (1982). Foot care for the high-risk patient. *RN, 45*(11), 46–49.

Dychtwald, K. (1984). *Body–mind.* New York: Jove.

Exton-Smith, A. N. (1981). Hypothermia. In D. Coakley (Ed.), *Acute geriatric medicine.* Littleton, MA: PSG.

Felig, P. (1981). Exercise. In M. Winich (Ed.), *Nutrition and the killer diseases.* New York: Wiley.

Fitzgerald, M. G. (1978). Diabetes. In J. C. Brocklehurst (Ed.), *Textbook of geriatric medicine and gerontology* (2nd ed.). Edinburgh, London: Churchill Livingstone.

Fox, R. H., Woodward, P. M., Exton-Smith, A. N., Green, M. F., Donnison, D. V., & Wicks, M. H. (1973). Body temperature in the elderly: A national study of physiological, social, and environmental conditions. *British Medical Journal, 1,* 200.

Fuller, E. (1982). Exercise: Getting the elderly going. *Patient Care, 16*(17), 66–70, 73, 76–78, 80, 82, 84, 88, 91–92, 94–95, 99, 103, 106, 109–110.

Getchell, B. (1979). *Physical fitness: A way of life* (2nd ed.). New York: Wiley.

Graham, J. L. (1984). A Mayo Clinic podiatrist reviews the most commonly diagnosed—and most commonly misdiagnosed—diabetic foot problems. *Transition, 2*(6), 39–45.

Green, M. F. (1981). Metabolic emergencies. In D. Coakley (Ed.), *Acute geriatric medicine*. Littleton, MA: PSG.

Harris, R. (1983). Exercise and physical fitness for the elderly. In W. Reichel (Ed.), *Clinical aspects of aging* (2nd ed.). Baltimore: Williams & Wilkins.

Holm, K., & Kirchhoff, K. T. (1984). Perspectives on exercise and aging. *Heart & Lung, 13*(5), 519–524.

Horowitz, M. (1970). *Image formation and cognition*. New York: Appleton-Century-Crofts.

Hughes, B. (1987). Diabetes management: The time is right for tight glucose control. *Nursing, 87, 17*(5), 63–64.

Jasmin, S., & Trygstad, L. N. (1979). *Behavioral concepts and the nursing process*. St. Louis: Mosby.

Jenkins, D. J. A., Wolever, T. M. S., Taylor, R. N., Barker, H., Fieldin, H., Baldwin, I. M., Bowling, A. C., Newman, H. C., Jenkins, A. L., & Goff, D. V. (1981). Glycemia index of foods: A physiological basis for carbohydrate exchange. *American Journal of Clinical Nutrition, 34,* 362–366.

Jordan, J. (1982). Chronic complications. In D. W. Guthrie & R. A. Guthrie (Eds.), *Nursing management of diabetes mellitus* (2nd ed.). St. Louis: Mosby.

Kamenetz, H. (1976). A guide to geriatric rehabilitation. In M. W. Falconer, M. V. Altamura, & H. D. Behnke (Eds.), *Aging patients—A guide for their care*. New York: Springer.

Lamy, P. P. (1984). Modifying drug dosage in elderly patients. In T. R. Covington & J. I. Walker (Eds.), *Current geriatric therapy*. Philadelphia: Saunders.

Lemon, B. W., Bengston, V. L., & Peterson, J. A. (1972, October). An exploration of the activity theory of aging: Activity types and life satisfaction among in-movers to a retirement community. *Journal of Gerontology, 27*(4), 511–523.

MacBryde, C. M. (1964). The diagnosis of obesity. *Medical Clinics of North America, 48,* 1307.

Melmed, S., & Hershman, J. M. (1982). The thryoid and aging. In S. G. Korenman (Ed.), *Endocrine aspects of aging*. New York: Elsevier.

Nelson, R. L. (1984). Authoritative guidelines for the primary care physician who treats middle-aged patients with NIDDM. *Transition, 2*(6), 17–29.

Nemchik, R. (1982, November). A very different diet; A new generation of oral drugs. *RN, 45*(11), 41–45, 97–98.

Nickerson, D. (1982). Oral hypoglycemic agents. In D. W. Guthrie & R. A. Guthrie (Eds.), *Nursing management of diabetes mellitus* (2nd ed.). St. Louis: Mosby.

O'Dea, K., Nestel, P. J., & Antonoff, L. (1980). Physical factors influencing postprandial glucose and insulin responses to starch. *American Journal of Clinical Nutrition, 33,* 760–765.

O'Hara-Devereaux, M., Andrews, L. H., & Scott, C. D. (1981). *Eldercare: A guide to clinical geriatrics*. New York: Grune & Stratton.

Parte, D., & Halter, J. B. (1981). The endocrine pancreas and diabetes mellitus. In R. H. Williams (Ed.), *Textbook of endocrinology* (6th ed.). Philadelphia: Saunders.

Peterson, C. M. (1979). Assessing diabetic control with hemoglobin Alc. In Pfizer Laboratories (Ed.), *Individualizing therapy in maturity-onset diabetes*. New York: Science Medical Publishing.

Podolsky, S., & El-Beheri, B. (1984). Nutrition and the elderly diabetic. In J. M. Ordy, D. Harman, & R. B. Alfin-Slater (Eds.), *Nutrition in gerontology* (Vol. 26 of Aging Series). New York: Raven Press.

Rossman, I. (Ed.). (1986). *Clinical geriatrics* (3rd ed.). Philadelphia: Lippincott.

Runcie, J. (1978). Obesity in the aged. In R. B. Greenblatt (Ed.), *Geriatric endocrinology*. New York: Raven Press.

Samuels, M., & Samuels, N. (1975). *Seeing with the mind's eye*. New York: Random House.

Seltzer, H. (1972). A summary of criticisms of the findings and conclusions of the University Group Diabetes Program. *Diabetes, 21,* 976–978.

Shuman, C. R. (1984). Optimum insulin use in older diabetics. *Geriatrics, 39*(10), 71–89.

Simonton, O. C., Matthews-Simonton, S., & Creighton, J. (1979). *Getting well again*. Los Angeles: J. P. Tarcher.

Skillman, T. G. (1984). Oral hypoglycemic agents for treatment of NIDDM. *Geriatrics, 39*(9), 77–83.

Skyler, J. S., Beatty, C. M., & Goldberg, C. M. (1984). Managing diabetes: An updated look at diet. *Geriatrics, 39*(7), 57–68.

Stucky, V. (1982). The meal plan. In D. W. Guthrie & R. A. Guthrie (Eds.), *Nursing management of diabetes mellitus* (2nd ed.). St. Louis: Mosby.

Ullrich, I. H. (1984). Endocrine disorders. In T. R. Covington & J. I. Walker (Eds.), *Current geriatric therapy*. Philadelphia: Saunders.

Vestal, R. E. (1984). *Drug treatment in the elderly.* Australia: ADIS Health Science Press.

Williams, T. F. (1978). Diabetes mellitus in the aged. In R. B. Greenblatt (Ed.), *Geriatric endocrinology.* New York: Raven Press.

Williams, R. H., & Parte, D., Jr. (1974). The pancreas. In R. H. Williams (Ed.), *Textbook of endocrinology.* Philadelphia: Saunders.

Wolfsen, A. R. (1982). Aging and the adrenals. In S. G. Korenman (Ed.), *Endocrine aspects of aging.* New York: Elsevier.

Yen, P. K. (1983). Nutrition: A new look at obesity. *Geriatric Nursing, 4*(3), 184–189.

Yokay, L. C. (1973). *Oriented massage.* New York: Award Books.

10

RESPIRATORY CHANGES

Pulmonary disease is one of the most significant causes of morbidity and mortality in our society today. Because lung cancer and chronic pulmonary diseases are, for the most part, diseases of life-style, it is not surprising that these diseases are escalating rapidly. Asthma, or reversible airways disease, and pneumonias are still quite prevalent, while tuberculosis is on the decline in many areas of the United States. Pulmonary disorders such as chronic lung disease and lung cancer often remain unrecognized until very late in the course of the disease. Hence, they often complicate other physiological problems before they are recognized. If this is not the case, the client with chronic lung disease often gradually reduces activity and life-style without realizing, or at least admitting, that he or she has a physical problem. Certainly educating clients to be alert to symptoms of pulmonary disease is as important a part of the nurse's instructional and case finding efforts as educating clients with known pulmonary disease.

The lungs are very fragile organs. They are also an important part of the body's defense system. Their health and function are among the most vital of body processes. Some mild changes in lung structure and function occur as the body ages, but these usually do not cause physical difficulty in the individual whose lungs have not been damaged by tobacco or air pollution and who does not suffer from a disease such as asthma. Persons whose lungs are compromised have many pulmonary and physical problems as they age. Indeed, they may seem to age more rapidly than their peers and have a markedly shortened life-span as a result. Their quality of life is often greatly reduced by the presence of obstructive airway diseases and/or lung cancer.

This chapter explores the major changes in lung structure and function that accompany the aging process, the most common lung diseases affecting the elderly, the primary risk factors for lung disorders, and the principal drug therapy for lung disorders. Emphasis in each case is on pathology, assessment, diagnostic procedures, and medical and nursing management. The major therapeutic modalities for most lung disorders are discussed together because they are commonly applied to clients with a wide variety of lung disorders. Education and support for life-style change are especially important in the management of long-term pulmonary diseases. Although these changes usually do not prolong life, they greatly improve the quality of life that remains for both client and family.

AGING OF THE RESPIRATORY SYSTEM

As with other areas of the body, some changes in the respiratory system occur with aging. These can be roughly divided into four categories: airway clearance, immunity/defense mechanisms, physical properties, and respiratory control.

Airway Clearance

During most of an individual's life, the majority of the foreign material that reaches the lungs is removed by the mucociliary escalator. This system is composed of hair-like cilia and a thin blanket of mucus lining the airways. If a particle enters the respiratory tree, it comes into contact with the mucous blanket and is trapped. The cilia wave continually moves that mucus toward the mouth. Normally about 10 ml of sputum is raised in this manner each day. It is usually reflexly swallowed without any awareness on the part of the individual. With aging and continual exposure to harmful substances, the cilia gradually are damaged so that they become less flexible (Bowles, Portnoi, & Kenney, 1981). There is also some degeneration of the bronchial epithelium and mucus glands (Adams, 1981). These changes impair the ability to clear the airway effectively and increase susceptibility to infection.

Along with the changes in the mucociliary escalator, aging leads to a decrease in the muscle strength of the diaphragm and chest wall. The extent of the change depends upon many factors, among which are nutritional state, general activity, and general muscle strength. The changes that occur diminish respiration efficiency and reduce the effectiveness of the cough, thus increasing the susceptibility to respiratory problems.

Immunity/Defense Mechanisms

The body's immune responses generally decrease with age, and the immune defenses of the lung are no exception. One specific immune complex that is rendered less effective is the macrophage, a phagocyte on the alveolar surface whose duty it is to attach to and engulf tiny particulate matter (Bowles et al., 1981). Cellular and humoral immunity is also generally decreased (Pierson & Hudson, 1981). These changes leave the respira-

tory tract more susceptible to infection and other problems.

Physical Properties

The lung's physical construction changes in several ways with aging. Normally, as a person breathes, the chest wall expands easily (is compliant). This expansion pulls the lung structures open, reduces intrathoracic pressure, and leads to inhalation. When one exhales, the muscles of the chest wall relax, allowing the lung to return to its original size by virtue of elastic recoil of the lung structures. With aging, some of this elastic recoil is lost, thus reducing the lungs' ability to return to their original resting size. The result is a tendency to retain or "trap" air and a diminished ability to exhale fully. Although the total amount of air in the lungs [total lung capacity (TLC)]

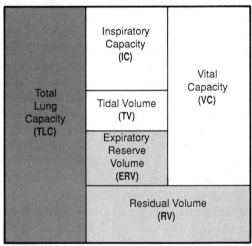

LEGEND:

▓ Volume unchanged

☐ Volumes which increase

☐ Volumes which decrease ERV + RV = FRC

Figure 10-1. Changes in lung volume with aging. TLC does not change with aging. As the amount of air trapped increases, the amount of air that is moved by breathing is decreased.

does not change, the amount of air retained [residual volume (RV) and functional residual capacity (FRC)] increase. The amount of air moved with each breath [vital capacity (VC)] is somewhat reduced (Fig. 10–1). Also, as the alveoli expand, some of their walls are destroyed. In fact, by age 90, most lungs have enough alveolar destruction to meet the strict criteria for a diagnosis of emphysema (Pierson & Hudson, 1981).

The tendency to lung expansion and loss of elasticity is offset somewhat by a tendency to lung fibrosis and stiffening (Adams, 1981) as fibrous tissue replaces some alveolar tissue. As a person ages, reduction of chest wall compliance also combats the tendency to excessive lung expansion. Osteoporosis and costal cartilage calcification stiffen the chest wall as they take their toll. The vital capacity, therefore, gradually diminishes, so that, by age 70, the predicted vital capacity is about 70% of its predicted value at age 20 (Pierson & Hudson, 1981).

In addition to moving somewhat smaller volumes of air each year, other processes also affect the diffusion of oxygen. As a person ages, the number of small airways that remain closed during quiet breathing increases. Also, as fibro-

tic tissue replaces some alveolar tissue, oxygen diffuses less easily. Therefore, the effective gas exchange rate decreases slightly each year, resulting in an average fall in arterial oxygenation (Po_2) of 4 mm Hg per decade. Levels of pH and carbon dioxide do not change. By age 80, the approximate normal arterial oxygenation level is 70 mm Hg (Pierson & Hudson, 1982).

Respiratory Control

As a person ages, control of respiration becomes less precise. Both peripheral receptors and chemoreceptors respond less readily to changes in the level of respiratory gases, specifically oxygen and carbon dioxide. In the "normal" older person, this should not be problematic under usual circumstances. It could, however, result in one's being less able to adjust his or her ventilation to situations of exercise or other increased demand. In the presence of such a complication as chronic obstructive pulmonary disease (COPD), it contributes to a tendency to retain carbon dioxide. Even normal older individuals have less predictable respiratory patterns than younger people. In fact, some older persons with no pulmonary pathology have difficulty with sleep apnea (Pierson & Hudson, 1981).

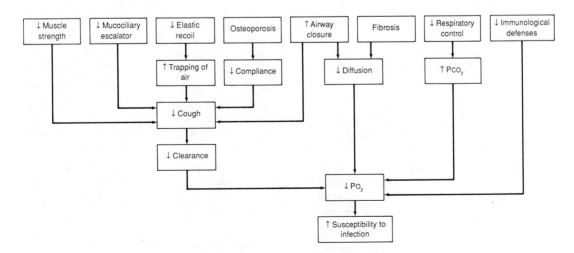

Figure 10-2. Aging of the Respiratory System and Its Consequences.

Cumulative Respiratory Changes of Aging

The results of the changes discussed above are minimal in the healthy aging person. Clinical evidence may be totally unapparent. However, if the person becomes ill or has other risk factors present (most notably, smoking), he or she is much more susceptible to respiratory problems and complications than a younger person. The changes also increase his or her susceptibility to the side effects of drug therapy, such as respiratory depression (Fig. 10–2).

THERAPEUTIC MEASURES

Oxygen Therapy

Oxygen may be inhaled in various concentrations for the purpose of improving arterial oxygenation, reducing cardiac or ventilatory work, or any combination of these. Oxygen is administered only with a physician's order or standing order. In an emergency, the gerontological nurse practitioner can, if institutional policy permits, start low-flow oxygen pending arterial blood gas results and a physician's order.

The term *low-flow oxygen* refers to administration of oxygen at a flow rate of 5 L/min or less. It is important that administration begin with low-flow oxygen when there is a possibility of carbon dioxide narcosis.

Carbon dioxide narcosis is the principal danger of oxygen therapy. Normally, carbon dioxide accumulation is a major stimulator of the cerebral respiratory center. However, some older persons and persons with chronic respiratory disease develop a chronic tendency to hypoventilate and retain carbon dioxide. Gradually, the respiratory center loses its sensitivity to the elevated carbon dioxide level. As a result, the major stimulator of respiration becomes low oxygen, or hypoxemia. That is, when arterial oxygenation falls to a certain level, the person is stimulated to breathe. If too much supplemental oxygen is given, it can raise the arterial oxygena-

tion (P_{O_2}) above the level needed to stimulate respiration. The breathing becomes further depressed until the P_{O_2} falls to a level that stimulates respiration. In severe cases, a respiratory arrest could occur. It is, therefore, imperative to avoid excessive administration of oxygen. Arterial blood gas measurements must be used as a guide to oxygen therapy. It is also important to remember that, even in the case of respiratory distress in the person who retains carbon dioxide, increasing the oxygen flow can be quite harmful.

For many persons with chronic lung disease, normal P_{O_2} may be between 60 and 80 mm Hg. The nurse can observe for carbon dioxide narcosis by examining the trend of the carbon dioxide level (P_{CO_2}). If the P_{CO_2} is rising as the P_{O_2} rises, respirations are being depressed and carbon dioxide narcosis may be impending.

Oxygen is not a PRN drug. The client either needs it or does not. On a short-term basis, no one can tell if a client needs supplemental oxygen. In general, if arterial blood gases drawn at rest show the need for supplemental oxygen, the client needs supplemental oxygen all of the time. When the pulmonary status improves and the client no longer needs additional oxygen, this is demonstrated by the blood gas results.

For some persons, there are times of special oxygen need. These persons may be able to maintain a marginally adequate P_{O_2} at rest without requiring supplemental oxygen. However, if physical or metabolic demands are put on the body, the oxygen supply to the tissues may become inadequate. During these times, supplemental oxygen (usually 1–3 liters) is needed. These times of special oxygen need include exercise and eating. Digestion requires much oxygen.

Some persons may be able to maintain a marginally adequate P_{O_2} when they are awake, but the more shallow respirations during sleep will cause the P_{O_2} to fall below acceptable levels. There is then a need for oxygen therapy during sleep. Orders for supplemental oxygen at these special times (exercise, sleep, and eating) are *not* PRN orders. The order will state a specific oxygen flow rate for each activity. Often one oxygen flow rate is needed at rest and a higher one is needed for exercise. Use of oxygen at these times is not optional. All these orders are determined by arterial blood gas measurements.

Oxygen may be administered in a variety of ways, each carrying certain advantages and disadvantages. The most common and easy to use method is the nasal cannula (nasal prongs). The nasal cannula is comfortable and does not interfere with movement, eating, or talking. Despite the fact that the oxygen is humidified prior to administration, this method tends to dry the nasal mucosa. This dryness can be combated by lubricating the inside of the nose with water-soluble jelly or a saline solution. If jelly is used, take care to avoid clogging the outlets of the nasal cannula.

It is perfectly acceptable for a mouth breather to use the nasal cannula. There are a few potential problems with its use, however. These include the fact that the amount of oxygen that is delivered is somewhat low and unpredictable. The amount of oxygen to use with each cannula is determined by blood gas results. The cannula cannot be used if a bilateral nasal obstruction is present. If the strap of the apparatus is pulled too tightly, skin breakdown over the cheeks and ears may occur. The most common problem with the nasal cannula is that the client either removes it from the nose or inadvertently turns it so that the nasal prongs are directed toward the nasal tip, thus occluding the air flow.

A variety of masks (Mims, 1987) are available for administering oxygen. These provide a more reliable oxygen flow and can deliver more humidity than the nasal cannula. In general, however, masks are hot, uncomfortable, and poorly tolerated. They also interfere with eating, drinking, and talking, causing the client to remove them frequently and thus depriving him or her of the supplemental oxygen. A nasal cannula should be provided for the client to wear while eating so that the mask can be removed. If the

client persists in removing the mask at other times, a cannula would provide a more consistent oxygen supply.

For maximum effectiveness, masks must fit the face tightly, but a tight fit is difficult to achieve and maintain. If the strap or mask is too tight, skin breakdown will occur. The mask should be removed and the skin washed and dried every 2 hours. The mask itself should be washed with water every 8 hours.

Oxygen may be used in the home as well as in the hospital. Gas and liquid oxygen are the two types of home oxygen delivery systems currently available. Both of these are normally used with the nasal cannula. If the oxygen is supplied as a gas, large tanks are delivered to the client's home. Long tubing is used to enable the client to move about the house while using the oxygen. A small portable oxygen tank on a special cart is available for use outside the house.

A more convenient system for home use is liquid oxygen. With this system, there is a large "mother tank" of liquid oxygen to which the client may connect the tubing when at home. There is also a small tank that weighs 8–12 pounds and can either be carried on a shoulder strap or pushed on a cart. This tank is filled from the mother tank and holds an 8-hour supply of oxygen.

A newer choice of home oxygen systems is the oxygen concentrator. Two types of concentrators are available. One uses a permeable plastic membrane that separates oxygen and water vapor from other gases in the air. The client receives about 40% oxygen at any designated flow between 1 and 10 L/min. No separate humidity source is needed because the water vapor from the air is supplied along with the oxygen (Karasov, 1982).

Another type of concentrator uses molecular sleeves that absorb the nitrogen from the entering air, leaving the oxygen. The concentration of oxygen the client receives with this device depends on the flow rate. Concentrations range from 80 to 100% with flow rates of 1–8 L/min (Karasov, 1982).

Oxygen concentrators are bulky and not yet portable. There is a trend toward miniaturization, however; within a few years, it is likely that oxygen concentrators will be as portable as gas and liquid oxygen portable systems are now. The problem in reducing concentrator size, at present, is that the oxygen output of the smaller models may be less predictable and/or lower than with present models.

Any of these oxygen systems may be rented from a company that provides the services of a respiratory therapist. The therapist will explain how to use the system, how to care for it, and how to recognize when the oxygen supply is low and when it is necessary to reorder.

The choice of a home oxygen system depends on cost and on the client's life-style. The client is charged for oxygen cylinders on the basis of the number of cylinders used per month, whereas oxygen concentrators are rented for a fixed monthly rate. If a person uses oxygen only a few hours a day or is out of the house using portable oxygen sources several hours daily, the gas or liquid oxygen systems would probably be more economical. If the client usually remains at home, the oxygen concentrator is probably the better choice economically. Another consideration with concentrators is their dependence on electricity; they would not be a wise choice where electrical outages are frequent.

The client who uses home oxygen therapy should be encouraged to travel normally. When traveling by airplane, the client must use the plane's oxygen system because the home portable systems are not properly pressurized for use during flight. An oxygen system will be made available for use at the flight destination on request. When traveling by car, arrangements can be made to have oxygen available at a motel. If traveling by car or bus, a route should be planned that avoids areas of high elevation, which exacerbate respiratory difficulty.

There are many hazards of oxygen therapy; these are well described in basic nursing texts, which may be consulted for additional information.

Exercise

Many older persons tend to reduce their activity for a variety of physical and psychological reasons. It is well documented that this tendency to a sedentary life-style adversely affects their physical and psychological well-being. A regular program of aerobic exercise offers many advantages to the older person. The best known of these is the improvement of cardiopulmonary fitness and stamina. The deep breathing associated with exercise also protects against one of the hazards of the sedentary life-style: hypostatic pneumonia. Moreover, a regular exercise program helps to improve psychological well-being.

Another advantage of exercise is its effect on the muscles. Muscle tone and stamina of all muscles, including the respiratory muscles, improves with exercise. Improving the tone of the respiratory muscles also helps to improve the effectiveness of the cough. Exercise is also very important in reducing the oxygen consumption of the muscles. When a muscle is well conditioned, it consumes less oxygen per unit of work than when it is deconditioned (Moser, Archibald, Hansen, Ellis, & Whelan, 1980). As a result, the muscle becomes fatigued less quickly. Cardiopulmonary work is also reduced because the exercising muscles are less demanding of oxygen. Another important facet of a muscle conditioning program is the need for adequate nutrition. Without this, it is impossible to condition muscles properly.

Exercise in the Presence of Respiratory Disease

Persons who have respiratory disease or other conditions that cause dyspnea often must severely limit their activity. This causes their muscles to become deconditioned and demand more oxygen per unit of work. Unable to generate the added work with their deconditioned respiratory muscles, they must further restrict their activity. As a result, they rapidly become deconditioned, lose muscle mass, and may become dyspneic on the slightest exertion. Often the term *respiratory cripple* is applied to persons in this debilitated state.

Exercise training will not improve lung function per se, but it will enable the person to tolerate more activity with less oxygen consumption than before the training began (Traver, 1982). Exercise training is often begun in the hospital and then continued at home on a long-term basis. Training is not restricted to persons with pulmonary disease but can be applied to anyone who has been deconditioned for any reason.

The training program usually begins with evaluation of the person's exercise tolerance. Even before the individual is ready for formal testing, the nurse can observe and describe exactly what activity is tolerated and what breathing patterns and reactions are displayed at the onset of dyspnea. It is not enough to record that the client "ambulated" and did or did not "tolerate" it. A more meaningful statement is "ambulates 25 feet very slowly before the onset of dyspnea. Becomes panicked at onset of dyspnea and can control respirations only with specific directions." It is also fairly simple to apply the standard classification of dyspnea (Table 10–1).

Before testing or beginning an exercise program, it is essential to teach diaphragmatic breathing and pursed lip breathing. These breathing patterns should be used to gain control at any time of distress as well as during exercise. In times of distress secondary to pulmonary disease, most persons can gain control using this method within 1 minute. If the dyspnea is due to a cardiac problem, it usually takes a little longer to gain control. Once the client understands and

has mastered the breathing, he/she should practice resting during inhalation and performing simple activities during exhalation. This method prevents breath holding (a common problem) and promotes the maximally efficient use of the respiratory muscles. For example, many men become short of breath during shaving because of breath holding. This simple change in breathing patterns will enable shaving without distress. Another problematic activity is tying the shoes. The client should inhale and then bend down from a sitting position to tie one shoe while exhaling through pursed lips. Then, the shoe tying process can be repeated after sitting up and inhaling.

When the client is able, rest and exercise testing is done, normally using a stationary bicycle or treadmill. For client protection and for maximal evaluation, cardiac monitoring and ear oximetry (to monitor oxygenation) are used throughout the testing.

Based on the results of the testing, an individualized aerobic exercise program is planned. Usually, a target pulse rate is calculated and the client is taught to exercise within the target range.

Pulse rate is a much better guide than dyspnea for evaluating the amount of energy expended during exercise, but the client will probably need to be convinced of this. Most respiratory clients begin to panic at the first sign of dyspnea. They need to learn that breathlessness is a part of exercise for everyone, that it is not harmful, and that it need not be a cause for panic. Thorough instruction and practice in the breathing techniques are essential to maintaining respiratory control during exercise. The use of inhaled bron-

TABLE 10–1. CLASSIFICATION OF DYSPNEA

Grade I	Can keep pace walking on the level with a normal person of similar age and body build, but not on hills or stairs.
Grade II	Can walk a mile at own pace without dyspnea, but cannot keep pace with a normal person.
Grade III	Becomes breathless after walking about 100 yards, or for a few minutes on level.
Grade IV	Becomes breathless while dressing or talking.

Modified from Committee on Diagnostic Standards, American Thoracic Society, 1962.

chodilator drugs just prior to exercise can also increase the ability to exercise without undue dyspnea. As previously discussed, some clients will need to use oxygen while exercising.

Early exercise periods are often conducted with the cardiac monitor and ear oximeter in place. Other important observations during exercise include pulse, dyspnea, color, and the presence of coughing or wheezing. The most popular exercises are walking, stair climbing, and bicycling, although any aerobic activity is appropriate. It is important that the exercise be regular, gradually increased according to a specified plan, and carefully monitored so that the person does not overexercise on days of feeling particularly good. The program should have realistic goals and be started slowly, as is true of any exercise program. In bad weather, exercise could be accomplished by walking about the house, using the stationary bike, or walking in a shopping mall.

Activities of Daily Living

The more activities of daily living that the person can perform independently, the better the quality of life will be. The same breathing techniques used in exercise should be applied to the activities of daily living. Some specific activities should be carefully timed with breathing. For example, the client should pull the vacuum cleaner toward himself or herself upon inhalation and push it away upon exhalation. Washing dishes can be done by leaning the elbows on the sink so as to stabilize the shoulder girdle and permit the use of the accessory muscles of respiration. The hands are then free to wash the dishes. Just as the cardiac client should use all possible means to conserve energy, so should the person with pulmonary disease. It is also important to avoid bending, squatting, and straining, as these actions require a great deal of energy and are often done with unconscious breath holding. Isometric exercise is also usually done with breath holding and should be avoided.

Pulmonary Hygiene

Keeping the chest free of secretions and/or other debris is very important in preventing respiratory infections. There are several methods of accomplishing this, some of which are used only for clients who are ill and some of which are appropriate for all older persons.

Turning and Moving

For the person who is at risk for or has atelectasis, moving, turning, and coughing remain popular methods of reducing the risk. The ideal method, of course, is ambulation and activity. If a person is ill, early ambulation is one of the most effective means of preventing atelectasis.

If a small airway is obstructed by secretions, atelectasis develops quickly in the alveoli served by that airway. Therefore, during periods of illness, a person should be turned at least every 2 hours and preferably more often as a means of mobilizing secretions and reducing the risk of airway obstruction by mucus and mucus plugs.

A newer method of accomplishing the same thing is to place high-risk immobilized clients on a kinetic bed. This is a motorized bed that turns from side to side continually and seems to be quite beneficial in preventing atelectasis. It cannot, however, be used for orthopnic persons such as with COPD, as they cannot tolerate the flat position.

Coughing

Along with moving the client, frequent coughing exercises will help to clear the airway. The cascade cough is the optimal method of accomplishing this. The cascade cough is performed by coughing several times during a single exhalation. In this way, a person does not inhale the sputum which has just been coughed part of the way up the airway, but it continues to be worked up and out of the airway. If secretions are extremely tenacious and the client is unable to clear them adequately, a bronchoscopy is sometimes performed for the purpose of removing secretions. Postural drainage and percussion, which are discussed later in this chapter, also assist the client in clearing the airway by coughing.

Hydration

Coughing is most effective if the secretions are thin and easy to expectorate rather than being thick and tenacious. The best expectorant is a high intake of fluids, excluding milk. Milk and milk products tend to thicken the secretions and should, therefore, be limited. All older persons should have a high fluid intake within the limits of their cardiovascular tolerance. Eight 8-oz glasses of fluid should be the minimum daily intake for those with normal cardiovascular systems. If the sputum thickens, the fluid intake should immediately be increased.

Breathing Exercises

Two types of clients can benefit from breathing exercises. One is the client with chronic respiratory disease who needs to gain control over respirations and breathe in the most efficient manner possible. The other is the individual who has been or is at risk for an acute ventilatory problem, such as the client who is immobilized or recovering from surgery. The principles and advantages of deep breathing for these persons are well described in basic nursing texts.

Breathing exercises should be practiced at a time when the chronic lung client is physically comfortable. It is important to be relaxed during the exercises. Often, teaching relaxation techniques as well as breathing techniques can be quite helpful. Gentle back massage and other such aids to relaxation may also be used. If possible, the client should be sitting up during the practice sessions.

The client must learn to breathe deeply, using the diaphragm. Many clients unconsciously develop a habit of breathing very shallowly and moving only the upper chest. This

contributes to an increased amount of dead space with each breath, poor respiratory muscle tone, and uneven ventilation with poor air mixing. It can make the person feel far more short of breath and instinctively breathe even more rapidly and shallowly.

To learn diaphragmatic breathing, the client should sniff two or three times while the hands are placed over the diaphragm to get the feel of diaphragmatic movement. The sniffing can then be expanded to slow inspiration. The hands should feel the movement at the waist.

After that, the client should place one hand on the chest and one on the abdomen. With deep breathing, abdominal movement should be felt while the chest remains still. After mastering this, the client can learn to contract the abdomen to aid expiration and relax it to aid inspiration.

Pursed lip breathing is often instinctively discovered by persons in respiratory distress. To accomplish pursed lip breathing, the client inhales slowly through the nose and exhales slowly through pursed lips. Exhalation should be twice as long as inhalation. The client can do this more easily by mentally counting to two on inspiration and four on expiration. This breathing pattern reduces the dead space with each breath, facilitates control of respirations, slows respirations, and prevents instinctive breath holding.

It is important not to expect anyone to use these breathing techniques constantly. Dyspnea is defined as an awareness of breathing. Therefore, if someone concentrates on breathing at all times, he is, by definition, dyspneic. Clients should be encouraged to practice the techniques several times a day so that their use will be instinctive when the need arises.

Incentive Spirometry
This is a very helpful way to promote deep breaths in those who need extra reinforcement or direction. Spirometers raise a ball or turn on a light as the person takes a deep breath through the mouthpiece and holds it. For the immobilized or postoperative client, a goal of ten spi-

rometry breaths per hour is appropriate (Spearing & Cornell, 1987).

Intermittent Positive Pressure Breathing (IPPB)

IPPB is defined as "the use of a pressure-limited respiratory to deliver a gas with humidity and/or aerosol to a spontaneously breathing client for periods of less than twenty minutes each several times a day" (American Thoracic Society [ATS] Respiratory Care Committee, 1978). IPPB machines have been popular methods of preventing postoperative atelectasis for many years. Instead of allowing the client to inspire actively, the IPPB machine applies positive pressure at the mouth to give a passive inspiration. The use of IPPB is now controversial. Whether or not it is the optimal method of achieving stated goals for a given client has not been determined. Studies have not shown it to be more effective than spontaneous deep breathing, and, in fact, many persons have been shown to take a deeper breath without it. It has also not been shown to deliver a drug any more effectively than simply providing the drug in a nebulized mist that the client breathes in any comfortable pattern (Petty, 1974). Those physicians who use IPPB believe that it may do any or all of the following:

1. Mobilize secretions and improve the cough effort
2. Provide deeper breaths than the client takes unaided
3. Prevent or reduce atelectasis
4. Deliver aerosolized medications
5. Temporarily reduce the work of breathing
6. Temporarily reduce hypoxemia and hypercapnia
7. Provide subjective improvement

IPPB may be useful for the person who is too weak to do breathing or coughing exercises or is unconscious. For maximum benefit, the objectives for using IPPB should be clearly defined and the treatment tailored to the client.

In order to use IPPB properly, the client must be coached before and during the procedure. It is important that the client relax and coordinate his breathing with the machine, breathe as slowly as possible with a pause after each inspiration to maximize drug delivery, and be sitting upright during the treatment.

IPPB has many disadvantages, including the fact that it is expensive and there is a likelihood of cross-contamination if the same machine is used between clients. Some clients will have difficulty in coordinating respirations with the machine. The energy expended during the treatment may increase the work of breathing and leave the client exhausted. Even when the treatment is optimal, there is no long-term effect on the work of breathing, lung function, or oxygenation.

The tidal volume delivered by IPPB varies with each breath. Any resistance by the client or secretion accumulation will cut off the air flow prematurely. Even when appropriate tidal volumes are delivered, the gas flow tends to follow the path of least resistance and is, therefore, more likely to inflate already open lung areas than areas of atelectasis.

IPPB reduces hypoxemia and hypercapnia only for the duration of the treatment. This may or may not be in the client's best interest. If the client is a carbon dioxide retainer, the treatment can cause carbon dioxide narcosis, as was discussed earlier in this chapter. Though IPPB has been used extensively for chronic lung disease in the past, studies have not shown that these clients live longer or more comfortably than those who have other methods of bronchodilator delivery. There has, however, been some documentation of psychological improvement in persons who have used IPPB for some time.

If IPPB is used at home, the client or a family member must learn to care for and clean the equipment. This is a complicated procedure, the performance of which should be checked periodically by the health care team.

IPPB must be given with a bronchodilating drug if it is to be of value. If normal saline is used alone, the treatment actually increases bronchospasm (Petty, 1974). When IPPB is used, its use should be re-evaluated periodically to determine if a simpler, less costly alternative would be more appropriate (ATS Respiratory Care Committee, 1978).

IPPB is contraindicated in situations where increased intrathoracic pressure is a hazard. These include increased intracranial pressure, reduced cardiac output, and actual or potential tension pneumothorax.

Nebulization

As described in the previous section, an easier and less expensive alternative to IPPB is nebulization. Both bronchodilating drugs and mists for the purpose of hydration and liquefaction of sputum can be delivered in this manner. The client breathes the mist using whatever respiratory pattern is comfortable. As with IPPB, the treatment is more effective if the client is in an upright position while it is given. The major precaution is that some clients will have so much sputum mobilized by the hydrating mist that they may not be able to handle it effectively. If this is the case, the nurse may need to suction the client.

Chest Physiotherapy

Chest physiotherapy (CPT), or postural drainage and percussion, uses the "catsup-bottle" theory to aid in secretion removal. When catsup sticks in the bottle, people often turn the bottle upside down and pound on it to remove the catsup. CPT uses the same principle to remove sputum from the airways—the client is positioned for gravity drainage and then percussion and vibration loosen the sputum so it can be coughed out (Carroll, 1987).

The number of times per day that CPT is performed depends on the client's condition and the reason for the CPT. In any event, the treatment is most effective if the airways are as open as possible. Therefore, CPT should follow the use of an inhaled bronchodilator. During times of production of large amounts of sputum, CPT is usually performed four or more times daily. This amount of treatment, however, is not compatible with life-style during times of less sputum production. Therefore, it is appropriate to ask the client to choose the time of day that sputum is the most problematic and to perform CPT at that time. Many clients will add a second treatment on their own, but this is their choice and not that of the health care team. If the sputum increases or thickens, this is a sign of potential infection. The client should then increase both CPT and hydration as well as consult a physician.

To maximize comfort and minimize danger, CPT should be performed at least 45 minutes before meals or not less than 1 hour after meals. The actual procedure is well described in basic nursing (McHugh, 1987) and physical therapy texts and is beyond the scope of this discussion. Auscultating just after the treatment is somewhat misleading, because the procedure will stimulate temporary bronchospasm. Some clients produce little sputum during the procedure but will have a great deal of sputum "slide" out easily about 1 hour after the procedure. Either result is normal.

DISEASE PROCESSES

Pneumonia

Pneumonia is a major health problem in the elderly; if not quickly and vigorously treated, it may be fatal. It is estimated that, of the cases of pneumonia that are serious enough to require hospitalization, 50% occur in persons who are over 60 years old (Hill & Stamm, 1982).

Pneumonia is generally defined as an inflammation or infection of the lungs. Pneumonia is classified in a number of ways (Table 10–2). It occurs in acute, subacute, or chronic forms, with acute and subacute pneumonia being most prevalent among the elderly. The cause of pneumonia may be infectious and noninfectious, such as aspiration or hypostatic pneumonia. The causative agents may be bacterial or nonbacterial. The bacterial causes predominate and may

TABLE 10–2. WAYS IN WHICH PNEUMONIAS ARE CLASSIFIED

Acuity: Acute, subacute, or chronic

Transmission: Infectious or noninfectious

Acquisition: Community acquired or hospital acquired

Agent: Bacterial (aerobic or anaerobic)
    Nonbacterial (viral, chemical, or fungal)

Distribution: Lobar, lobular (bronchopneumonia),
    or interstitial

include both aerobic and anaerobic bacteria (Hill & Stamm, 1982). Nonbacterial causes include viruses, fungi, and chemical irritants.

Pneumonia may also be categorized according to the lung structures that are affected. Lobar pneumonia, if allowed to progress untreated, will ultimately involve the entire lobe by direct spread through the alveoli. Fortunately, most cases of pneumonia are no longer allowed to progress to this extent. Lobar pneumonia or bronchopneumonia spreads to the alveoli via many of the airways, and thus shows a patchy distribution. Interstitial pneumonia is variable in its extent. The interstitial tissue of the lung is first attacked and then the disease spreads to the alveoli by destroying the alveolar walls (Clark, 1975–1976). Pneumonia can also be classified as to whether it is acquired in the hospital or in the community. This is an important distinction since the causative organisms are very different in the two groups.

Risk Factors

In addition to age, there are many other factors that put a person at risk for pneumonia. These include chronic illness, debility, immobility, and immunosuppression. The elderly who live in groups, such as in nursing homes, are particularly vulnerable. Smokers and persons with already compromised cardiopulmonary systems are at risk. Alcoholics and drug abusers are at risk both because of debilitation and the increased danger of aspiration. Aspiration is itself a risk for many others as well. Epileptics or anyone with a compromised swallowing or gag reflex is at risk, as is anyone with major dental infections. Aspiration is not usually a problem in normal persons unless they have been anesthetized.

Causative Organisms

Almost any organism can cause pneumonia. Often a mixture of organisms are responsible, with one or more organisms predominating. *Pneumococcus* organisms cause over 50% of the bacterial pneumonias. However, those caused by the *Staphylococcus* and gram-negative rods are more serious (Harvey, Johns, McKusick, Ownes, & Ross, 1980). Viral pneumonias are common as well. In addition, pneumonia is not uncommonly the first presenting sign of carcinoma of the lung or of tuberculosis. When the pneumonia is cleared, the chest x-ray reveals the underlying tumor or cavity that precipitated the inflammatory response of pneumonia.

Prevention

Pneumonia can be prevented with basic nursing measures such as promoting mobility, good general health, optimal cardiopulmonary function, and avoiding upper respiratory infections. Vigorous attention to preventing aspiration, treatment of predisposing diseases, and prevention of cross-contamination of respiratory organisms is important. Respiratory depression should be avoided. Use of prophylactic antibiotics is not helpful. Persons who are at high risk for pneumonia should receive both influenza vaccine and pneumococcal vaccine. The pneumococcal vaccine has been proven safe and confers immunity to about 14 strains of organisms for 3–5 years (Hill & Stamm, 1982).

Assessment Parameters

There are four classic signs of pneumonia that are generally required for a diagnosis: (1) new infiltrate on the chest x-ray; (2) cough productive of purulent sputum, (3) leukocytosis, and (4) fever (Clark, 1975–1976). There are many other signs and symptoms generally associated with pneumonia, but these are also found with many other conditions. The four major signs, taken in combination with each other, are almost always diagnostic of pneumonia. Other findings associated with bacterial pneumonia include dehydration, confusion, stupor, delirium, tachypnea, cyanosis, dyspnea, shortness of breath, inspiratory pain, pleuritic pain, tachycardia, shaking chills, congestive heart failure, and blood-flecked or "rusty" sputum. The person with viral pneumonia gives a history of an antecedent flu or upper respiratory infection and complains of myalgias and headache. The sputum may or may not be purulent. With interstitial pneumonia, there is abrupt onset of fever and a nonproductive hacking cough. Chest examination in interstitial pneumonia may or may not be normal (Harvey et al., 1980).

Chest examination may reveal bronchial breath sounds, rales, ronchi, and sometimes wheezing. There may be signs of consolidation, such as increased tactile fremitus, whispered pectoriloquy, and egophony ("E to A" change). There may be a pleural friction rub or evidence of pleural effusion (dullness upon percussion).

Unfortunately, many elderly persons do not exhibit the classic signs and symptoms of pneumonia. Thus, the diagnosis may be missed. Commonly, the elderly have little or no fever. They may have chills, vomiting, altered level of consciousness, stabbing chest pain, lethargy, dyspnea, and a productive cough (Futrell, Brovendu, McKinnon-Mullet, & Browder, 1980). The matter is complicated further in that alcoholics and immunosuppressed clients also present unusual symptoms—most commonly fever and prostration out of proportion to the apparent physical status (Harvey et al., 1980). Persons who have chronic obstructive pulmonary disease (COPD) may be quite ill and even have respiratory failure from an upper respiratory infection without actually having pneumonia. A new infiltrate must be present on the chest x-ray for a diagnosis of pneumonia in this client (Harvey et al., 1980).

A high index of suspicion is very helpful, as pneumonia can mimic a variety of other conditions. Some historical data that are helpful in making a diagnosis include a description of the onset and duration of illness (it varies with the different types of pneumonia), any concomitant underlying disease, immunological status, whether any condition makes the client prone to aspiration, and whether there has been recent antibiotic therapy (Gerding, 1981).

The workup of all clients suspected of having pneumonia should include a Gram stain of the sputum, cultures of the blood and sputum, a white blood cell (WBC) count with differential, and a chest x-ray. The Gram stain and cultures should be obtained before antibiotics are administered. If the client is seriously ill, the arterial blood gases should be monitored as a guide for oxygen therapy.

The Gram stain is a rapid and effective means of determining the causative organism of pneumonia. It is important that the specimen be sputum rather than saliva. Hopefully, the client will be able to cough up a good sputum specimen. If not, it can usually be collected following treatment with a bronchodilator or CPT. If these fail, more invasive procedures such as transtracheal aspiration or bronchoscopy may be indicated.

Both sputum and blood cultures are collected, but these take considerably longer than the Gram stain to evaluate. Often, they are negative due to the difficulty of culturing many of the causative organisms of pneumonia. If the causative agent is a virus, the culture will be negative as well. Ideally for diagnosis, both the sputum and blood cultures will be positive for the same pathogen. Broad-spectrum antibiotics are usually begun after the samples are obtained. Treatment can be refined and individualized once the results are known.

In most types of pneumonia, there is a pronounced leukocytosis with a left shift. This might not occur in the alcoholic or immunosuppressed client. It is sometimes absent in the client who has an infection that is so severe that the body defenses are overwhelmed and no longer able to respond; it may also be absent in some viral pneumonias.

Nursing Care and Medical Management

The management of pneumonia involves both the treatment of the causative organism and symptomatic care and support of the client. Viruses do not respond to pharmacological intervention, so there is no specific antibiotic treatment for viral pneumonia, but other care as described herein is appropriate. Generally, viral pneumonia tends to be milder than bacterial pneumonia, but it can be serious and even fatal.

The first management goal is to combat the causative organism if possible. Broad-spectrum antibiotics are begun early and then, once the organism has been identified, specific drugs are chosen. The nurse must check for allergy prior to administering drugs such as the penicillins and must be alert for allergic reactions, side effects, and toxic effects with any of the drugs that are used. In addition to the penicillins, gentamycin and erythromycin are commonly used drugs. If the antibiotic therapy is effective, the client should begin to show improvement within 48 hours. The drugs should be continued for several more days or even a few weeks, depending on the severity of the disease and the client's response to it.

Adequate ventilation is the second goal. To achieve this, the client should receive both inhaled and systemic bronchodilators. These open the airways and thus aid oxygenation. Frequently, arterial blood gas studies indicate the need for oxygen therapy as well. Rarely, clients will need tracheostomy or mechanical ventilation.

Airway clearance is a major goal. A great deal of sputum is produced in all types of pneumonia, with the exception of interstitial pneumonia, in which sputum production is unpredictable. Many persons require assistance in clearing the sputum from the respiratory tree. As discussed earlier, hydration is of utmost importance, as it will thin the sputum and make it easier to expectorate. Hydration may be delivered by the oral or intravenous route or a combination of the two, depending on the client's ability to drink adequate fluids. Mist therapy may also be used as a hydration measure.

A productive cough is essential to airway clearance. Therefore, cough suppressants are contraindicated in most cases of pneumonia. Many elderly persons already have a reduced cough efficiency and will require aid to clear the airway. Chest physiotherapy or suctioning, or both, may be necessary.

A further goal is the appropriate treatment of any underlying or pre-existing disease. This is especially true of compromised cardiopulmonary systems. Optimal function of these systems is an essential part of the treatment of pneumonia.

Another important goal is to reduce cardiopulmonary work. This can be accomplished in part by reducing the metabolic demands of the body. The client should be on bed rest, and the time permitted for talking and socialization should be restricted, as these activities increase the need for oxygen. The gerontological nurse practitioner must be careful to assure turning, coughing, and deep breathing on a regular basis and to prevent other hazards of immobility during this time. The diet should consist of nutritious foods that are light and easily digested (as digestion requires a tremendous amount of oxygen). Anything that depresses respiration, such as sedatives and hypnotics, should be avoided. Fever places great metabolic demands on the body. Therefore, fever and chills should be prevented if possible and promptly treated if present. On a long-term basis, the client will probably be allowed out of bed within a few days, but should plan on a long convalescence with much extra rest.

Adequate nutrition is an essential goal. Without its achievement, the body's ability to combat the disease will be lessened, as will respiratory muscle strength.

Another goal is optimal fluid and electrolyte status. Many clients who have pneumonia develop fluid and electrolyte imbalances. These must be monitored and treated on an individual basis. Accurate intake and output records are essential, as is monitoring of laboratory studies and clinical signs for indications of altered fluid and electrolyte status.

Many persons with pneumonia experience chest pain. This may be muscle pain secondary to excess coughing, pleuritic pain due to pleural irritation, or a combination of both. Individuals experiencing chest pain usually splint their respirations when breathing is painful. This splinting is certainly antagonistic to the client's need for optimal ventilation. Therefore, mild analgesia should be used to keep the client as comfortable as possible. Narcotics must not be used, however, as they suppress respirations or cough.

Monitoring client status is essential. This includes physical assessment of the neurological and cardiopulmonary status, evaluation of the quantity and quality of the sputum, serial chest x-rays, and arterial blood gases. The health care team should also watch for early signs of complications, which may include delayed resolution, superinfection of bacteria over a viral infection, acute respiratory failure, shock, pulmonary edema, pleural effusion, sepsis, otitis media, herpes simplex, and gastrointestinal problems.

A final goal is to prevent the spread of the infection, both to other areas of the client's body and to other persons. Thorough hand washing, both by the gerontological nurse practitioner and the client, is essential. The client should be taught the proper care and disposal of sputum and tissues. Oral hygiene should be given frequently so that the organisms coughed up will not cause oral infections. Also, the taste and smell of the sputum are noxious to the client. Oral hygiene, therefore, improves comfort and confers a sense of well-being. If the client is at home, dishes should either be scalded or washed in the dishwasher. In the hospital, other elderly, debilitated, immunosuppressed, or cardiopulmonary clients should not share the room with a client who has pneumonia.

Obstructive Airways Disease

The term *obstructive airways disease* refers to conditions in which there is obstruction to airflow upon expiration. Normally, the airways open somewhat upon inspiration and partially close on expiration. In the absence of pa-

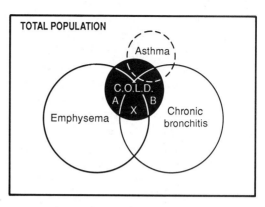

Figure 10-3. Triad of Obstructive Lung Diseases. (Reprinted with permission from Burrows, B., Knudson, R. J., & Kettel, L. J. (1975). *Respiratory insufficiency*. Chicago: Year Book.)

thology, the airways do not close upon expiration to such a degree as to obstruct airflow. In the presence of obstructive pulmonary disease, however, the airways do close to the extent that the air that was inhaled cannot be exhaled without difficulty. Sometimes, the airways close totally upon expiration.

There are two major types of obstructive airway disease: acute or reversible airway obstruction (asthma) and chronic airway obstruction (emphysema and chronic bronchitis). These diseases usually do not exist in their pure forms, but in some combination with one another (Fig. 10–3). Any combination of them can and does exist, although they can occur in isolation. The existence of one of the diseases does not necessarily lead to or predispose to the development of the others.

Acute Airways Obstruction (Asthma)

Asthma is an episodic airways obstruction that occurs in response to stimuli that in normal individuals would not provoke this response and that cannot be ascribed to underlying heart disease or any other cause. Between exacerbations of asthma, the lungs are theoretically normal or nearly so (West, 1977). In actuality, some clients feel very normal between attacks while others continue to show some respiratory compromise.

The causes of asthma may be divided into two major categories: extrinsic or intrinsic. Though its mechanism is not yet understood, extrinsic asthma is basically an immune response in which an allergen such as pollen or animal dander causes the production of histamine and other chemicals by the lung. The airway responds to this in three ways: (1) bronchospasm, which is the rhythmic squeezing of the airways by their own muscle bands; (2) production of large amounts of thick mucus or sputum; and (3) inflammation, which leads to mucosal swelling or edema. The edema and mucus production obstruct the airway from the inside, and the bronchospasm obstructs it from the outside.

Extrinsic asthma may affect persons of any age group. The victim often has a personal and/or family history of allergy, hives, rashes, or eczema. Skin tests in children and young people are often positive for specific allergens (West, 1977). Skin tests are less reliable in adults and may not even be done.

Intrinsic asthma involves the same three airway responses and affects adults more often than children. Attacks are caused by such factors as respiratory tract infection, exercise, or emotional upset. Infection is an especially important precipitator of attacks. Many persons with intrinsic asthma never wheeze unless they have a respiratory infection, at which point they are very ill.

Few asthmatics have one cause alone as the basis for the attacks. Many mechanisms are often involved. Whatever the cause, once bronchospasm in precipitated, airway response to superimposed stimuli is greatly increased. For example, the person who is having mild bronchospasm in response to pollen might become emotionally upset. Because the airways have already been compromised by the pollen, the airway response to the emotions may be greatly magnified. It is important to note that, without the physical tendency to bronchospasm, no amount of emotional upset, pollen, or other stimuli will cause the wheezing of asthma. Therefore, to say that asthma is due to emotions alone is incorrect,

irresponsible, and destructive. It needlessly causes the asthmatic and family to feel guilty and may also prevent the asthmatic from receiving the proper medical therapy for the attack.

Bronchospasm is not always due to asthma. Some other phenomena can cause wheezing as well. Unilateral localized wheezing may be caused by the aspiration of foreign bodies or by the obstruction of an airway by a tumor. The wheezing is the result of air moving past the narrowed or obstructed portion of the airway. Other possible causes of wheezing are pulmonary emboli, infections, left ventricular failure (pulmonary edema), cystic fibrosis, immunologic deficiency, and viral respiratory illnesses.

Assessment Parameters

Because the major symptom of asthma is wheezing, it is important to ask clients when they wheeze and what causes them to wheeze. For example, do they wheeze only when they have a respiratory infection, only when they are lying down on their backs, or only when they exercise or do certain types of work? They may wheeze with any combination of these activities. Also, it is important to determine what they do to relieve the wheezing.

Asthma in adults is frequently part of a triad of asthma, aspirin intolerance, and nasal polyps. Because of this phenomenon, it is usually advisable for asthmatics to avoid taking aspirin.

Although allergies can cause adults to experience symptoms of asthma, skin tests in adults are often inconclusive, and hyposensitization may not be helpful. Inhalation challenge sometimes helps to diagnose the offending allergens, but the procedure is difficult, and factors such as bronchial irritability, infection, medications, and emotions may alter the results. The easiest way to determine an allergic basis for adult asthma is in the history. The gerontological nurse practitioner should ask questions such as "what happens when you are around someone who is mowing a lawn?" Find out what happens upon exposure to flowers, pollens, dust, animals, and cigarette, cigar, or pipe smoke. Inquire about chemicals, including common household products and possible exposure in the workplace. If the client describes consistently occurring wheezing, sneezing, coughing, dyspnea, chest tightness, or other such symptoms upon exposure to pollens and irritants, an allergic or irritative basis for the asthma should be strongly suspected. The occurrence of seasonal symptoms will further substantiate this theory. Because various trees and plants pollinate, bloom, or seed at specific times of the year, ascertain how the client usually feels during each season of the year. A laboratory test that will further help to determine an allergic basis for symptoms is the eosinophil count, which is usually elevated in the presence of allergy.

The health history should also explore the possibility of exercise-induced asthma. The health care professional should ask exactly what the client is able to do, what is difficult, and what changes have occurred over a period of months or years. The gerontological nurse practitioner should find out specifically about the client's tolerance for each daily activity. These are critical baseline data. To know that the individual can climb stairs is not enough. Can it be done without stopping to rest? Is the client able to climb, but only very slowly? How much walking, running, or swimming is necessary to cause wheezing? In the laboratory, exercise-induced asthma may be evaluated by bicycling or free running. Free running is considered the more reliable test if the client is able to accomplish it.

Frequently, the victim of an asthma attack waits several days before seeking emergency treatment. When care is finally sought, the client is often in severe respiratory distress. Assessment findings include dyspnea, audible wheezing, orthopnea, tachycardia, and apprehension. Complaints include chest tightness and inability to take a deep breath. The client will sit upright, using the accessory muscles to breathe. There may or may not be cyanosis, coughing, or diaphoresis. Intercostal retractions may or may not be present. There is often dehydration because the respiratory effort of the past days has caused the client to greatly limit any activity

that interferes with breathing, including taking fluids.

On auscultation, the gerontological nurse practitioner will find greatly reduced, harsh breath sounds. If it is still early enough in the attack, there will be expiratory wheezing throughout the chest. As the attack progresses and the airways narrow, the wheezing occurs both on inspiration and expiration. If there is little or no wheezing, the airways may be so narrow that very little air is being moved. The examiner may find the chest sounds quiet and tight. This indicates that there is no longer enough air moving to cause breath sounds or wheezing. This client needs immediate aggressive treatment.

Nursing Care and Medical Management

Management of an acute asthma attack is directed at relieving signs and symptoms by combating the pathological changes. The bronchospasm is treated with intravenous aminophylline for a period of 30 minutes to 1 hour and repeated every 4–6 hours. Sometimes, the aminophylline drip is continuous after the initial bolus as described above. Other routes of aminophylline administration (oral, rectal) are contraindicated, as they will not rapidly achieve and sustain the necessary aminophylline blood level. Often subcutaneous terbutaline is also given for its synergistic action with the theophylline. The client will receive a nebulized bronchodilator as well. This should be given by aerosol nebulizer rather than IPPB in order that the client may breathe in a comfortable pattern. Persons in respiratory distress do not tolerate IPPB treatments well. The nebulized bronchodilator is given by the unassisted method every 3–6 hours during the day and at night if the client wakens with symptoms of respiratory distress. The unassisted method means the client can breathe a mist of the drug in his or her own breathing pattern. In the acute phase of bronchospasm, the client should be in high Fowler's position with the arms supported.

Because of the increased work of breathing and the compromised oxygenation, the vital signs should be closely monitored. The vital signs reflect the amount of respiratory work the client is doing and the cardiac response to it. The arterial blood gases are an important parameter of the effectiveness of that work—they reflect how much air is actually being moved by each breath. The nurse cannot assess the effectiveness of ventilation by observing the client because a person who appears to be working very hard to breathe may actually be moving very little air. A rising P_{CO_2} reflects a reduction in the amount of air being moved. As long as the blood gases show the client hyperventilating in order to maintain oxygenation, the client is considered to be stable. However, as the client begins to tire, less air is moved with each breath. This is manifested by a rising P_{CO_2}. Clients experiencing an asthma attack whose blood gases show a normal or elevated P_{CO_2} should be admitted to the hospital, as there is danger of their becoming so fatigued that they could develop respiratory failure. These clients will need intubation and mechanical ventilation. During the attack, a client needs continuous oxygen therapy in order to reduce ventilatory work and to better supply tissue oxygen needs. The nasal cannula is usually the most easily tolerated method of oxygen administration. The oxygen demand should be reduced as much as possible by reducing the demand for self-care, eating, drinking, and talking.

The client must be helped to clear the thick sputum from the chest in order to facilitate air exchange. Hydration is the most effective way to thin the sputum and facilitate its clearance. In the person without cardiac compromise, intravenous fluids should be infused rapidly—up to 200 ml/hr for at least 24 hours. If the cardiovascular system is compromised, fluid intake should be decreased accordingly; diuretics may be used along with giving fluids. It is important to give fluid and not restrict it even if diuretics must be used to help deal with the excess. In any case, the gerontological nurse practitioner should watch for signs of fluid overload, as well as for improved sputum mobiliza-

tion. CPT also helps clear the chest of sputum and is generally performed after the inhaled bronchodilator has opened the airways.

The client is treated for infection only if infection is present. Therefore, early in the illness, sputum should be collected for such tests as culture, Gram stain, and wet prep. Daily observations of quality and quantity of sputum should be charted.

Intravenous steroids in high doses are very helpful in reducing the inflammatory response of asthma. As the client improves, the steroids may be given orally. The dose is gradually decreased as appropriate. The health care team must avoid tapering the dose too rapidly, as the inflammatory response may again increase. Inhaled and oral steroids are not effective during the very acute phase of the asthma attack.

As the client improves and the airways become more open, it is helpful to document this change. An objective method of obtaining this documentation is the use of daily vitalographs (simple spirometry). This is a simple one-breath test with the expiratory airflow recorded on a sheet of paper. On a long-term basis, more complex pulmonary function testing is an important monitoring method, although this is not usually done during the acute episode.

Above all, it is important to avoid sedating the asthmatic. A maximal respiratory drive is critical to survival during an asthma attack. The asthmatic can better be calmed by the continuous presence of the gerontological nurse practitioner and the prompt administration of vigorous therapy. As respirations improve, anxiety will decrease.

Once the client has passed the very acute phase of the attack, but while he or she is still hospitalized, therapy should be directed at the same pathology. Much of this therapy can be continued after the client has returned home. Aminophylline and terbutaline can be given orally. The client may remain on nebulized bronchodilators for a few days before beginning to use a hand-held bronchodilatory aerosol in preparation for discharge. Often, asthmatics are advised to use this inhaler on a regular basis (two to four times daily). The danger of overuse should be emphasized, along with instructions to contact the physician if more frequent use seems necessary. It can also be helpful to use the inhaler just before performing activities that normally cause wheezing.

The client will continue to receive oxygen until the arterial blood gases indicate that it is no longer needed. Weaning from oxygen is then necessary. Arterial blood gases should be the sole guide for oxygen therapy in the respiratory client. At least 65 ounces (about 2 L) of fluids should be given daily if the cardiovascular system will tolerate it. Diuretic therapy may be necessary along with this for some clients. The client should continue to observe the sputum for quantity and character. Steroids will gradually be tapered. Some clients are discharged on continuing low doses of oral steroids. Many others can use beclomethasone (Vanceril) instead. This topical steroid is inhaled and does not cause the side effects that plague long-term users of oral steroids. Vanceril should be used after the inhaled bronchodilator so that the airways are as open as possible to receive it. The client should develop a normally active life-style, with good rest, exercise, and dietary habits. Prescribed medications should be taken on a regular basis regardless of how the client is feeling. Stopping one or more medications can cause another attack. It is important that clients learn to consult the physician for early signs of bronchospasm or change in the color, character, or quantity of sputum. Of course, smoking and exposure to allergens and irritants are discouraged.

Chronic Obstructive Lung Disease

Chronic obstructive lung disease (COLD) is similar to asthma in that there is obstruction to expiratory airflow and that there are exacerbations and remissions. The acute (reversible) and chronic diseases differ in that the lungs of the chronic clients do not return to normal between exacerbations. Instead, the disease slowly progresses. These clients do have times when they

feel better and times when they feel worse. The most common problems that worsen their symptoms and may even cause them to be hospitalized with respiratory failure are infections and exposure to very strong airway irritants.

The term *COLD,* or chronic obstructive pulmonary disease (COPD), refers to "persistent airways obstruction of uncertain etiology" (Burrows, Knudson, Quan, & Kettel, 1983). Usually, the term refers to emphysema or chronic bronchitis. Some other types of COLD are bronchiectasis, cystic fibrosis, and pneumoconiosis (black lung or coal miners' lung).

The incidence of COPD is now second only to heart disease as the largest cause of disability in the United States (Burrows et al., 1983). It is a major financial drain, with about 5% of those on Social Security suffering from emphysema (American Lung Association [ALA], 1971). It is also a major psychosocial problem, having been likened to a "living hell" by many of its victims. Presently, men are affected more than women, but this is changing rapidly as increasing numbers of women smoke. Irreversible small airway changes are now thought to begin after only 20 pack years of smoking, although most victims of COPD do not recognize symptoms at that time. (A pack year is one pack per day times 1 year. For example, two pack years of smoking could be accumulated by smoking two packs per day for 1 year or by smoking one-half pack per day for 4 years.) Most persons with COPD first experience difficulty, which they may or may not deny, beginning between the ages of 45 and 64 after many more than 20 pack years of smoking.

Emphysema

Emphysema is the destruction of the alveoli that support the airways and serve as a diffusing surface for oxygen and carbon dioxide. Therefore, both air exchange and airway support are diminished. The airways thus have an increased tendency to collapse during expiration and impede airflow (Eggland, 1987). Although much is still unknown about emphysema, it seems to be due to many separate injuries of smoking and air pollution that occur over a long period of time. Nearly all emphysema clients are or have been smokers; rarely, however, emphysema can result from infection or genetic causes.

Assessment Parameters.

In its early stages, which may last for years, emphysema may be asymptomatic or its symptoms may go unrecognized by the client. Often, even middle-aged persons attribute emphysema symptoms to aging and just gradually reduce their activity level. Typically, these persons continue to smoke and do not seek medical help until the disease is well advanced and the quality of life has deteriorated. The history should include a smoking history and assessment of exercise tolerance. To assess exercise tolerance, the gerontological nurse practitioner should ask specific questions such as, "Can you climb a flight of stairs without stopping to rest?" "How fast can you climb the stairs?" "When was the last time you were able to climb stairs?" "Can you keep up with persons your age when you are walking, playing golf, etc.?" "Can you use a vacuum sweeper, make a bed, or carry groceries?" "How far can you walk before you must stop to rest?" "How fast are you walking at the time?" Exercise tolerance can be further assessed using a stationary bicycle or a treadmill, if the client is able to tolerate these tests.

A history of respiratory infections should be discussed. It is common for the client to report an increasing number of infections each year for several years, with the infections tending to become more severe and to last longer. Exacerbations of acute respiratory failure that are very similar to asthma attacks without wheezing may be reported. Common causes of these exacerbations are infections and airways obstructed by mucus plugs.

Persons who have pure emphysema generally do not wheeze. However, the possibility of wheezing should be investigated, as was de-

scribed for the client with asthma. Other symptoms that should be investigated include orthopnea, cough, sputum production, dyspnea, and chest pain. The symptoms of cor pulmonale should also be included. These are discussed later in the chapter.

Physical findings may include cough, sputum, dyspnea on exertion or at rest, orthopnea, and diaphragmatic flattening. Often, the victim uses a tripod position to breathe, that is, leaning on the arms to aid chest expansion. The gerontological nurse practitioner should question clients about what makes them cough, when they cough, and about sputum production. Typically, persons with emphysema do not produce sputum except during periods of acute respiratory infection. The level of orthopnea should be ascertained. For example, can clients lie flat on their backs with one pillow or do they need to lie on their side, lie on their back with several pillows, or even sit up in a chair to sleep? Do they use pursed lip breathing and if so, when? The gerontological nurse practitioner should check the client's technique for pursed lip breathing. Some clients use their own methods, which vary a good deal from the accepted and most useful pursed lip breathing techniques. Chest percussion will reveal hyperresonance and reduced diaphragmatic excursion. Breath sounds will be diminished, probably with bibasal rales. There will be marked expiratory slowing. There may or may not be an increased anterior–posterior diameter or "barrel chest." Air trapping will cause a flat diaphragm to be present on the lateral chest x-ray even if the anterior–posterior diameter is normal. Pulmonary function tests will show increased residual volume with total lung capacity either normal or elevated. Airflow tests (spirometry) will show varying degrees of expiratory airflow obstruction.

Nursing Care and Medical Management.

Acute and long-term management of emphysema is very similar to that of asthma and is directed at the pathology of the disease. It is extremely important that the client stop smoking, although many clients find this to be a difficult task. The care for the client with emphysema in an acute episode of respiratory failure is the same as for the asthmatic in an acute exacerbation of asthma: bronchodilators given by the intravenous, subcutaneous, and inhaled routes, CPT, hydration, oxygen, treatment of infection, intravenous steroids, avoidance of sedative or depressant drugs, promotion of rest, and reduction of metabolic needs. Diuretics are likely to be needed for clients with emphysema because they are likely to have right-sided heart failure and fluid retention. (See discussion of cor pulmonale.) The oxygen airflow is usually less for the client with emphysema than it is for the asthmatic. Theoretically at least, the asthmatic has normal lungs between attacks and usually has normal blood gases (Po_2 in the 90s and Pco_2 about 40 mm Hg). Clients with emphysema usually have a much lower Po_2 as their normal and may or may not have a higher Pco_2 than normal. Oxygen should be given only as needed to maintain gases that are normal for a particular client. For example, if the normal Po_2 for a client is 70 mm Hg, that is what should be maintained with oxygen. Giving a higher oxygen level could depress respirations and cause the client to retain more carbon dioxide. In fact, if the Pco_2 is rising along with the Po_2, this indicates the oxygen is being administered at too high a level. For this reason, flow rates of oxygen for the client with emphysema, even if very acutely ill, are generally limited to 1–5 L/min. The physician will also be less eager to use mechanical ventilation for the client with emphysema who is in respiratory failure. There are two reasons for this reluctance. The first is that clients with emphysema have learned to tolerate lower blood gases than asthmatics and compensate for them. Therefore, they will survive lower blood gases than would asthmatics. The second reason is that the respiratory muscles of the client with emphysema tend to be in extremely poor condition. When the ventilator takes over all or part of the respiratory work, these muscles decondition quickly, making it notoriously difficult to wean COPD clients from the ventilator.

As clients improve, they will change to oral and inhaled drugs, as described for the asthmatic. A major difference is that clients with emphysema usually do not need long-term steroid therapy with Vanceril as do many asthmatics. The asthmatic has an inflammatory disease of the airways, whereas the main problem in emphysema is destruction of the alveoli. Relaxation therapy, breathing retraining, and graded exercise programs are important as well. Home oxygen therapy is often necessary in the late stages of the disease. Infections and acute exacerbations are treated aggressively in the same manner as asthma. The client should maintain good health habits, avoid upper respiratory infections, smoking, and other irritants, and maintain a light, nutritious diet. The key to coping is education in the areas discussed at the beginning of this chapter. This is where the gerontological nurse practitioner can make a significant difference in the client's ability to cope with the disease.

The management described here does not prolong life or improve pulmonary function, but the increased oxygenation on a daily basis improves function of all other body systems and thus enables the client to pursue a more normal life-style. Each client's potential for progress is individual and depends on the extent of the disease, the cessation of smoking, and adherence to other areas of the therapeutic regimen.

Chronic Bronchitis

Chronic bronchitis is almost always caused by smoking, although it can also result from repeated severe respiratory infections. In contrast to the alveolar changes of emphysema, the pathological changes of chronic bronchitis involve inflammation of the airways. Mucosal edema leads to narrowing of the airway and the production of large amounts of sputum that further obstruct the airway. The result is expiratory airflow obstruction and a symptomatology and progression similar to emphysema. Chronic bronchitis is more likely than emphysema to occur in association with asthma, in which case it is called asthmatic bronchitis.

The definition of chronic bronchitis reflects the major difference between chronic bronchitis and emphysema. Chronic bronchitis is said to be present when the person produces sputum for 3 months of the year for two consecutive years. The 3 months do not have to be consecutive. Although sputum production is never normal, many smokers feel that the production of white sputum is "normal" for them and thus ignore the presence of chronic bronchitis for several years. As in emphysema, the onset is insidious, with frequent respiratory infections that gradually increase in length and severity. Also as in emphysema, the activity tolerance decreases gradually and insidiously.

Assessment Parameters and Management.

Assessment parameters and management for chronic bronchitis are essentially the same as those for emphysema on both an acute and long-term basis, with two major differences. Because chronic bronchitis is an inflammatory process, steroid therapy may be more important than in emphysema. The person with chronic bronchitis also needs daily CPT. The client needs to develop long-term control of the CPT because it will become a major element in the client's life-style. Clients with asthma and emphysema, in contrast, need CPT only when they are producing large amounts of sputum (as in a time of infection). In order to incorporate CPT into the life-style, the chronic bronchitic can be taught "Plan A" and "Plan B." In Plan A, the client identifies the time of day in which there is the most difficulty with sputum. That is the time of day when CPT should always be done. Later, the client and the gerontological nurse practitioner can discuss the result and decide whether to also perform the CPT at another time of day when sputum is troublesome. The client should remain on Plan A along with the other management techniques as long as his or her condition remains stable. At the first sign of infection or respiratory difficulty, however, the client should switch to Plan B, which includes increasing the CPT to four to six times daily, further increasing the fluid intake, and drug therapy as prescribed. Doing CPT this often will take most of the day, but the results in reduced severity of illness will justify the effort. In order to make clients more independent with CPT, some physicians will allow them to do their own CPT with a hand-held vibrator rather than always depending on a family member to perform this service for them.

Tuberculosis

Tuberculosis is a disease for which management and prognosis have changed radically. Now, the client can expect to be fully cured without fear of a relapse, and can expect to accomplish this with very little change in life-style during the course of the illness. What has not changed is the fact that tuberculosis is still a very significant health problem. Presently, about 28,000 new cases are diagnosed annually in the United States (Pritzker, 1981).

The disease is caused by the *Mycobacterium tuberculosis*. Nicknamed the tubercle bacillus, the organism is a hardy spore-forming organism. Although tuberculosis may be transmitted in a variety of ways, it is almost always transmitted as airborne droplet nuclei when the victim coughs, laughs, sneezes, or talks. The organisms stay airborne for several hours. The danger of spread is directly related to the number of organisms that infect the respiratory secretions. If the concentration of organisms is very high, the person is very infectious. If the victim does not cough or if the sputum is negative or only lightly infested, the victim is much less infectious or not infectious at all. The client is most infectious prior to diagnosis and treatment and converts quickly once therapy is begun.

When tubercle bacilli are inhaled, the larger ones are trapped by the mucus blanket and are expectorated. Only the smaller ones find their way to the alveoli. If a person has not previously been infected, the bacilli multiply unhindered in the alveoli as a very minute tuberculosis pneumonia. The victim is asymptomatic at this time and is not infectious. During this period, the organisms move into the blood and lymph glands and potentially can be seeded in other body organs. Only a small percentage of persons actually develop extrapulmonary tuberculosis, however. If the person has a normally active immune system, multiplication of the organisms is eventually suppressed and the area is sealed off by a granuloma, a process that takes up to 10 weeks. Prior to the formation of the granuloma, the person is said to have primary tuberculosis. This is not synonymous with active tuberculosis. In fact, the asymptomatic primary infection can increase immunity to reinfection, although the untreated person is at risk for exacerbation of the tuberculosis for the remainder of his or her life (Glassroth, 1981). Eventually, the granuloma may calcify.

If the body defenses are inadequate and the tuberculosis is not walled off, the incubation period for the disease is about 6 months. Only about 5% of individuals who are exposed actually develop active tuberculosis at this time. Most active cases develop many years later. About 90% of the cases of active tuberculosis are reactivation of the old walled-off organisms (Glassroth, 1981). This is called postprimary tuberculosis. Occasionally, the area of pneumonia of the primary phase extends to a more extensive pneumonia or to a disseminated miliary tuberculosis, but this is rare.

Persons at risk for postprimary tuberculosis are those whose body defenses are compromised for any reason. Individuals who are alcoholic, malnourished, poor, or live in crowded conditions are at risk, although reactivation can occur in persons of any socioeconomic status. Immunosuppression for any reason can precipitate the breakdown of the granuloma and the liberation of the organisms. For example, persons receiving long-term steroid therapy or radiation therapy or have immunological diseases are among those at risk. Those with silicosis are at high risk and should be on lifelong tuberculosis pro-

phylaxis. Thoracic surgery also increases the risk of tuberculosis.

Assessment Parameters

A high level of suspicion is very helpful in the diagnosis of tuberculosis because the early symptoms are often vague and could be the result of any number of problems. The history should ascertain whether any family members or close friends had tuberculosis when the client was a child. Many of today's older persons were exposed to tuberculosis in this way as children. Because prophylactic treatment was unavailable until the 1950s, these individuals are at risk for granuloma breakdown and active disease.

After the history and physical examination are completed, skin testing is the first diagnostic study to be undertaken. A positive skin test will occur following completion of the primary phase of the disease. A positive test does not mean that active disease is present, but rather that the primary immune response has occurred.

Skin testing, although valuable, is not without its problems. False positives may occur if the client has been given bacillus Calmette–Guerin (BCG) vaccine or has had another *Mycobacterium* disease. False negatives may occur if insufficient time has elapsed for the primary phase to be completed, if the test was improperly administered, or if the client has taken steroids, had a recent immunization, or a recent viral disease. If the client is malnourished or immunosuppressed, the immune system may be incapable of responding to the skin test. False negatives or positives may also result from reading the test improperly.

Another source of error has to do with the fact that sensitivity to the skin test diminishes with time. Hence, a person may have a minimal reaction to the test if the primary episode was many years earlier. If the test is repeated soon after the first skin test, the second test will be more positive as a result of the body defenses reacting to the first test. This is known as the booster phenomenon and may lead to false-positive interpretations.

A newly positive skin test should be followed up with chest x-rays and sputum smears and cultures. Aerosol or nebulization therapy is often used to aid the client in raising a deep sputum specimen. If these methods are unsuccessful, other methods of obtaining sputum, such as a bronchoscopy, may be necessary. The sputum smear offers a quick indication of whether tuberculosis might be present, but because some other organisms stain acid fast, it does not provide a definitive diagnosis. The culture takes up to 6 weeks because tuberculosis is a comparatively slow-growing organism. Therefore, if the smear, the x-ray, and other clinical data suggest a diagnosis of tuberculosis, treatment is begun while the results of the culture are awaited.

The assessment should address signs and symptoms commonly displayed by individuals with tuberculosis, the most common symptom being a chronic cough. Other symptoms include fatigue, indigestion, anorexia, late afternoon and evening fever, night sweats, amenorrhea, and hemoptysis. Hemoptysis that occurs in the absence of an apparent cause (such as pneumonia) should be investigated by bronchoscopy. It is a common presenting sign of both tuberculosis and carcinoma of the lung.

Nursing Care and Medical Management

In the absence of acute illness, there is now no reason to hospitalize the client for diagnosis or management of tuberculosis. Most clients remain at home during the entire course of diagnosis and therapy with little or no change in lifestyle. Once therapy is begun, the client is usually noninfectious within 1 week and feels well, so there is no need for isolation.

If, for some reason, the client is hospitalized for initial diagnosis and management, it is important to protect others who are ill from exposure to tuberculosis. The tuberculosis client should be housed in a private room with ultraviolet light and nonrecirculated air. (This is a system whereby air from this room does not mix with the air being circulated throughout the hospital.) The door to the room should remain closed. When entering the room, the gerontological nurse practitioner should wear a mask. The client should wear a mask when leaving the room for procedures such as x-ray. Tissues and secretions should be disposed of in a closed bag. Upon the client's discharge, the room needs only routine cleaning.

The major breakthrough in the management of tuberculosis has been in the area of drug therapy. Unlike the previous long-term therapy, excellent results are now being accomplished in as little as 9 months of therapy with a combination of isoniazid (INH) and rifampin (RIF). INH, which is bacteriocidal, has been a first-line prophylactic and treatment modality for tuberculosis for many years. Only recently has it been routinely teamed with RIF, an antibiotic that is chemically different but also bacteriocidal for tuberculosis. Used together and correctly, they accomplish a cure without the fear of relapse.

Treatment involves 2 weeks to 2 months of daily doses of the drugs (INH 300 mg and RIF 600 mg daily). Ethambutol (EMB) is added if the client has emigrated from or resides in an area with a history of high drug resistance to INH or has received previous chemotherapy for tuberculosis. After the initial treatment phase, clients continue self-administration of the drugs at home on a daily basis if they can be expected to be compliant. For convenience, INH and RIF are supplied in a single capsule. If the client is believed to be unreliable, a somewhat higher dose of the drugs is administered twice weekly at a public health clinic. This allows ingestion of the medication to be supervised. In either case, administration can be monitored with indicators such as clinic attendance, pill counts, and sputum examination. Treatment is continued until at least 6 months have elapsed after the sputum cultures have converted from positive to negative. Because more than 90% of the clients on this therapy convert within 3 months, treatment lasts about 9 months. If there are compliance problems or evidence of complications or disseminated disease, treatment may continue longer. Clients are monitored 3, 6, and 12 months after the completion of treatment because relapses, if they occur, usually do so within that time. Follow-up after 12 months is not usually needed (Iseman, Albert, Locks, Raleigh, Sutton, & Farer, 1980). A summary of the drugs, their effects, and monitoring is found in Table 10–3.

In some cases, the INH and RIF combination is not the most appropriate therapy, even though these are the primary drugs for tuberculosis, are the most effective, and are the least toxic. If the client is drug resistant, has been treated for tuberculosis before, or has complications, other drugs may be added. At least one of the two primary drugs should be in the combination at all times, however. The secondary drugs are somewhat less effective and more toxic, whereas the tertiary drugs are the least effective and the most toxic. In retreatment, it is usually best to select two drugs to which the client has not been exposed. Adding one new drug to a regimen that is failing or has failed only increases the chances of multiple drug resistance (Glassroth, 1981). Fortunately, resistance to RIF and EMB is rare (Glassroth, 1981), so these two drugs can usually be included in a treatment program.

Adherence to drug therapy is the major problem in the management of tuberculosis because clients usually feel good very quickly. Because they do not perceive themselves as being ill, they often forget or do not understand the need to continue regular medication. If they have other problems that they consider to be of greater importance, they may take medications for these and exclude the tuberculosis therapy (Pritzker, 1981). Thorough teaching and close follow-up is, therefore, essential for all clients during the complete course of therapy.

Nursing care of tuberculosis is symptomatic. Because most clients feel good, attention should be focused on the drug therapy and good daily health habits, including rest, nutrition, and exercise. Babies and young children are very susceptible to the disease and should be kept away from the infectious person.

Prevention

INH can be used effectively as prophylaxis in persons who have had the primary tuberculosis episode and are, therefore, at risk for developing active tuberculosis. Usually, 5 mg/kg body weight of INH is given to adults for 1 year. This protects the person for up to 16 years. Usually the therapy is innocuous, but occasionally hepatotoxicity or hepatitis develops. This problem increases with age, peaking with an incidence of 2.3% in persons 50–64 years of age. Alcohol use on a daily basis appears to add to the likelihood of hepatotoxicity. Indications for using INH prophylaxis are summarized in Table 10–4.

Cancer of the Lung

Tumors of the lung may be either benign or malignant, but the majority of them are malignant. Rare as recently as a generation ago, lung cancer is now the most fatal malignancy in both men and women. It was estimated that in 1985 there would be 144,000 new cases of lung cancer and 126,000 deaths resulting from it (American Cancer Society, 1985).

Risk Factors

Vastly more important than other risk factors for lung cancer is cigarette smoking. The risk is dose and time related, so that the heavier and the longer a person smokes, the higher are the chances for developing cancer of the lung. Heavy smokers are about five times more likely to develop lung cancer than are nonsmokers, with this risk increasing to ten times for persons over 65 who have been smoking since they were in their 20s (Geschickter, 1973). If a person stops smoking, the lung cancer risk gradually decreases; after about 13 years of nonsmoking it is reduced to about that of the person who has never smoked

TABLE 10-3. TREATMENT OF TUBERCULOSIS IN ADULTS AND CHILDREN

	Dosage[a]		Most Common Side Effects[a]	Tests for Side Effects[a]	Remarks[a]
	Daily	Twice Weekly			
			Commonly Used Drugs		
Isoniazid	10–20 mg/kg up to 300 mg PO or IM	15 mg/kg PO or IM	Peripheral neuritis, hepatitis, hypersensitivity	SGOT/SGPT (not as a routine)	Bactericidal. Pyridoxine 10 mg as prophylaxis for neuritis: 50–100 mg as treatment
Ethambutol	15–25 mg/kg PO	50 mg/kg PO	Optic neuritis (reversible with discontinuation of drug; very rare at 15 mg/kg), skin rash	Red-green color discrimination and visual acuity[b]	Use with caution with renal disease or when eye testing is not feasible
Rifampin	10–20 mg/kg up to 600 mg PO	600 mg PO	Hepatitis, febrile reaction, purpura (rare)	SGOT/SGPT (not as a routine)	Bactericidal. Orange urine color. Affects action of other drugs
Streptomycin	15–20 mg/kg up to 1 g IM	25–30 mg/kg	8th nerve damage, nephrotoxicity	Vestibular function, audiograms; [b]BUN and creatinine	Use with caution in older patients or those with renal disease
Pyrazinamide	20–40 mg/kg up to ~2 g PO		Hyperuricemia, hepatotoxicity	Uric acid, SGOT/SGPT	Under study as First-Line Drug in short-course regimens

Less Commonly Used Drugs

Drug	Dose		Remarks
Capreomycin	15 mg/kg up to 1 g IM	8th nerve damage, nephrotoxicity	Vestibular function, audiograms: [b]BUN and creatinine	Use with caution in older patients. Rarely used with renal disease
Kanamycin	15 mg/kg up to 1 g IM	Auditory toxicity, nephrotoxicity, vestibular toxicity (rare)	Vestibular function, audiograms[b]: BUN and creatinine	Use with caution in older patients. Rarely used with renal disease
Ethionamide	15–30 mg/kg up to 1 g PO	GI disturbance, hepatotoxicity, hypersensitivity	SGOT/SGPT	Divided dose may help GI side effects
Para-amino-salicylic acid (aminosalicylic acid)	200–300 mg/kg up to 12 g PO	GI disturbance, hypersensitivity, hepatotoxicity, sodium load	SGOT/SGPT	GI side effects very frequent, making cooperation difficult
Cycloserine	10–20 mg/kg up to 1 g PO	Psychosis, personality changes, convulsions, rash	Psychologic testing	Very difficult drug to use. Side effects may be blocked by pyridoxine, ataractic agents or anticonvulsant drugs

[a]Check product labeling for detailed information on dose, contraindications, drug interaction, adverse reactions, and monitoring.
[b]Initial levels should be determined upon start of treatment.
Used with permission from Farer, Laurence S. (1982). Tuberculosis: What the physician should know. New York, American Lung Association and American Thoracic Society, p. 11.

223

TABLE 10–4. GUIDELINES FOR THE USE OF ISONIAZID AS PREVENTIVE THERAPY

Indications

Household members and other close associates of newly diagnosed patients
Newly infected persons
Significant tuberculin skin test reactors with abnormal chest roentgenogram
Significant tuberculin skin test reactors with special clinical situations (steroids, diabetes, silicosis, gastrectomy, etc.)
Other significant tuberculin skin test reactors up to age 35
Other significant tuberculin skin test reactors over age 35 only in special epidemiologic situations

Contraindications

Progressive tuberculosis disease (more than one drug needed)
Adequate course of INH previously completed
Severe adverse reaction to INH previously
Previous INH-associated hepatic injury
Acute liver disease of any etiology

Special Attention

Concurrent use of other medications (possible drug interactions)
Daily use of alcohol (possible higher incidence of INH-associated liver injury)
Current chronic liver disease (difficulty in evaluating changes in hepatic function)
Pregnancy (prudent to defer until postpartum unless contact, new infection or other urgent indication)

Used with permission. From Farer, Laurence S. (1982). Tuberculosis: What the physician should know. *New York, American Lung Association and American Thoracic Society, p. 12.*

(Rodescu, 1977). The smoker who is exposed to other risk factors has an even greater risk of lung cancer. These factors include air pollution and exposure to uranium, chrome, nickel, gold, arsenic, or asbestos. The smoker also increases the cancer risk for others. Secondhand smoke, or the smoke that goes into the air as the cigarette or cigar burns, is inhaled by those in the room with the smoker. Studies now show that the nonsmoking spouses of smokers have a much higher cancer risk than do the nonsmoking spouses of nonsmokers (ALA, *Second Hand Smoke*).

Other risk factors include age, sex, heredity, pre-existing pulmonary disease, economic status, and urbanization. The most common age for the occurrence of lung cancer is 35 to 75. Mortality rises sharply when the cancer occurs after the age of 55 (Tashkin & Cassan, 1978). Heredity involves both the tendency to smoke (which may, in fact, be an environmental rather

than a hereditary factor) and the tendency to develop cancer when risks are present. It is interesting that only a relatively small percent of those who are at high risk for lung cancer actually develop it. This means that there is probably some (as yet unknown) factor that promotes or retards a person's ability to tolerate the insults of smoking and other risks.

Pre-existing pulmonary disease is a very important risk factor. Lung cancer victims often already are suffering from diseases such as tuberculosis, pulmonary fibrosis, pleural diseases, old pulmonary emboli, bronchiectasis, or chronic bronchitis. A Philadelphia study showed that 55% of the lung cancer victims studied had one or more of these pre-existing conditions (Rodescu, 1977). Persons of lower economic status tend to be at higher risk for lung cancer. This is probably due to lower general body resistance. Urbanization is an important risk in that it greatly increases exposure to irritants and pollutants. The lung cancer rate is higher in urban than in rural areas.

Types of Lung Cancer

About 95% of lung cancers originate in the airways and are, therefore, classified as bronchogenic cancers. These include squamous-cell or epidermoid carcinoma, small-cell or oat-cell carcinoma, and bronchiolar or alveolar carcinoma (the adenocarcinomas). The remaining 5% of the cancers arise in the alveoli and bronchioles. These include adenomucoid, adenocystic, giant-cell carcinoma, and melanoma. Though their origin is somewhat different, they have much the same result for the client in terms of symptoms, diagnostic studies, management, and prognosis.

The most common type of bronchogenic carcinoma is the epidermoid or squamous-cell type. The tumor is dense, hard, and slow to grow and metastasize. It usually grows endobronchially and leads to obstructive atelectasis and pneumonia relatively early. A slowly resolving pneumonia or pneumonitis may be the first symptom of this or of some of the other types of lung cancer. Cavitating pulmonary lesions on x-ray may also be an early feature of this type of carcinoma.

Oat-cell or undifferentiated carcinoma, in contrast to the epidermoid type, grows rapidly and metastasizes quickly. Often fatal in less than 1 year, it infiltrates under the bronchial mucosa so that bronchial obstruction, if it occurs at all, is a very late feature.

The prefix *adeno* means gland. Adenocarcinoma of the lungs, therefore, shows a cellular organization that is similar to the bronchial glands and may even contain mucus. This type is usually located in the periphery of the lungs. It grows rapidly but does not spread as quickly as the oat-cell variety. By the time this type is discovered and the client goes to surgery, about 40% of the tumors have already metastasized to the lymphatic system.

Assessment Parameters

The signs and symptoms of lung cancer are usually late and nonspecific. No typical pattern has been identified, other than that the cancer usually remains asymptomatic until well advanced. By the time symptoms become apparent, there is often extensive spread or metastasis. The earliest symptoms include persistent pneumonitis, persistent cough with or without sputum production, hemoptysis, chest pain, progressive weight loss, and "arthritis" of the shoulder or other joints (Geschickter, 1973). Dyspnea or low-grade fever may also be present. Other findings may include lung abscess, palpable lymph nodes in the neck or axilla, unilateral vocal cord paralysis or diaphragmatic paralysis, pleural effusion, or metastases to other organs. Because smokers often already have respiratory symptoms such as cough, excessive production of sputum, and dyspnea, the symptoms of lung cancer tend to be overlooked. Any change in these symptoms, therefore, bears investigation. Late signs and symptoms of lung cancer include clubbing of the fingers, loss of the voice, severe shortness of breath, and persistent headaches and nausea (Rodescu, 1977). Mediastinal involvement may lead to pericardial effusion, tamponade, and arrhythmias.

Lung cancers may stimulate the pituitary–adrenal system, so that endocrine symptoms are also a part of the late picture of these diseases. There may be increased plasma corticoids and adrenocorticotrophic hormone (ACTH), leading to Cushing's syndrome, inappropriate secretion of the antidiuretic hormone (ADH), hyperparathyroidism with hypercalcemia, and gynecomastia. This endocrine response can be used as a method of monitoring the response of the lung tumor to therapy (Greifzu, Crebase, & Winnick, 1987).

In contrast to bronchogenic carcinoma, the alveolar cell carcinomas originate in the lining of the alveoli or bronchioles. These are far more rare cancers, with no apparent geographic, racial, or sexual differences in risk. There is no direct relation to smoking or air pollution and the victims are often young—under 40. There is an insidious onset that resembles chronic pulmonary insufficiency with a gradually increasing cough, which is usually productive, weight loss, weakness, low-grade fever, and pneumonitis. Hemoptysis usually does not occur, nor does pain.

Diagnostic Procedures

Although the chest x-ray alone is not diagnostic of lung cancer, it is a very important screening and evaluation device. Anyone who has a cough or a major change in his or her cough for more than 4 weeks or who has hemoptysis for no apparent reason (such as pneumonia) should have a chest x-ray. Typical findings of an early lung cancer include the peripheral coin lesion, so named because it is an isolated round lesion that looks like a coin. There may also be pneumonia with lobar collapse, a rounded mass adjacent to the hilum or in the apex, a lung abscess, or cavitary lesions. Sometimes the only finding is pleural effusion. Other possible findings on x-ray include rib destruction, elevated diaphragm, and enlarged mediastinal lymph nodes.

The definitive diagnosis of lung cancer is made by identification of malignant cells. Sputum is collected for cytological examination in an attempt to recover and identify tumor cells. Often, however, the cells are not coughed out in the sputum. Then a biopsy becomes necessary. The method of biopsy that is performed depends on many factors, especially the expected location of the tumor. Biopsy may be done via bronchoscopy, mediastinoscopy, thoracentesis, lymph node biopsy, or open lung biopsy. Other tests that may also be part of the workup include bronchograms, angiograms, lung scans, sedimentation rate (which may be elevated), and hemoglobin and hematocrit (which may be low).

Nursing Care and Medical Management

As yet, the only real cure for lung cancer is surgical resection. However, detection is often so late that survival rates are depressingly low.

Presently, only 9% survive for 5 years after diagnosis and treatment. Early detection elevates the survival rate to about 39%, but only about 20% of lung cancers are discovered early enough to fall into this category (Rodescu, 1977). Factors that are considered in the choice of treatment include the type and extent of the tumor and the client's ability to withstand surgery. Because many lung cancer clients have other pulmonary disease, many of them are poor risks. Usually, clients who can tolerate a standardized exercise test can tolerate surgery (Rodescu, 1977). Other evaluative procedures include arterial blood gases, pulmonary function tests, lung scanning, and measures of pulmonary artery pressure. Serious cardiac, renal, or liver disease, severe anemia, and unstable metabolic conditions are contraindications for surgery.

Resectability of the tumor is determined in large part by measuring its rate of growth. This is expressed as volume doubling time, which can be measured on serial chest x-rays. Although the volume doubling time for lung cancer as a whole is 103–107 days, small-cell carcinoma doubles in about 33 days. More than 70% of the clients who have small-cell carcinoma, therefore, already have extrathoracic metastases at the time they are diagnosed. Forty percent of these clients die within 1 month of diagnosis. Surgery is obviously contraindicated (Rodescu, 1977). In other types of cancer, contraindications to surgery include the involvement of the hilar lymph nodes, pleural effusion, and extension of the tumor to the ribs, chest wall, arm, or other structures (Rodescu, 1977).

The surgery for lung cancer is the removal of the affected area, which usually involves at least a lobectomy. Often, a pneumonectomy is necessary. Preoperative radiation therapy has not been shown to increase the resectability of the tumor. However, radiation therapy or chemotherapy is sometimes used as a palliative measure postoperatively or in nonresectable tumors. If the tumor is nonresectable, palliative therapy may reduce symptoms such as cough, hemoptysis, bronchial obstruction, superior vena cava syndrome (obstruction of the vena cava), or pain. The therapy can relieve symptoms and prolong life for only a few months. Even with optimal surgical treatment, the prognosis for lung cancer remains poor. The lung cancer victim with the best prognosis is the one who has a coin lesion that is detected incidentally on a routine examination before symptoms occur.

Cancers That Metastasize to the Lungs

The lungs are a common site for metastases from cancer of other areas of the body, probably because of their function as a filter. About 50% of the clients with all types of cancer have lung metastases at autopsy. This rate is exceeded only by metastases to the lymph nodes and to the liver. The pleura and ribs are frequently involved. Symptoms of metastasis to the lungs are similar to the late symptoms of primary lung cancer.

Nursing Care and Medical Management

Nursing care of the person with lung cancer involves all the considerations for anyone who has a cancer or catastrophic illness. The client will also need care that is specific to the condition, surgery, or testing procedures. All the measures discussed in this chapter, with the exception of CPT, may be employed to aid the respiratory effort. If pleural effusion is a problem, frequent thoracenteses may be indicated to drain the fluid. A chest tube may also be necessary. Occasionally, tetracycline is instilled into the pleural space in an attempt to fuse the pleura together and stop the pleural fluid accumulation that is compromising respirations.

ENVIRONMENTAL RISK FACTORS

Although air pollution is a very important health problem, it is difficult to study and quantify. One reason for this is the overwhelming influence of smoking, which has many of the same effects as air pollution. Because the air is never the same in any two places, and because many of the effects of air pollution may accumulate over a lifetime, it is difficult to ascertain the exact effect of any particular pollutant (Shy, Goldsmith, Hackney, Lebowitz, & Menzel, 1978). Other factors that influence study results and that are also difficult to quantify are the influence of aging, occupational exposure, housing, medical care, and urbanization. There is also a problem in measuring and quantifying levels of pollution because many of the measures currently available were developed when fossil fuels were used for home heating and were therefore the major pollutants. Now, different pollutants are problematic and as such may not be precisely measured by the monitoring equipment (Shy et al., 1978). Thus, though many studies have been conducted with reference to air pollution, their results are often confusing, inconclusive, or contradictory.

In spite of the problems in studying pollution, some things are known. Pollutants fall into four general categories: (1) the fossil fuels, (2) vehicle emissions, (3) miscellaneous, and (4) pesticides. The miscellaneous pollutants are emitted from smelters, refineries, and manufacturing and include such substances as arsenic, asbestos, beryllium, cadmium, hydrogen sulfide, lead, and mercury. Possible industrial sources of asbestos exposure include asbestos mines, shipyards, and fabricating plants. Asbestos is now being found in the bodies of persons who were not exposed to it occupationally; this is a special cause for concern. Sources that may be contributing to this asbestos exposure include automobile brake linings, fire retardant sprays, rock mixtures that are spread on roadbeds, building insulation, and the demolition of asbestos-containing buildings. Pesticides are a category of pollutants about whose effects we still have little data. In regard to all pollutants, safety thresholds are difficult to determine. It is well accepted, however, that the effects of pollutants are dose related, that is, the higher the exposure to the pollutant, the more likely that adverse effects will occur (Shy et al., 1978).

There are additional risk factors associated

with pollution. Individuals at the extremes of age—children and the elderly—are especially vulnerable to the effects of pollution. Those with pre-existing cardiopulmonary disease or an altered immune status also have more problems with the effects of pollution than other groups (Cortese, 1981). The effects of pollution also seem to be increased if any one of three coexisting factors are present: if the temperature is especially cold during the period that the person is exposed to the pollutants; if it is windy during this time; or if the person is exercising when the exposure occurs (Shy et al., 1978). Persons at risk are asked to remain inside and not exercise unduly during periods of air inversion or other episodes of very high pollution.

Physiological Effects

A wide variety of adverse physical reactions in adults have been attributed to pollutants. These range from merely annoying irritation to disease, disability, and even death. Many of the documented effects are on the cardiopulmonary systems, with the most serious effects occurring in persons with pre-existing cardiopulmonary disease.

The local effects of pollution can be summarized as follows:

1. Certain irritants can slow or even stop the action of cilia. This leaves the underlying cells without protection. The cilia and their underlying cells may even be destroyed (Corman, 1978). Ciliary destruction allows any irritant or pollutant prolonged contact with the lung tissues because the mucociliary escalator is unable to do its job of cleansing the airway. For example, the effects of smoking may be worsened because the airways become less able to protect themselves, and potential carcinogens or bacteria that would otherwise have been removed are allowed prolonged contact

2. The pollutants may cause the production of increased thickened sputum. This sputum is difficult to cough out and thus obstructs the airway, leading to reduced oxygenation and the increased hazard of infection. Persons exposed to high levels of pollution are definitely more susceptible to respiratory infections than those who are not (Corman, 1978)

3. Pollutants can cause constriction of the airways (bronchoconstriction). This is intended as a protective reflex to narrow the airways and allow less of the pollutant to enter the body (Shy et al., 1978). However, it also interferes with gas exchange and can lead to altered body levels of oxygen and carbon dioxide and to air trapping

4. Pollutants can immobilize the body's immune defenses (Corman, 1978). This greatly increases susceptibility to infection as well as to whatever specific hazard is posed by the particular pollutant to which the person is exposed

5. Pollutants can cause edema or hyperplasia of the cells lining the airways (Corman, 1978). This reduces airway caliber and thus interferes with gas exchange. It may also alter the activity of the specific cells involved, such as to alter mucus production

These pathological alterations from air pollution can result in any combination of increased risks for the exposed individual. One of the best known is the increased mortality in times of air stagnation or inversion. The deaths are more frequent in individuals above 45 years of age and in those with pre-existing cardiopulmonary disease. The victims usually die of cardiopulmonary causes, including pulmonary edema, but can die of other problems, such as hepatotoxicity (Shy et al., 1978).

A second result of pollution is increased COPD morbidity. Pollution may either increase the pathology or actually cause some pathological changes of COPD. It definitely has either an additive or synergistic interaction with smoking, the major cause of COPD (Shy et al., 1978). Many studies have demonstrated that persons with COPD have increased difficulty with their disease when pollution levels are high. One study compared autopsies of 300 persons who lived in St. Louis, which is heavily polluted, with those of 30 inhabitants of Winnepeg, Canada. The study found four times as much emphysema among the cigarette smokers in the St. Louis group. Even the St. Louis nonsmokers were affected. There was three times as much mild to moderate emphysema in the St. Louis group as in the Winnepeg group. Thus, in St. Louis, emphysema appears to develop earlier and progress more rapidly than in Winnepeg (Corman, 1978). It is likely that air pollution is at least partially responsible.

Exacerbations of asthma are a well recognized result of air pollution. Persons with pre-existing asthma are quite susceptible to any assault on the airway, even if the exposure is on a short-term basis. Just as other factors that increase airway reactivity increase the asthmatic's response to subsequent noxious stimuli, so air pollution increases the likelihood that the asthmatic will react to other stimuli in the environment. Even in the nonasthmatic, chest tightness, cough, and wheezing may result from exposure to air pollution.

The incidence of acute respiratory disease seems to increase in the presence of air pollution. These include such conditions as colds, acute bronchitis, and pneumonia. Pollution does not cause the infections per se, but it does seem to lower body resistance so that the person is more susceptible to infection.

Cancer of the lung has not yet been proven to be a result of air pollution, but the data are highly suspicious. Although smoking remains the most important cause of lung cancer, it seems pollution appears to be involved as well. Agents that are proven carcinogens for laboratory animals are documented to exist in polluted urban air. Other agents that are not carcinogens may play a role by interrupting or immobilizing the mucociliary escalator and allowing the carcinogens more prolonged contact with the respiratory tissues. A study by the National Cancer Institute found a higher incidence of cancer deaths in areas near copper, lead, and zinc smelters, where arsenic is the major suspected pollutant, and around asbestos factories than in other areas.

Air pollution seems to exacerbate pre-existing cardiovascular disease. Hemoglobin, which normally transports oxygen to the body cells, has a higher affinity for carbon monoxide, a major pollutant, than for oxygen. As a result, carbon monoxide replaces oxygen in combination with hemoglobin and less oxygen is carried to the body cells. The person with cardiovascular disease is unable to compensate for hypoxia by either increasing cardiac output, increasing tissue perfusion, or both. As a result, the symptoms of cardiovascular disease such as angina or reduced exercise tolerance occur earlier than otherwise would have been the case, and more cardiovascular fatalities occur (Shy et al., 1978). Carbon monoxide is discussed below in more detail as a consequence of smoking.

There are many miscellaneous effects of air pollution. Burning and irritation of the eyes, nose, throat, and/or chest are warnings that should be heeded (Anderson, 1978). Some pollutants alter nerve conduction and may also alter levels of coordination. Many of them may be absorbed and alter body biochemistry as well (Shy et al., 1978). The liver and kidneys may be damaged as they attempt to deal with the offending chemicals. Leukemia is now recognized to be a consequence of exposure to some pollutants. Skin cancer is a hazard posed by the weakening of the protective ozone shield around the earth caused by fluorocarbon pollution. It is estimated that a 5% reduction in this protective layer could result in 30,000 additional cases of skin cancer annually (Costle, 1977). There are other serious consequences of pollution for young children and nursing mothers, but these are beyond the scope of this discussion.

Dealing with pollution remains a major challenge for our society. Air quality standards are currently set in many areas at levels estimated to protect the majority of the population from significant impairment. These levels may or may not be adequate to protect more sensitive persons and those at higher risk (Shy et al., 1978). The public should constantly be vigilant in protecting these standards. The standards are vulnerable in each session of legislative bodies when special interest groups, economic needs, or other factors seem to take priority over them and tempt legislators to ease the standards. Even where there are standards, not every area has the necessary monitoring and inspection bodies to uphold them (Costle, 1977).

A major problem associated with pollution is the fact that much of the public is still unaware of the risks to which it is exposed. Therefore, people do not pressure their legislators to protect them from pollution. Other individuals are not aware that they are victims of pollution and continue to be exposed. This is because some consequences of pollution may not appear until long after exposure, by which time extensive damage has been done. The problems of multiple pollution hazards are very real. Few persons are exposed to only one pollutant or only a predictable combination of pollutants. The risk of damage increases as the number of pollution hazards to which a person is exposed increase and as exposure lengthens. It is, therefore, incumbent upon all citizens to keep their pollution exposure as low as possible and to avoid smoking, which only complicates the problem (Anderson, 1978).

Smoking

Each year 3 million Americans die prematurely from the effects of smoking. Millions more live on with health problems that are created or aggravated by smoking. The facts are no longer debatable: *smoking is hazardous to your health*. Tobacco is used in several ways: as cigarettes, pipes, cigars, and as snuff. Smoking as a class also includes hallucinogenic drugs. These are known to be harmful, but are not included in the focus of this discussion.

Physiological Effects
Three major agents are released as tobacco is smoked: tars, nicotine, and carbon monoxide.

The smoker also encounters other hazards as inhaling burning debris and exposure to excessive heat. The heat is a special problem for pipe smokers, who tend to always place the hot pipe in the same spot on the lips. Users of snuff or smokeless tobacco tend to get cancer of the mouth, so careful oral examinations on a routine basis are in order for them.

One of the most hazardous effects of smoking is the exposure to carbon monoxide. Carbon monoxide appears to affect the body in two ways. First, as discussed above, it competes with oxygen for hemoglobin receptor sites. Second, once the body's oxygenation level is lower, the work load of the heart and lungs increases in order to oxygenate the body more effectively. The carbon monoxide level is not changed by using filtered cigarettes (McIntosh, Entman, Evans, Martin, & Jackson, 1978).

Smoking also interacts with air pollution, as was discussed above. Crowded highways are major sources of carbon monoxide. One study of this interaction showed that London cab drivers who smoked had a 2% higher level of carbon monoxide in their blood than nonsmoking London cab drivers. Another study showed nonsmoking industrial workers to have a carbon monoxide level of 0.78% while their smoking counterparts had levels of 1.38% (McIntosh, et al., 1978). In addition to interacting with air pollution, carbon monoxide has some other effects similar to pollution. It impairs psychomotor performance and judgment, may cause psychological stress, and may cause physical distress in those with a sensitivity or pre-existing disease.

Nicotine has long been blamed for smoking's most harmful effects. It increases the heart rate, causes peripheral vasoconstriction, and increases cardiac work load as a result of its stimulating effect on the sympathetic nervous system. There is some speculation that this sympathetic stimulation effect decreases with heavy smoking and is indeed more pronounced in the light smoker. Because it is known that heavy smoking is statistically linked to higher death rates than is light smoking, one could speculate that nicotine is the major cause of death as the result of smoking (McIntosh et al., 1978).

Smoking affects the lung tissues much the same way as does air pollution. It reduces and may stop ciliary action. It alters the bronchial epithelium in several ways: (1) hyperplasia (an increase in the number of cells due to irritation), (2) loss of ciliated columnar cells with consequent loss of mucociliary activity, and (3) potentially precancerous changes in the cell nuclei. These precancerous lesions seem to be particularly concentrated at airway bifurcations, where the tars, debris, and other products of smoking accumulate. The difference between these cells and actual cancer cells appears to be that the precancerous lesions have not yet broken through the basement membrane. Apparently, the process is reversible if the person stops smoking before the breakthrough occurs. Lung tissues can be destroyed as in emphysema, possibly due to severe cough efforts to clear the airways. There is also fibrous thickening of the alveolar and capillary walls, with a resultant increase in the work load of the right heart as the pulmonary vasculature is disrupted (Hammond, 1962).

Statistics show much higher death rates for smokers than for nonsmokers or those who have stopped smoking for over 1 year. The death rate increase correlates roughly with the number of cigarettes that are smoked each day; for example, the mortality of two and one-half pack per day smokers is 225% that of nonsmokers. Cigar and pipe smokers do not have a higher death rate in relation to lower respiratory tract problems, because they do not inhale. However, their death rate is much higher in relation to cancers of the mouth, tongue, lips, larynx, pharynx, and esophagus because these tissues are directly exposed to the smoke and heat (Hammond, 1962). Snuff and smokeless tobacco also carry a high incidence of oral cancer as well as gum and tooth diseases.

In addition to being the major cause of emphysema, chronic bronchitis, and lung cancer, smoking is also closely related to heart disease, to an increased incidence of respiratory infections, to carcinoma of the bladder, and to cirrhosis of the liver. It is closely linked to Buerger's disease, which may completely disappear when the person stops smoking. Smoking may or may not cause gastric and duodenal ulcers, but it certainly intensifies symptoms and increases the mortality from ulcers. Though smoking does not cause atherosclerosis, it compounds problems related to it and increases the chance of a myocardial infarction. Smoking increases the hazards of pulmonary complications from anesthesia and potentiates the peripheral vascular complications of diabetes.

Secondhand Smoke. There are two kinds of smoke from cigarettes, pipes, or cigars. Mainstream smoke is what the smoker inhales. Sidestream, or secondhand smoke, is what escapes from the burning end of the cigarette, pipe, or cigar into the environment. Cigarette smokers take about eight or nine puffs of smoke from a cigarette, for about 24 seconds of exposure to mainstream smoke. Meanwhile, the cigarette burns for about 12 minutes, continuously polluting the atmosphere. Cigars and pipes burn longer. The pollution lingers after the burning ceases. The sidestream smoke contains higher concentrations of noxious compounds than the mainstream smoke—up to twice as much tar and nicotine, three times as much benzpyrene (a suspected carcinogen), five times as much carbon monoxide, and fifty times as much ammonia. There is also a high proportion of cadmium in sidestream smoke. This is thought to be a major cause of emphysematous lung damage. We know that the nonsmoker is physically affected because, after only 30 minutes in a smoke-filled room, the carbon monoxide level in the nonsmoker's blood rises, as does his or her blood pressure and heart rate. Once nonsmokers have left the smoky environment, it takes several hours to clear the carbon monoxide from the blood. After 3–4 hours, half of the carbon monoxide is still present in their bodies. Studies also show that children who live with smokers have about twice as many respiratory illnesses as children who do not live with smokers (ALA, *Second Hand Smoke*).

Stopping Smoking. Smoking is a powerful habit and cannot be easily given up. The American Lung Association, American Heart Association, and American Cancer Society all have resources and programs that are designed to assist persons who want to stop smoking. These are either free or available at very low cost, in contrast with many commercially available programs, which are no more effective and may be hazardous, as well as expensive.

If a person is highly motivated to stop smoking, there are several things the gerontological nurse practitioner can do to assist in this effort. For example, it may be helpful for the smoker to analyze the reasons for smoking. The American Cancer Society has identified four types of smokers: those who smoke for a positive pleasurable effect, those who use smoking as a crutch, those who are psychologically addicted, and those who smoke from habit without being aware of the act itself. Once the smoker discovers reasons for smoking, it may become easier to make a conscious decision to continue to use smoking in this way or to stop. Some techniques may be useful for the smoker who decides to quit. For example, if smoking is used as a crutch so that the hands are occupied or as a way to gain thinking time, other appropriate activities can be deliberately chosen to meet those needs.

Often it is also helpful for the person to decide when smoking is most pleasurable. Perhaps there are two to four times during the day (such as after meals) when smoking is especially enjoyable. A good goal to start with is to smoke only at those times. Once that goal has been achieved, the smoker can then work toward stopping completely. Other persons may be better able to stop ''cold turkey.'' A variety of other techniques are also available. The smoker can learn them from the previously mentioned voluntary agencies. There is also a new product

which is available, Nicorette Gum. It is used by the smoker in place of cigarettes as he or she withdraws from smoking. The gum has a much lower nicotine content than cigarettes and does not have the other noxious chemicals, such as carbon monoxide. It is available by prescription only and has been helpful to some smokers who are unable to withdraw from the nicotine abruptly.

It is important that the cigarette smoker not switch to pipes or cigars as a substitute for cigarettes. Most smokers will continue to inhale and so will be no better off. Neither should they use eating as a means of oral gratification.

It is important that the smoker who is attempting to quit realize that his or her airway will attempt to clear itself of accumulated debris and sputum when it is no longer constantly being insulted by cigarettes. This means that cough and sputum production will probably be worse after smoking stops and may continue to be so for 3 months to 1 year. Many smokers resume smoking at this time as a way of controlling the cough, so they need to be cautioned beforehand about what will happen and why.

Above all, the person who is attempting to stop smoking needs a great deal of support, encouragement, and understanding from the nurse, significant others, and associates. It will be helpful if family members and associates who smoke either agree to stop or to at least refrain from smoking in the presence of the person trying to quit. Stopping is quite difficult—there are no simple solutions.

DRUG THERAPY

The major classes of drugs used to treat respiratory disease are bronchodilators, steroids, anticholinergics, antibiotics, diuretics, potassium supplements, and oxygen. Only the bronchodilators, anticholinergics, and steroids are discussed here, as information regarding the other drugs is widely available and oxygen has been discussed previously in this chapter. The drugs are summarized in Table 10–5.

Bronchodilators

The airways are encircled by bronchial muscles that have tone and that control the airway size. Normally, these muscles maintain the airways in a state of slight bronchoconstriction. However, bronchial tone may change with either the situation or pathology. The bronchial muscle tone comes under the control of that segment of the sympathetic nervous system called the adrenergic receptors.

The adrenergic receptors can be subdivided into several sections, the functions of which are not limited to the airways. A drug that primarily affects one subsegment of the organs served by the adrenergic receptors, therefore, usually affects the other organs served as well, leading to that drug's major side effects. Two of the most important subsets of the adrenergic receptors are the beta-1 and beta-2 receptors. Beta-2 receptors are found primarily in the airways, though they also play some part in cardiac stimulation, vasodilation, anxiety, nervousness, insomnia, tremors, and glucogenesis. Their primary function, when stimulated, is to relax the airways (bronchodilation). Beta-1 receptors, on the other hand, are found primarily in the heart. Their stimulation can lead to increased cardiac output, tachycardia, and a tendency to cardiac irritability and arrhythmias. Beta-1 receptors are found to a lesser extent in bronchial muscle, but play a minor part in bronchial muscle tone (Ziment, 1978). It is much more therapeutic to use beta-2-stimulating drugs and beta-2 agonists for bronchodilation than beta-1-stimulating drugs because beta-2 drugs affect the receptors that are most prominently located in the airways. Beta-2 drugs affect the heart to a lesser extent, with cardiac stimulation as one of their side effects. Using beta-1 drugs for bronchodilation can result in a hazardous level of cardiac stimulation because a large amount of the drug is necessary to achieve bronchodilation, their primary action

is cardiac stimulation, and they are very short acting so must be repeated at short intervals to maintain bronchodilation.

Bronchodilators may be given as intravenous, oral, or inhaled (topical) preparations. The intravenous and oral preparations should be used on a regular basis to maintain therapeutic blood levels. The topical drugs may be used on a regular basis, PRN prior to activities that cause shortness of breath or wheezing, or as immediate treatment for these symptoms. Care should be taken to avoid overuse of bronchodilators, as this can lead to paradoxical bronchoconstriction.

The topical bronchodilators are provided both as convenient cartridge (metered-dose) inhalers and as solutions for use in intermittent positive pressure or nebulization devices. Some clients may have difficulty using the inhalers because they require some muscular coordination. These persons may find it easier to use the nebulizer to deliver the topical bronchodilators.

The theophylline group forms the basis for all bronchodilator therapy and is the most important category of bronchodilators. For the usual pulmonary client, one of the theophyllines is given along with a beta-2 agonist such as terbutaline, alupent, or albuterol. A topical bronchodilator is also prescribed. Theophylline can be supplied as a rectal suppository but its absorption is erratic and this preparation is best avoided. The metabolism of theophylline is very individual so that monitoring of theophylline blood levels is necessary to adjust the dose correctly. This is especially important in the older client who may also have impaired liver function (Ziment, 1981). Instructions for use of the cartridge inhalers, which should be carefully followed, but often are not, may be found in Table 10–6. The gerontological nurse practitioner should check periodically to see that the client is using the inhaler properly.

Anticholinergics

Bronchospasm can be stimulated by the cholinergic receptors via stimulation of the mast

TABLE 10–5. SUMMARY OF MAJOR DRUG THERAPY IN RESPIRATORY DISEASE

Therapeutic Actions	Drug Examples	Side and Toxic Effects	Precautions, Nursing Implications
		Bronchodilators: Methylxanthines (theophyllines)	
Potent bronchodilation Increased ciliary beating	Aminophylline IV: 250–300 mg tid Tabs: 100–200 mg 4–6 times/day Theodur (Aminodur) 100–200 mg 2–4 times/day Elixophyllin 100–200 mg 2–4 times/day Choledyl (oxtriphylline) 200 mg Slo-phyllin 125–250 mg Aerolate SR 65–260 mg Bronkodyl 200 mg Aminophylline Suppositories	Low incidence Gastric discomfort common. Prevent by taking with food and perhaps smaller divided doses Side effects: polydipsia, dizziness, tachycardia, mild diuresis Toxicity: N/V, seizures, hematemesis, hypotension, coma, arrhythmias, flushing, headache, delirium Excess caffeine intake may add to side effects	Contraindications: peptic ulcer Infants and debilitated, especially with liver or heart disease, at special risk for toxicity IV drug's half-life increased in CHF and decreased in smokers Absorption of suppositories unreliable Intolerance to one xanthine does not necessarily mean intolerance to another Must be taken regularly to maintain blood level; only IV preparation is PRN drug Must dilute IV drug well and give slowly Minimum dose: 20 ml over 20 minutes Must individualize dose If theophylline blood level to be drawn, draw 1 hour before next scheduled dose Therapeutic range: 11–20 mg/dl
		Bronchodilators: Beta-2 Agonists	
Bronchodilation	Bronkosol (Isoetharine) Inhalation every 4 hours	Cardiac and stimulating effects	Usually dilute with 3 parts saline or water Should not be used with epinephrine but can be used alternately
Bronchodilation Decreases airway resistance	Metaproterenol (Alupent) Inhaled, tabs, elixir	Excess use can lead to paradoxical bronchial constriction	Contraindications: pregnancy, under 12 years old, drug allergy Caution: hypertension, coronary artery disease, CHF, diabetes Use inhaler PRN for shortness of breath, wheezing, and before problematic activities as well as regularly as ordered Use inhaler no more than every 3 hours
Bronchodilation	Terbutaline (Brethine, Bricanyl) inhaled Tabs: 2.5–5 mg 2–4 times/day S.Q.: 0.25 mg every 8 hours	Nervousness, weakness, drowsiness, tremor, headache, nausea, vomiting, hypotension	If tremors extremely problematic, may reduce dose; tremors usually decrease after a few weeks on the drug Lasts about 4 hours
Bronchodilation	Proventil (Albuterol) Inhaled or tabs	Same as terbutaline but with much less nervousness and tremor. Unusual taste or irritation of mouth. Reported nausea, excess CNS or CV stimulation	Should last about 6 hours Caution: coronary insufficiency, hypertension, hyperthyroidism, diabetes mellitus

Bronchodilators: Sympathomimetic Amines (Adrenergic)

Bronchodilation Improve effect of xanthines	Ephedrine (Bronchaid tabs) (OTC)	Bronchial irritation and edema Dried secretions, mucus plugs GI stimulation and irritation, nausea, tachycardia, palpations, hypertension, tremor, headache, flushing, anxiety, dizziness High incidence of prostatic hypertrophy and urinary retention in elderly males	Short duration Rebound bronchospasm with overuse
Primary cardiac stimulant Secondary bronchodilator	Epinephrine (Adrenalin) Nebulized forms: Micronephrine, Vaponephrine, Primatine (OTC), Bronkaid Mist (OTC)	High incidence of cardiovascular side effects	Very short action Usually repeated in about 20 minutes

Steroids

Anti-inflammatory Decrease airway obstruction and improve responsiveness to bronchodilators	Solu-Medrol IV: 60–80 mg tid in acute phases Prednisone/prednisolone 5–60 mg daily or in divided doses Long term: qod if possible	Short term: stress ulcer Long term: adrenal suppression, abnormal fat deposits, osteoporosis, growth suppression, myopathy, hypertension, diabetes, peptic ulcer, cataracts, electrolyte imbalances, easy bruising, lower resistance to infection, increased appetite, altered mentation (euphoria, psychosis) Signs of steroid withdrawal: malaise, headache, N/V, anorexia, backache, joint pain, emotional instability, increased allergic symptoms, and bronchospasm	Caution: peptic ulcer, diabetes, cardiovascular disease, hypertension, TB, chronic infection, psychological disorders If steroid dependent, must increase dose during stress Do not use alone—only with bronchodilators If long term, give qod or daily as single dose in early morning Taper—do not discontinue suddenly If changing to Vanceril, overlap with oral steroid Steroid-dependent person should wear identification bracelet to that effect Skin test for TB before starting long course of steroids Former TB patients on long-term steroids should also get INH
Topical steroid action	Bechlomethasone (Vanceril) 2 puffs 2–4 times a day	Sore throat. Occasional candida infection of mouth Increased nasal congestion or nasal polyps may occur after ceasing oral steroid	Must take regularly—not a PRN drug Use inhaled bronchodilator about 3 min before Vanceril Rinse mouth well after use

Anticholinergic

Reduce bronchospasms	Atropine inhaled	All side effects and precautions as with systemic atropine	Helpful only for selected patients May excessively dry secretions

TABLE 10–6. HOW TO USE CARTRIDGE INHALERS

1. Exhale slowly and completely
2. Place mouthpiece loosely in mouth. Do not close mouth around it
3. Begin a slow deep inspiration and deliver the drug just as that inspiration begins
4. After inspiring as deeply as possible, hold breath for 5–10 seconds
5. Exhale. Wait 1 minute before taking the second puff
6. Keep the mouthpiece clean. Shake inhaler well before using

cells. When the mast cells are stimulated, they release mediators such as histamine that precipitate minor bronchospasm and also stimulate the vagus nerve. The vagal stimulation in turn can lead to profound bronchospasm. Although little is yet known of the mechanism, it is known that hypersensitivity is one possible stimulator of the cholinergic response. In younger asthmatic clients, cromolyn sodium is sometimes effective in preventing the onset of an asthma attack. Because this drug is not usually used for the elderly, however, it is not included in this discussion. For some clients of any age, however, atropine type drugs may block this type of response. The effect of the atropine is individual. The physician may, therefore, prescribe atropine as a part of the topical drug therapy and then withdraw it if it does not prove effective for that particular client.

Steroids

The steroid drugs are very important in the therapy of the inflammatory airway response. They may be administered intravenously, orally, or topically. Short-term use of steroids, either orally or intravenously, is absolutely necessary in acute exacerbations of emphysema, chronic bronchitis, and asthma. Used on this basis, the drugs carry few hazards other than increasing the risk of stress ulcer. Some clients require maintenance doses of oral steroids on a long-term basis, however, and are therefore prone to all the hazards of long-term steroid use. The particular problems of steroid use in the elderly include the tendency for osteoporosis, cataracts, fluid and electrolyte imbalance, increased appetite, lower resistance to infection, and mental status changes, including steroid psychosis. In many clients, these problems can be avoided by maintaining them on topical steroid therapy (beclomethasone [Vanceril]). Because the drug has only a topical effect, systemic steroid side effects are not a problem. The major hazard of topical steroid use is the potential development of oral candida if the mouth is not rinsed well after every use. The most important problem in using optimal steroids is the fact that the client cannot physically feel the effect. Hence, the drug may be abruptly discontinued and the client consequently predisposed to an acute episode of bronchospasm. Topical steroids are not effective during an acute asthma attack and should be replaced by oral or intravenous steroids during that time.

Hazardous Drugs

Sedatives and hypnotics can pose problems when they are administered to any elderly client. They are especially dangerous when administered to the elderly client who has a respiratory problem as they depress respirations. As a result, the client can become hypoxic, retain carbon dioxide, or both. Relaxation techniques are far safer than tranquilizers and sedatives for use in these clients. Haldol, in small doses, is often safe and effective.

Antihistamines

Antihistamines are a potential problem for the elderly pulmonary client as they dry secretions and therefore make it more difficult to clear them from the airways. Antihistamines are generally not used for pulmonary clients.

TABLE 10–7. COMBINATION BRONCHODILATORS

Drug	Contents	Duration of Action
Amesec	Aminophylline 130 mg Ephedrine 25 mg Amobarbital 25 mg	Short (capsule) Long (tablet)
Marax	Theophylline 130 mg Ephedrine 25 mg Hydroxzine Hydrochloride 10 mg	Short
Tedral	Theophylline 130 mg Ephedrine 25 mg Phenobarbital 8 mg	Short
Tedral SA	Theophylline 180 mg Ephedrine 48 mg Phenobarbital 25 mg	Long
Quibron	Theophylline 150 mg Glycerol guiacolate 90 mg	Short

Combination Drugs

A variety of available drugs combine a small amount of theophylline with ephedrine as a bronchodilator and then add a sedative preparation to reduce the side effects of the ephedrine. In addition to the fact that these combination drugs are more expensive than single drugs, there are several additional reasons to avoid them. First, the amount of theophylline contained in these combinations is too small to be effective (Table 10–7). Second, ephedrine is much less effective than the aforementioned bronchodilator drugs. It also has some troublesome side effects, the most important of which is the potential of urinary retention in elderly males. Acute reactions to ephedrine result in such problems as severe hypertension, pulmonary edema, and cardiac arrhythmias. Ephedrine also interacts with other drugs, such as antagonizing the antihypertensive effects of guanethidine. The ephedrine may be less effective if the client is taking reserpine or methyldopa. If the client is taking monoamine oxidase (MAO) inhibitors, the pressor effects of ephedrine are compounded. Finally, the fixed combination of ephedrine and theophylline is potentially more toxic than if the drugs are administered separately (Webber-Jones & Bryant, 1980). Moreover, a sedative agent is added to the drug combination in order to reduce the many side effects of ephedrine; the resulting sedative effect is of no help and of possible harm to the client.

Over-the-Counter Preparations

Both oral and inhaled bronchodilators are available as over-the-counter (OTC) drugs and are heavily advertised. The inhaled preparations are usually epinephrine (Adrenalin), whereas the oral drugs may be either epinephrine (Adrenalin) or ephedrine. Adrenalin preparations should be avoided: they are primarily beta-1 drugs and therefore are less than maximally effective as bronchodilators; they are also short acting and therefore are frequently overused to the point where dangerous cardiac stimulation occurs. Cardiac arrest is not infrequent as a result of the use of these preparations to treat acute episodes of bronchospasm and shortness of breath. Some theophyllines are also used in OTC preparations, but should be taken only under the supervision of a physician. OTC preparations should not be used in addition to prescribed drugs. The most important advice about OTC drugs is that, if a person is experiencing sufficient respiratory distress to need OTC preparations, a careful evaluation by a pulmonary physician is warranted.

SUMMARY

This chapter has explored the physiological changes associated with aging of the lungs, the major pathological lung disorders, and the common therapeutic modalities for lung disorders. In terms of morbidity and mortality, lung disease is among the most important diseases in the United States today. Often unrecognized until very late, diseases of the lung comprise a large portion of the caseloads of many home health care nurses. It is, therefore, critical that the gerontological nurse practitioner who works with the elderly either in the acute or home care setting be thoroughly acquainted with the most common lung diseases and their management.

REFERENCES

Adams, G. F. (1981). *Essentials of geriatric medicine* (2nd ed.). Oxford: Oxford University Press.

American Cancer Society. (1985). *1985 cancer facts and figures*. New York: American Cancer Society.

American Lung Association. (1971). *Air pollution primer*. New York: American Lung Association.

American Lung Association. *Second Hand Smoke*. (Pamphlet).

American Thoracic Society Respiratory Care Committee. (1978). Intermittent positive pressure breathing. *ATS News. 4*(3), 5–6.

Anderson, J. M. (1978). You may get more than you can see or smell. *American Lung Association Bulletin, 64*(5), 2–8.

Bowles, L. T., Portnoi, V., & Kenney, R. (1981). Wear and tear: Common biologic changes of aging. *Geriatrics, 36*(4), 77–86.

Burrows, B., Knudson, R. J., Quan, S. F., & Kettel, L. J. (1983). *Respiratory disorders*. Chicago: Year Book.

Carroll, P. (1987). The right way to do chest physiotherapy. *RN, 50*(5), 26–29.

Clark, D. F. (1975–1976). *Management of pneumonia*. Pulmonary Fellows Presentations. University of Arizona. Unpublished.

Corman, R. (1978). *Air pollution primer*. New York: American Lung Association.

Cortese, A. D. (1981). *The health basis for clean air*. *American Lung Association Bulletin, 63*(6), 3–6.

Costle, D. M. (1977). A report from the new EPA Administration. *American Lung Association Bulletin, 63*(6).

Eggland, E. T. (1987). Teaching the ABCs of COPD. *Nursing 87, 17*(1), 61–64.

Farer, L. S. (1982). *Tuberculosis: What the physician should know*. New York: American Lung Association and American Thoracic Society, pp. 11–12.

Futrell, M., Brovendu, S., McKinnon-Mullet, E., & Browder, H. T. (1980). *Primary health care of the older adult*. North Scituate, MA: Duxbury Press.

Gerding, D. N. (1981). Etiologic diagnosis of acute pneumonia in adults. *Postgraduate medicine, 69*(4), 136–150.

Geschickter, C. F. (1973). *The lung in health and disease*. Philadelphia: Lippincott.

Glassroth, J. (1981). Tuberculosis: A review for clinicians. *Clinical Notes on Respiratory Diseases, 20*(2), 5–13.

Greifzu, S., Crebase, C., & Winnick, B. (1987). Lung cancer: By the time it's detected, it may be too late. *RN, 50*(3), 52–58.

Hahn, K. (1987). Slow-teaching the C.O.P.D. patient. *Nursing 87, 17*(4), 34–41.

Hammond, E. C. (1962). The effects of smoking. *Scientific American, 207*(1), 39–51.

Harvey, A. M., Johns, R. J., McKusick, V. A., Ownes, A. H., & Ross, R. S. (1980). *The principles and practice of medicine* (20th ed.). New York: Appleton-Century-Crofts.

Hill, C. D., & Stamm, W. E. (1982). Pneumonia in the elderly: The fatal complication. *Geriatrics, 37*(1), 40–50.

Iseman, M. D., Albert, R., Locks, M., Raleigh, J., Sutton, F., & Farer, L. S. (1980). Guidelines for short-course tuberculosis chemotherapy. *American Review of Respiratory Disease, 121*(3), 611–613.

Karasov, D. (1982). A closer look at oxygen concentrators. *Respiratory Therapy, 12*(3), 91–96.

McHugh, J. (1987). Perfecting the three steps of chest physiotherapy. *Nursing 87, 17*(11), 54–57.

McIntosh, H. D., Entman, M. L., Evans, R. I., Martin, R. R., & Jackson, D. (1978). Smoking as a risk factor. *Heart and Lung, 7*(1), 145–149.

Mims, B. C. (1987). The risks of oxygen therapy. *RN, 50*(7), 20–25.

Moser, K., Archibald, C., Hansen, P., Ellis, B., & Whelan, D. (1980). *Better living and breathing: A manual for patients*. St. Louis: Mosby.

Petty, T. L. (1974). A critical look at IPPB. *Chest, 66*(1), 1–2.

Petty, T. L. (1981). Home oyxgen therapy for COPD. *Postgraduate Medicine, 69*(4), 102–113.

Pierson, D. J., & Hudson, L. D. (1981). Pulmonary problems. *Geriatrics, 36*(4), 45–47.

Pritzker, D. (1981). There's a greater chance for permanent TB cure with short-term drug therapy. *American Lung Association Bulletin, 67*(3), 2–7.

Rodescu, D. (1977). Lung cancer. *Medical Clinics of North America, 61*(6), 1205–1218.

Shy, C. M., Goldsmith, J. R., Hackney, J. D., Lebowitz, M. D., & Menzel, D. B. (1978). Health effects of air pollution. *American Thoracic Society News, 4*(2), 22–63.

Spearing, C., & Cornell, D. J. (1987). Incentive spirometry inspiring your patient to breathe deeply. *Nursing 87, 17*(9), 50–51.

Tashkin, D. P., & Cassan, S. M. (1978). *Guide to pulmonary medicine*. New York: Grune & Stratton.

Traver, G. A. (ed.). (1982). *Respiratory nursing: The science and the art*. New York: Wiley.

Webber-Jones, J. E., & Bryant, M. K. (1980). Over-the-counter bronchodilators. *Nursing 80, 10*(1), 34–39.

West, J. B. (1977). *Pulmonary pathophysiology: The essentials*. Baltimore: Williams & Wilkins.

Ziement, E. (1981). How to select an appropriate respiratory drug. *Geriatrics, 36*(5), 89–101.

Ziment, I. (1978). *Respiratory pharmacology and therapeutics*. Philadelphia: Saunders.

11

CARDIOVASCULAR CHANGES

The frequency of cardiovascular diseases in the elderly is high. These diseases are not a part of the normal aging process, as much of the general population believes, but are due to pathological processes. The normal changes that accompany increasing age, however, create an environment in which pathological processes may progress more readily, especially if an individual has certain risk factors. In this chapter, the normal changes of aging in the cardiovascular system are discussed. The risk factors that speed the development of pathological processes in the cardiovascular system are discussed separately, along with how they can be altered. The following cardiovascular diseases occur frequently in the elderly: ischemic disease, including angina, myocardial infarction, cerebral vascular accident, and peripheral vascular disease; congestive heart failure; and anemia. Each of these is discussed along with assessment parameters and commonly used health care management modalities.

AGING OF THE CARDIOVASCULAR SYSTEM

Some physiological changes that occur in the cardiovascular system are due to the aging of the body and are independent of pathological processes. These physiological changes affect the efficiency with which the cardiovascular system functions and alter the function of the whole body. The cardiovascular system is the link to providing the oxygen and nutrients needed by the body tissue for metabolic requirements. Therefore, changes in it affect the whole.

The physiological changes that normally accompany aging occur at different rates in every individual. The rate of the aging process is dependent on an individual's life-style, environment, and heredity. Normal changes are unmodifiable and are considered intrinsic (Ebersole & Hess, 1981). Later, in the "Maintenance of Wellness" section, the extrinsic factors are discussed.

Changes in the Heart and Vessels

The size of the heart does not change significantly during the aging process (Denham, 1980), although there is an illusion of enlargement. This illusion is caused by changes in the dimensions of the thoracic cavity that occur with age. In truth, the heart remains about the same size throughout the life-span if pathological factors are not presented or if there is no change in the individual's activity level (Ebersole & Hess, 1981). However, a nonpathological decrease in the size of the heart may occur in many aging individuals; this is due to disuse atrophy of the myocardium resulting from a decrease in a person's activity level. The heart, like any muscle, will decrease in size when used less.

The cardiac output is decreased by the aging process. Cardiac output is measured by the amount of blood ejected by the heart per minute and is derived from the number of beats per minute and the stroke volume, which is the amount of blood ejected with each beat. Stroke volume is dependent on the size of the heart chambers, filling time, and the strength of the heart muscle for contraction. With aging, the efficiency and strength of the heart muscle are decreased, resulting in decreased stroke volume and, thus, decreased cardiac output. The heart rate has been found to remain unchanged throughout the lifespan or to be slightly decreased at the resting rate. This, coupled with the decreased stroke volume, means that there is a decrease in the cardiac reserve available to meet an increased demand for oxygen. The cardiac reserve is defined as the heart's ability to increase its pumping capacity. When a stressor presents itself to an aged person, diminished cardiac output becomes a significant factor. It makes no difference if the stressor is physiological or psychological—due to illness, activity, excitement, or worry—the heart is not able to meet the body's need for oxygen as quickly and efficiently as in previous years. Pulse rate increases with the presentation of the stressor, but the response rate is slower and the degree of increase is less than in the young adult. When the stressor is gone, the heart is much slower to return to the previous resting rate, putting an additional energy drain on the heart itself and the entire body (Forbes & Fitzsimons, 1981; Malasanos, Barkauskas, Moss, & Stoltenberg-Allen, 1981; Yurick, Robb, Spier, & Ebert, 1980). Some individuals may even develop congestive heart failure as a result of the body's attempt to compensate for an increased oxygen demand (Yurick et al., 1980). The valves of the heart also undergo aging changes, thickening and becoming somewhat rigid due to sclerotic changes (Denham, 1980; Malasanos et al., 1981; Yurick et al., 1980). These alterations account for the heart murmurs found in many aging clients. These murmurs are usually heard as a soft systolic ejection murmur (Forbes & Fitzsimons, 1981, Malasanos et al., 1981).

The vessels of the cardiovascular system also undergo changes as a result of aging. Arteries lose elasticity (Forbes & Fitzsimons, 1981) because of the decreased amounts of elastin and fragmentation of the elastin that is present (Malasanos et al., 1981). There is also an increase in the collagen present that further decreases the elasticity of the arteries (Forbes & Fitzsimons, 1981), causing dilation and elongation in the larger arteries (Malasanos et al., 1981). Additionally, deposits of calcium and fat are laid down along the intima of the vessels. These deposits are believed to occur without the presence of the pathological process of arteriosclerosis, but nonetheless cause a narrowing of the lumen of the arteries and further decrease the ability of the artery to expand and stretch with changing tissue needs. Therefore, an increase in peripheral resistance occurs, leading to a reduction in the circulatory perfusion of the tissues distal to the narrowed arteries and a slight increase in the blood pressure (Forbes & Fitzsimons, 1981). It is not uncommon to find systolic pressures of 150–155 mm Hg in elderly clients. If possible, the pressure should be lowered, but this is difficult because of physiological changes in the elderly person (American Heart Association [AHA], 1980). As the vessels lose elasticity, they may also become dilated and elongated, resulting in tortuous vessels (Malasanos et al., 1981).

The fewest changes in perfusion occur in the brain and heart, whereas the greatest number of perfusion changes occur in the kidney and liver (Ebersole & Hess, 1981). Perfusion changes that take place throughout the body account for many of the various system changes that are attributed to aging. One such example is in the cardiovascular system itself, as the incidence of varicose veins is increased in the aged. This is due to the physiological loss of elasticity and elongation of the vessels. The baroreceptor sensitivity is also blunted with age (Malasanos et al., 1981).

Changes in the Respiratory System Affecting Oxygen Absorption

The aging process in the lungs also contributes to the problems that result from aging in the cardiovascular system. Maximum breathing capacity decreases, resulting in a decrease in the arterial blood oxygen level (Ebersole & Hess, 1981). In the lungs, as in the cardiovascular system, there is a loss of elasticity. There are also fewer alveoli, and their size is increased (Forbes & Fitzsimons, 1981) due to a degeneration of the intraalveolar septi and fusion of adjacent alveoli to form large alveolar sacs (Forbes & Fitzsimons, 1981; Malasanos et al., 1981). The new alveoli sacs take on the characteristics of emphysematous sacs in that they have an increased residual volume (Forbes & Fitzsimons, 1981; Yurick et al., 1980). The alveoli membranes also becomes thickened (Yurick et al., 1980). These changes result in an alteration in the exchange process of oxygen and carbon dioxide. The end result of the pulmonary changes of aging is that the arterial oxygen level is decreased, meaning that less oxygen is available to be delivered to the tissues. This is especially true when the individual is in the recumbent position. The decreased arterial oxygen levels help to explain the periodic confusion experienced by some aged persons at night (Yurick et al., 1980).

Cardiovascular Changes in the Genitourinary System

Vascular changes also occur in the renal arteries. The result is an impairment in the reabsorption of fluid and solids (Forbes & Fitzsimons, 1981) and a decrease in the glomerular filtration rate (Forbes & Fitzsimons, 1981; Lindeman & Klinger, 1981). Impairment in reabsorption is further increased because of the changes that occur specifically to the renal system. These include a loss of nephron mass and degenerative

changes in the remaining nephrons (Forbes & Fitzsimons, 1981).

MAINTENANCE OF CARDIOVASCULAR SYSTEM WELLNESS

To maintain the highest possible state of wellness of the cardiovascular system, or what is known by the American Heart Association as "heart healthy," an individual must have a "healthy" life-style (AHA, 1981). The first step is to be familiar with the risk factors that contribute to cardiovascular disease. The generally accepted risk factors include the following:

1. Family history of heart disease
2. Increased age
3. Sex (males have higher rates than females before menopause)
4. Psychological factors (type A personality and stress)
5. Cigarette smoking
6. Diet that is high in lipids and sodium
7. Obesity
8. Sedentary life-style
9. Hypertension
10. Diabetes

This list identifies risk factors that one should consider when attempting to maintain a state of wellness of the cardiovascular system. The first three risk factors are unalterable. A strong family history of heart disease has been shown to increase an individual's risk of developing cardiovascular disease. The aging population is obviously affected by the second and third factors. Aging is a risk factor in itself because the aging process alters the base of normal physiology, so that pathological processes progress more easily. After menopause, females have coronary disease almost as frequently as males (AHA, 1981). This is believed to be due, in part, to a decrease in the estrogen level. Estrogen has been shown to increase the level of high-density lipids in women before menopause, so it acts as a protective factor (Bullock & Rosendahl, 1984; Gresham, 1980).

Risk factors four through eight are considered the alterable risk factors. Ideally, changes should be made in these risk factors when an individual is in childhood. Research has shown that coronary heart disease begins in childhood, with symptomatology caused by the cumulative effects of years of risk factors being present (Gresham, 1980). Unfortunately, the young have difficulty realizing the long-term effects that their actions, or lack thereof, have on their bodies. Long-term use and abuse of the body through accidents, physical and psychological stress, and/or neglect in care of general health and nutrition take their toll on the body's condition for aging (Ebersole & Hess, 1981). It has been found that most people are not willing to make changes in life-style until there are positive signs that the pathological process is already present.

Whether the actions to decrease the alterable risk factors are taken when the person is young or old, the actions are the same. The outcome of altering these risk factors depends on the amount of damage already incurred by the cardiovascular system. Although current research has not shown conclusively that the pathological process can be stopped in all people, it appears that the process can be slowed; in some retrospective research, if the alteration of the risk factors is great enough, early enough (i.e., before the lesions become fibrotic), and consistent over a sufficiently long period of time, circulation has been shown to improve (Brocklehurst, 1985; Gresham, 1980). All the actions for altering the risk factors fall within the realm of self-care. This means that the individual must wish to make the changes and be willing to alter the activities of daily living. The reward is a general feeling of wellness and the knowledge that the individual is acquiring more control over his or her body.

Each of the alterable risk factors is discussed separately along with the actions needed

to alter them. The last two risk factors on the list, hypertension and diabetes, are considered controllable risk factors. It is important that these risk factors be controlled if the frequency and severity of the complications of cardiovascular disease are to be reduced. Studies performed by the Veterans Administration Cooperative Group on Antihypertensive Agents in 1967 and 1970 have shown that hypertension that is kept within normal ranges decreases the mortality from coronary heart disease (Fardy, Bennett, Reitz, & Williams, 1980). Hypertension is discussed further in the section on cardiovascular disorders. Diabetes has among its many complications an increased rate of cardiovascular diseases. Information on diabetes is included in Chapter 9.

Psychological Factors

An increased emotional stress level places physiological stress on the cardiovascular system and increases the risk for developing cardiovascular disease. Emotional stress can be due to the lifestyle and environment or to the personality type. The pace of today's life-style creates an environment of high stress. The individual's personality type, if it is Type A, can create stress itself. A Type A personality is one who is always pushing oneself and is often impatient. This person creates his or her own stress.

Personality is probably the most difficult of the risk factors to alter. Elderly persons are often very resistant to change. In order to change a personality type, methods of coping with stress, big or small, internal or external, need to be changed. For much of the aging population, altering their coping mechanisms to any great extent is unrealistic. The appropriateness of altering the coping mechanisms must be carefully and individually assessed. When an individual is found to exhibit anxiety or increased stress levels, a variety of methods are available to have the person decrease the anxiety level without changing the personality. Anything from yoga to redirecting energy to a creative project can be a successful relaxation technique. If the aged client has never practiced any form of relaxation technique, the gerontological nurse practitioner can teach the client imagery. The time taken to create a pleasant mental picture can itself provide the client relief from the stress. Physical exercise should also be kept in mind for the aged. This is an excellent way to relax mentally while promoting circulation and loosening joints (Ebersole & Hess, 1981).

While assessing a person's stressors and coping mechanisms, environmental stressors must also be assessed. At times, a change to decrease the stressors of the environment can be more readily instituted than a change in the aged client's way of dealing with the stressor, i.e., the coping mechanism. An example of this might be a client living in a setting that requires one to prepare one's own meals, though this is difficult. A referral to a local agency could give periodic relief from this stressor without uprooting the client and yet assist in providing part of the nutritional needs.

Cigarette Smoking

Cigarette smoking is a significant risk factor that the individual can alter. The earlier in life it is altered the more significant are the results. The risk of cardiovascular disease increases with the number of cigarettes smoked. The death rate due to coronary heart disease is nearly as low for cigarette smokers who have stopped as it is for people who have never smoked. However, the Framingham Study and other references speak of a decline in smoking's impact after the age of 65 (Dawber, 1980; Rowe & Besdine, 1982; Schrier, 1982). It seems that the difference between the number of smokers and the number of nonsmokers that develop cardiovascular disease narrows with age, especially after the age of 65. The narrowing of the gap is not as great when it comes to the incidence of sudden death and peripheral vascular disease. In these two areas, smoking definitely increases the incidence, even after the age of 65. There is also a very slight correla-

tion between strokes and smoking in the aged (Dawber, 1980).

The Framingham Study cites two possible reasons for the decline in importance of cigarette smoking with the aged. One is that with age there is a higher incidence of the other risk factors, reducing the relative impact on health and wellness of cigarette smoking (Dawber, 1980). The other is that those people whose heart and cardiovascular systems were susceptible to the effects of cigarette smoking would have already developed the disease and thus have been removed. This would leave those people who were not as susceptible and, therefore, the smoking and nonsmoking groups would be close to equal in developing disease (Dawber, 1980).

The physiological effects of cigarette smoking are multiple. Smoking depletes the body of nutrients. It stimulates the release of catecholamines in the body, bringing about an increase in the heart rate that places an added strain on the entire system (Fardy et al., 1980). There is also a slight increase in blood pressure and some increase in cardiac output. An increase in the frequency of premature beats is also a danger (Dawber, 1980). Considering that the aging circulatory system already has a higher pressure and is unable to increase its heart rate and cardiac output as much and as quickly as is often needed with stress, adding the nicotine to the body puts an even higher strain on the system. Additionally, with smoking, carbon monoxide is taken into the lungs. Because hemoglobin has a greater affinity for carbon monoxide than oxygen (Fardy et al., 1980), there is a decreased oxygen-carrying capacity at a time when the oxygen transport is already decreased due to the natural aging process.

Diet and Obesity

America is a nation of people who, as a whole, are overconsumers of calories, making the majority of people overweight, and a large percentage of these calories come from animal fats. The combination of these two facts contributes significantly to the amount of cardiovascular disease in this country (Fardy et al., 1980). This problem is further complicated for the aged because their overall caloric needs are decreased but their need for nutrients does not change. The number of calories needed is determined by physical activity level, general state of health, and lean body weight (Rowe & Besdine, 1982). There is about a 2% decrease in basal metabolic rate over the age of 51 years. The reduction in activity is usually about 200 kcal/day up to the age of 75 years and 500 kcal/day after the age of 75 years (Eisdorfer, 1982). Because of each person's individual differences, the decline in caloric needs must be individually determined (Harper, 1981). The diet for a healthy heart is lower in sodium and animal fats than the usual American diet and has the appropriate number of calories for body metabolism and activity level without a weight gain (Ebersole & Hess, 1981). There are three potential problems in a diet that may cause an increase in risk factors: (1) hyperlipidemia, (2) obesity, and (3) high sodium intake.

Hyperlipidemia can be diet-induced and refers to an excess level of cholesterol and/or triglycerides. Research currently shows that lipids can be divided into three main groups: the very-low-density lipoproteins (VLDL), low-density lipoproteins (LDL), and high-density lipoproteins (HDL). The VLDL carry most of the triglycerides in the body and a small amount of cholesterol. Hypertriglyceridemia is felt to be caused by a combination of life-style and diet. It is often associated with excessive intake of alcohol and sugar (especially simple sugars) and a sedentary life-style.

The LDL and HDL are both carriers of cholesterol but are thought to work in very different ways. The LDL are believed to carry the cholesterol to the peripheral tissues, including the arterial walls, where it infiltrates the vessel wall and leaves a fat deposit. Total serum cholesterol and LDL have been found to be elevated in the body by a dietary intake high in saturated fats. These are the meat and dairy product fats. It can likewise be lowered by a dietary intake of unsaturated fats incread of saturated fats. These are primarily vegetable oils, fish, and poultry. HDL are protective and decrease the problems that potentiate the development of artherosclerosis. At this time, it is believed that HDL transport the cholesterol from the tissue to the liver to be excreted. The amount of HDL can be increased by maintaining an ideal body weight and an appropriate percentage of adipose tissue to lean muscle and by maintaining an appropriate physical activity program (AHA Nutrition Committee, 1982; Fardy et al., 1980).

An increased cholesterol level is felt to have a greater impact on increasing the risk of coronary artery disease than does an increased triglyceride level. This may be due in part to the fact that the true effects of triglycerides have not been discovered, but it is still believed that triglycerides may play some role in the development of atherosclerosis. Therefore, cholesterol levels are stressed more frequently. Even with the new facts about HDL and LDL, total serum cholesterol is still considered clinically. This is because the bulk of the cholesterol is carried by LDL (Fardy et al., 1980). To date, no studies have shown significant changes in the elderly with decreased LDL levels, but the potential benefit makes it well worth the attempt to diminish LDL and to take actions to increase HDL, with the hope of inhibiting atherosclerosis (Rowe & Besdine, 1982).

Obesity is a risk factor for coronary heart disease because of the increased stress put on the heart and lungs by the excess body weight. First, the heart must pump blood through more tissue, thus increasing the work load of the heart. If the person is susceptible to hypertension, blood pressure is further increased. Second, obese persons have more difficulty moving about and often fail to attain the needed amount of exercise. So, weight reduction, even in the elderly, can be an important goal, not only for decreasing the risk of heart disease, but also because it is associated with degenerative joint disease, diabetes, and other disorders (Schrier, 1982).

High sodium intake results in a tendency to retain body fluids, thus increasing blood volume. This puts an increased work load on the heart and contributes to the development of hypertension. In individuals who already have hypertension, blood pressure is further increased (Fardy et al., 1980).

The Select Committee on Nutrition and Human Needs of the United States Senate in 1977 drew up the following dietary recommendations to reduce the risk of coronary heart disease (Fardy et al., 1980, pp. 179–180):

- Reduce fat consumption to 30% of total calories
- Reduce saturated fat consumption to 10% of total calories
- Balance monosaturated and polysaturated fat intake to 10% of total calories each
- Reduce cholesterol intake to about 300 mg daily
- Increase complex carbohydrate consumption to 48% of total calories
- Reduce sugar consumption to 10% of total calories
- Reduce salt consumption to about 5 g daily

Difficulty in having the aged person comply with a low-cholesterol and low-fat, low-sodium, or calorie-restricted diet is not unusual. In order to abide by the prescribed diet change, he or she must overcome long years of likes and dislikes, cooking habits, and often cultural influences. When providing client education on diet changes, the nurse practitioner must remember that moderate changes in dietary habits are better than no changes. Elderly persons may become involved in priority setting and negotiating compromises with the nurse practitioner, and this can result in a more thorough understanding of their diet and long-term moderate compliance (Eliopoulos, 1979).

Sedentary Life-Style

Inactivity in the elderly poses a major threat to loss of health and physical fitness and can contribute to an increase in some of the other risk factors of coronary heart disease (e.g., obesity, hypertension, hyperlipidemia and further decreased activity level) (Fardy et al., 1980) and is itself a risk factor for coronary artery disease. The key to physical fitness for the aged, as is true for all age groups, is to develop a regular and moderate exercise program that is tailored to fit an individual's needs, abilities, and interests. An individualized exercise program increases the person's general "fitness" level. Exercise increases cardiovascular and pulmonary function (Dawber, 1980; Ebersole & Hess, 1981). Thus, the person will feel like doing more and be able to do so without feeling overly exerted. This is extremely important for the elderly because the more they are able to do the better their chances are of keeping their independence.

The ability to perform more physical activity occurs because the individual is able to breathe more deeply and efficiently, taking more oxygen into the lungs and increasing the amount of oxygen available to the cardiovascular system. This accounts for the increase in the pulmonary function that comes with physical fitness. The cardiac muscle is also strengthened, allowing oxygen to be carried to the tissues with less work. The individual is then able to perform the same or an increased amount of activity with less strain on the heart than would have occurred before a physical fitness program. Systolic blood pressure will be lower with the same amount of activity. In some clients there will be a decrease in their resting heart rates and systolic blood pressure. The product of the heart rate times the systolic blood pressure is referred to as the double product. This measurement is an excellent gauge of what the myocardial demand is at a given time, so it can be used to determine how much cardiac work an activity uses (Fardy et al., 1980; Schrier, 1982). When an exercise program is followed consistently, there is an increase in the amount of oxygen uptake by the tissues, increasing the efficiency of the work done by both skeletal muscles and the myocardium (Fardy et al., 1980).

There are many benefits to maintaining a consistent, progressive activity program. In addition to reducing the work load of the heart, a decrease in other risk factors can be seen. Obesity, hypertension, and hyperlipidemia are all reduced and the HDL levels are increased. Additional benefits of attaining physical fitness are a better self-image, more self-confidence, an increased ability to cope with stress, better sleep patterns, better eating habits, and more flexibility of the joints with less discomfort (Ebersole & Hess, 1981; Fardy et al., 1980).

The appropriate way to increase physical fitness is through an endurance or aerobic activity program that pushes the heart rate to 70–85% of the person's demonstrated safe heart rate. A safe heart rate is one without any clinical signs or symptoms of cardiovascular stress and is determined through exercise testing (AHA, 1975). If stress testing is not available or appropriate, another way to set the exercise heart rate in the beginning of an exercise program is to keep the heart rate below 20–30% above the resting rate (Smith, 1982). This rate should be held for 30 minutes if possible, and the activity should be undertaken at least three to four times per week, with the ideal being every other day. The type of aerobic activity used depends on the individual's fitness status and mobility at the time the program is undertaken. For some aged people whose life-style has been sedentary for years, simple household chores may be the place to begin. Making a bed and sweeping a floor require the use of the large muscles in the body and can be quite exertional for some elderly. For the person who has mobility difficulties, exercises may be restricted to range-of-motion and/or resistance type exercises in a bed and/or chair. Both upper and lower extremities need to be exercised. For most relatively healthy aged persons, walking is an excellent aerobic activity. Other excellent forms of aerobic activity are dancing or swimming (Ebersole & Hess, 1981; Forbes & Fitzsimons, 1981). As the exercise program progresses, the person should be able to increase the intensity or speed with which he or

she exercises as well as the amount of time the exercise lasts. All activity sessions should consist of three segments: warm-up, activity, and cool-down. The warm-up should last about 5–15 minutes and consist of stretching exercise of the upper and lower extermities and the back. The activity phase should be whatever type of aerobic activity is assessed to be the safest for the individual and should last 30 minutes if possible. If 30 minutes is not safe, the time should be shortened to a time that is. As the individual progresses in the program, this time can be lengthened. The cool-down period should continue until the person's heart rate has essentially returned to its resting rate. Cool-down can be accomplished by slowing the pace of the activity, i.e., a slow walk after walking briskly, or performing the stretching exercises used in the warm-up.

Before the client embarks on an activity, the nurse practitioner should encourage a complete health assessment to determine what activity level is safe and to ensure there are no unknown health problems. The elderly client should also be taught the danger signals to watch for and what to do if these occur. The most important step is that exercise should be stopped immediately if the client experiences chest pain or tightness in the chest, severe shortness of breath, dizziness, loss of muscle control, or nausea. If the person experiences excessive fatigue, a feeling of exhaustion that requires bed rest, or fatigue preventing any activity after exercise, the exercise program is too vigorous for the individual's needs and should be reduced.

Another sign that the exercise is too vigorous is a delay in the time before pulse and respiratory rates return to normal. The pulse rate should drop to below 120 within 5 minutes (assuming that the rate during exercise was above this) and below 100 within 10 minutes. The respiratory rate should return to normal within 10 minutes. This is usually 12–16 respirations per minute (Cooper, 1981). It is best for elderly persons to learn to count their pulse rates accurately. Due to reduced vision and sensory and mental changes, this is not always feasible. In these cases, health professionals or a family member should check the person's pulse rates.

Whatever form of activity used, it must be done consistently and over an extended period of time to be beneficial. If for some reason the program is interrupted for a period of time, the individual should be reassessed by a physician and begun at a lower activity level than when the activity program was stopped.

CARDIOVASCULAR DISORDERS

Hypertension

Hypertension is a common problem in the elderly population. As previously discussed, the blood pressure increases due to a decrease in elasticity of the arterial walls from the normal aging process of the cardiac system. This, along with the changes in the aging kidneys that reduce the efficiency of filtering and increase the number of cardiovascular risk factors present in the elderly, accounts for hypertension being a frequent problem. Hypertension is defined here as a systolic blood pressure of 160 mm Hg or over, a diastolic pressure of 90 mm Hg or over, or both. There is no question that hypertension is a primary risk factor for cerebrovascular and cardiovascular mortality in the elderly as well as the younger population (Baldini, 1981; Joint National Committee on Detection, Evaluation and Treatment on High Blood Pressure, 1984; O'Brien & Pattee, 1981; Radin & Black, 1981).

Assessment Parameters
In the past it has been questioned whether a systolic pressure of 160 mm Hg and over and a diastolic pressure of 90 mm Hg and over should be considered hypertension in the elderly. It has also been questioned whether it should be treated even if it is considered hypertension. Current research indicates that the answer to both of these questions is "yes" (Joint National Committee on Detection, Evaluation, and Treatment

of High Blood Pressure [JNC], 1984). Much research has indicated that the key to successful control of hypertension in the elderly is to "go slow and start low" (Applegate, Zwaag, Dismuke, & Runyan, 1982; JNC, 1984; Libow & Butler, 1981; O'Brien & Pattee, 1981; Peitzman, Bodison, & Ellis, 1982; Radin & Black, 1981).

Once an elderly individual has been identified as hypertensive through several blood pressure readings with either systolic, diastolic, or both pressures being increased, a complete history and physical examination must follow. Data collected should include the individual's family history of cardiovascular or cerebrovascular disease, weight, normal exercise level, daily stress encountered, and normal dietary intake, especially the lipids, calories, and sodium content of the diet. The physical exam must include a funduscopic exam, chest x-ray, and electrocardiogram (ECG), as well as examination of the heart, lungs, and all pulses (Moser, Guyther, Finnerty, Richardson, Langford, Perry, Wood, Krishan, Branche, & Smith, 1977). Blood studies are needed to determine serum levels of sodium, potassium, triglycerides, and cholesterol.

Nursing Care and Medical Management
The primary reason for failure to control an individual's blood pressure is noncompliance with treatment plans. Noncompliance often results from a client's failure to understand the disease, its complications, and the treatment modalities chosen. Therefore, client understanding is of prime importance (Baldini, 1981). Clients must understand that hypertension is a lifelong problem and that the disease is usually asymptomatic. Explaining this to a client can be quite a challenge in itself, particularly when dealing with an elderly person who is resistant to change and who questions the purpose of making changes "this late in life." Having the individual understand is especially important because the first step in management of hypertension is usually making changes in weight, diet, exercise, and smoking to decrease risk factors.

In many clients this may be all that is necessary to bring their blood pressure within normal range (JNC, 1984; Libow & Butler, 1981; Moser et al., 1977; O'Brien & Pattee, 1981). The section on "Maintenance of Wellness" contains information on ways in which the client can be helped to make these changes.

If these changes are unsuccessful in bringing the blood pressure under control, medications will be added by the physician. If the blood pressure is extremely high when discovered, medications may be used at the beginning while modifications in weight, diet, exercise, and smoking are being made. Because elderly clients are very sensitive to medication and easily develop toxic levels, medications are begun well below what is usually considered the normal dose and increased very slowly as needed (Libow & Butler, 1981). This gradual increase reduces the likelihood of orthostatic hypotension by allowing the autoregulating mechanisms to adjust to changes in vessel pressures (O'Brien & Pattee, 1981).

The initial medication is normally a diuretic, frequently thiazide (Hill, 1987). The side effects of hypokalemia can usually be corrected with dietary supplements. Otherwise, a potassium supplement can be provided. For individuals on digoxin also, a potassium supplement is usually prescribed (JNC, 1984; Libow & Butler, 1981; O'Brien & Pattee, 1981; Radin & Black, 1981).

If the diuretic is unsuccessful in lowering the blood pressure to the desired level after about 1 month, a second medication is added to the diuretic. The second medication can be gradually increased until either the desired effects are attained, the maximum dose is reached, or an undesirable side effect develops. If the maximum dose is reached without side effects and the blood pressure is not lowered to the desired level, either another drug is used in place of the second drug or another medication is added. If side effects develop, another drug may be added in place of that medication or the dosage can be lowered to the point that the side effects are elim-

inated; another medication can be added to achieve the desired level of blood pressure. The medications most frequently used as the second step are adrenergic-inhibiting agents such as reserpine or methyldopa or a beta blocker (JNC, 1984; Reichel, 1983; Schrier, 1982). The nurse must watch carefully for side effects and teach the client to do so as well. With reserpine, the major side effect is depression. This may not occur when the client first begins taking the medication. Reserpine may also cause an alteration in central nervous system function. This could be experienced as drowsiness, fatigue, or decreased mental acuity (JNC, 1984; Libow & Butler, 1981; Reichel, 1983). The side effects of methyldopa are orthostatic hypotension, particularly if the dosage is too high for the client, and alterations of the central nervous system function (Denham, 1980; JNC, 1984; Reichel, 1983). Dry mouth, sodium and fluid retention, and sexual dysfunction may also result (Denham, 1980; JNC, 1984). The principal side effects of beta blockers can be brady arrhythmias and heart failure. Fatigue, mental depression, hallucinations, bronchoconstriction, sexual dysfunction or, in the diabetic client, hypoglycemia may occur (Denham, 1980; JNC, 1984; Reichel, 1983).

The drugs most frequently used in the third step are the vasodilators. The principal side effect of these medications is a reflex tachycardia that could precipitate angina. This reflex does not occur as frequently in the elderly, especially if the starting dosage is low (Denham, 1980; Reichel, 1983; Schrier, 1982).

Once blood pressure has been brought under control, the problem of long-term compliance must be addressed. The client needs to understand exactly how and when medications are to be taken. Close follow-up must be maintained in order to ensure that the client does not develop side effects and that the blood pressure continues to be controlled. When blood pressure does not remain under control, it is usually a result of one, or a combination, of the following: (1) failure to take the medications correctly, (2) a high sodium diet, and (3) use of competing medications, e.g., cold remedies (Futrell, Brovender, McKinnon-Mullett, & Brower, 1980; JNC, 1984).

For much of the elderly population economics are a concern, especially when close and frequent follow-up visits are necessary. One way to contain cost at a reasonable level is to have a gerontological nurse practitioner perform much of the initial assessment. The physician and nurse practitioner make a plan of treatment with the client. The nurse practitioner is then able to provide most of the follow-up checks. The physician periodically reviews the client's progress and sees the client when necessary. Current research has shown this method to be an effective way of providing successful treatment while containing cost (Futrell et al., 1980; Peitzman et al., 1982).

Ischemic Disease

Ischemic disease is any disease process in the cardiovascular system that is caused by a decrease in the amount of oxygen and nutrients provided to the tissues. The cellular response to deficits in oxygen and nutrients is essentially the same everywhere in the body. For the purpose of this chapter, the discussion is limited to the vessels in the heart, when discussing angina pectoris and myocardial infarction; the vessels in the brain, when discussing cerebral thrombosis, cerebral embolism, cerebral hemorrhage, and transient ischemic attacks; and the peripheral vessels, when discussing arterial and venous narrowing and occlusion.

In normal vessels supplying oxygen and nutrients to the tissues, a balance is maintained. Vessels constrict and dilate in order to carry the exact amount of blood needed to meet the tissue's need for oxygen and nutrients. In ischemic disease insufficient blood is carried to the tissues. This is due to a vessel's inability to dilate and carry more blood when the needs of a tissue are increased. This abnormality may be due to arteriosclerotic diseases, thrombosis formation,

emboli lodging in a vessel, or spasm of an artery. The chances of the last three of these events occurring are greatly increased by the development of the first event, arteriosclerotic disease.

Arteriosclerotic disease is used as an umbrella to cover three separate processes: Monckeberg's sclerosis, atherosclerosis, and arteriolosclerosis. More than one of these processes may be found in an individual, but it is believed that they occur independently of each other. Monckeberg's sclerosis is the accumulation of calcified salts within medium-sized arteries. At times these may be seen on x-rays but do not cause any narrowing and, therefore, are not clinically significant. Arteriolosclerosis is a process that causes thickening of the arterioles. This process is thought to prevent the vessel from performing its normal function of dilating in response to increased need (Price & Wilson, 1986; Underhill, Woods, Sivarajan, & Halpenny, 1982). Atherosclerosis is the major cause of cardiovascular diseases discussed in this chapter. It is the presence of plaque in the arteries. Plaque is composed primarily of fat that has been deposited along the artery wall. This causes narrowing of the lumen of the artery and prevents that portion of the artery from responding to the message sent by the nervous system to dilate when more blood is needed in the area distal to the plaque. The plaque begins in the inner layer of the vessel wall but extends to the media with growth (Price & Wilson, 1982; Underhill et al., 1982). Some of the principal areas that are prone to the development of plaque are the aorta, carotid, coronary, iliac, and femoral arteries (Bullock & Rosendahl, 1984; Lewis & Collier, 1983; Underhill et al., 1982).

When atherosclerotic and arteriolosclerotic diseases are present in the elderly client, the normal aging changes in the vessels are further augmented. It may require only minimal emotional or physiological stress to put the client in a compromised state. The possibility that an individual will develop atherosclerotic and arteriosclerotic disease can be predicted to some degree by the number of risk factors that are present. These risk factors are discussed in the "Maintenance of Wellness" section of this chapter.

Angina Pectoris

Angina pectoris is cardiac pain that results from a critical deficit in the amount of oxygen and nutrients received by a portion of the heart muscle. The pain is transient. It can usually be linked to increased amounts of physical or emotional stress and subsides when the stress is decreased. There are two common causes of angina pectoris. The most common one is narrowing of the coronary arteries from atherosclerosis, which prevents the vessels from dilating as tissue demand increases. Essentially, the pain occurs when the double product increases the myocardial demand for oxygen beyond the level that the individual is able to supply at that particular stage of atherosclerosis. It subsides when the double product declines to a level of myocardial demand that the vessels can meet. The other cause is a coronary spasm called Prinzmetal angina. This is a spasm of a coronary artery that results in a decrease in the size of the lumen. After the spasm stops the lumen returns to its previous size. Among other possible causes of angina pectoris are the following: anemia, which decreases the oxygen-carrying capacity of the blood; hyperthyroidism, which increases the heart tissue's need for oxygen, possibly beyond the level available; or any situation that causes an imbalance in supply and demand sufficient enough to cause ischemia, but not necrosis. In angina, there is no cellular necrosis. For an in-depth discussion of the pathological response of angina pectoris on a cellular level, refer to a pathophysiology text.

Assessment Parameters

The pain of angina pectoris is usually substernal. Some individuals describe the pain as radiating up the neck, to the jaw and/or to the left arm and hand. The pain is usually felt as a burning, squeezing, or pressure sensation and is often associated with shortness of breath and at times

with belching. On examination, the client may be found to be diaphoretic. The elderly client will express pain of lesser intensity than a younger client (Brocklehurst, 1985; Futrell et al., 1980; Eliopoulos, 1979). Alternatively, they may only experience shortness of breath, extreme fatigue, or syncope (Brocklehurst, 1985; Steinberg, 1983). This may be due in part to a decreased sensory ability. Given the variable ways in which the pain may present, angina pectoris is at times mistaken for indigestion, hiatus hernia, gallbladder disease, ulcer, or muscular pain.

Among the common precipitating factors that cause an increase in demand on the heart, resulting in angina, are exercise, overeating, emotional upset, or extremes in temperature. The pain usually lasts 10 minutes or less, and relief is coupled with withdrawal of the factor or factors that caused the increased demand. Other signs that may occur during the ischemic attack are an S3 or S4 and an ejection murmur on auscultation of the heart. On an ECG an S-T segment depression may be seen or, if the angina is due to a coronary spasm, an S-T segment elevation may be seen. These signs result from the tissue's response to the ischemic process and disappear with the pain. This is because the ischemic process does not allow the heart to perform in its usual manner. If the blood supply is decreased to a portion of the muscle that controls the closure of one of the valves, the valve is unable to open and close as normal. Therefore, a murmur is present. The same concept applies to the ECG changes. With a decrease in the blood supply, the conduction system of the heart cannot flow as normal. This alters the electrical pathways and changes the appearance of the ECG as well as interfering with the efficiency of the heart as a pump during the pain.

Angina pectoris caused by coronary spasm is slightly different from the usual angina in that the normal precipitating factors may be lacking. This form of angina frequently occurs at rest and may awaken the individual from sleep.

Angina pectoris is primarily diagnosed by

means of a thorough history and physical examination, assessment of signs and symptoms during a pain episode, and the ability of sublingual nitroglycerin to relieve a pain episode. If the pain is troublesome enough, a heart catheterization may be performed. During a heart catheterization, radiopaque dye is injected into the coronary arteries, allowing them to be visualized and the location and degree of narrowing to be determined. Heart catheterization usually carries a higher risk in an older person than in a younger client but may still be performed safely. One of the factors in the decision to perform a catheterization is whether the client is a good candidate for bypass surgery should a blockage be found (Bemis, 1981; Reichel, 1983; Schrier, 1982).

Nursing Care and Medical Management.

The treatment of angina pectoris is centered around counseling and health instruction to minimize risk factors to the extent feasible and the provision of appropriate medications. Most individuals quickly learn that the pain will be relieved in a few minutes after the precipitating activity is stopped. They also learn that they are usually able to avoid or postpone pain if that same activity is performed at a slower pace. Counseling and direction are needed by the client and family to plan daily activities. When dealing with elderly clients it is more important than ever to include family members in the instructions and planning of care. It is also very important to write down the plans so that the elderly client has something to which he or she can refer. Relying on memory is not effective.

The most frequently used medications for management of angina pectoris are nitrates. Nitrates dilate peripheral vessels, coronary arteries, and collaterals. Nitrates come in three forms, all of which are used for angina pectoris. Nitroglycerin sublingually is used for relief of acute angina pain and for prophylaxis against an attack before the client undertakes an activity that has been known to cause pain. Effective use

of this drug needs extensive instruction. The client should be instructed to stop activity with the onset of pain, to sit or lie down and to take the sublingual nitroglycerin. The tablet should not be swallowed and may even be removed if not dissolved after the pain is gone. The activity that precipitated the pain may be resumed at a slower pace after the pain subsides. The precaution of sitting or lying is used because many individuals respond to sublingual nitroglycerin by becoming hypotensive and faint if standing. The client should also be warned that a headache may develop with the medication, which should be relieved by an analgesic, such as Tylenol. Clients should be instructed to report headaches to their health care professional if they are severe. The dose of nitroglycerin may be too large, a problem that can be alleviated. The client should be instructed to keep the nitroglycerin with him or her at all times, to keep it in an airtight, dark container, and to obtain a fresh supply every 6 months, as the sublingual form of nitroglycerin loses its potency and effectiveness very quickly. The client must be reassured that it is not an addicting medication and that it must be taken with each onset of pain. The client should also be instructed that if the pain is not relieved with the first tablet of nitroglycerin, another tablet should be taken in 5–10 minutes. The client may use up to three tablets in sequence. If the pain is not relieved with three tablets, medical assistance should be sought immediately.

The oral nitrates are taken on a timed basis. They may serve the purpose of decreasing the number of pain episodes and decreasing the severity of those that do occur. The usefulness of oral nitrates has yet to be determined conclusively (Rodman & Smith, 1979; Selzer, 1983).

Nitrol ointment is used topically in measured doses and is absorbed readily through the skin. It is helpful in decreasing the number and intensity of episodes, and has been found to be especially useful in decreasing nocturnal episodes. The client must be taught to measure the dose on the calibrated papers that come with some brands of the medication or to peel the back off the premeasured types. The old site of the medication application must be washed off before a new dose is applied. The placement of the dose should be rotated. The site chosen should be relatively free of hair, and there should be good circulation to the area. This means that placement of the dose below the knees should be avoided in many elderly clients.

Propranolol (Inderal) is another medication that can be used to decrease the number of angina episodes. A beta blocker decreases the heart rate and cardiac output, thus reducing the demand of the myocardium for oxygen. Clients must be instructed to never stop taking this drug on their own. It must be withdrawn slowly to avoid possible precipitation of a myocardial infarction. It also must be used with great caution in clients who have asthma, heart block, sinus bradycardia, and congestive heart failure because it may precipitate a crisis situation (Futrell et al., 1980).

In the cases of angina pectoris that are caused by coronary spasm, the calcium antagonists may be used. This group of medications causes dilation of the coronary and peripheral vessels and a reduction of cardiac contractibility (Brocklehurst, 1985; Reichel, 1983; Selzer, 1983; Steinberg, 1983).

When medications are not successful in controlling angina pain, the client should be evaluated for bypass surgery. The mortality is significantly higher with bypass surgery in the elderly, but with careful selection of the clients, this surgery can be a very effective way to increase the quality of the individual's life and hopefully prevent an eventual myocardial infarction. Revascularization may relieve angina pain and provide an increased tolerance level (Schrier, 1982; Steinberg, 1983). This may mean the difference between maintaining independence in daily living and needing to move to a long-term care facility. If bypass surgery is performed on the elderly client, postoperative recovery occupies far more time than is required for their younger clients. It may take elderly clients as long as 6

months to return to their normal level of functioning (Reichel, 1983).

Myocardial Infarction

When the ischemia is extensive enough in the myocardium to cause necrosis, a myocardial infarction occurs.

Assessment Parameters.

The symptoms exhibited by the elderly can be different than those shown by younger clients. The principal change is the intensity of the pain, as it is with angina pectoris. Many elderly clients do not express a severe pain and, therefore, do not seek medical assistance as readily. Also, it is not uncommon to find during a routine examination, when an ECG is done, that the elderly client has experienced a silent myocardial infarction. The client may also seek medical assistance with symptoms other than pain, such as sudden onset of extreme dyspnea or symptoms of stroke (Brocklehurst & Hanley, 1981; Rowe & Besdine, 1982; Schrier, 1982; Steinberg, 1983).

Nursing Care and Medical Management.

The acute care of the elderly client with a myocardial infarction is no different than the care of the younger person, with the exception of a higher rate of complications and mortality (Reichel, 1983; Rowe & Besdine, 1982; Schrier, 1982; Steinberg, 1983). Care of the elderly may be further complicated by the coexistence of other pathological processes and the possibility of increased sensitivity to medications. This increases the incidence of toxic response in the elderly (Schrier, 1982). For extensive information concerning nursing and medical assessment and treatment of the acute myocardial infarction client, a general medical–surgical nursing text or critical care text should be consulted.

Long-Term Management or Rehabilitation.

Cardiac rehabilitation is an important component in care of the post-myocardial infarction elderly client. It should restore the elderly client to the highest level of functioning possible—physiologically, psychologically, sociologically, and vocationally if desired. It can mean the difference between the individual being able to return to independent living and needing to move to a care facility. Post-myocardial infarction cardiac rehabilitation in the elderly is implemented as discussed in the "Maintenance of Wellness" section for decreasing risk factors, with a few exceptions. The primary differences are due to the common occurrence of complications, especially those of congestive heart failure, immobility, and slowed healing of the elderly. Elderly clients are usually slower to progress to pre-myocardial infarction levels than are younger clients and at times they are unable to attain their pre-myocardial infarction level. However, they can usually reach a higher functional level than that of total dependence. Many individuals experience extreme frustration in not bouncing back. This further slows their progress and can stop it completely. Nursing and medical professionals must work with and encourage these clients.

Some factors are contraindications to the exercise portion of an outpatient rehabilitation program. Primary among them are unstable angina, severe ventricular arrhythmias, uncontrolled atrial fibrillation, second- or third-degree heart block, shortness of breath, drop in blood pressure with exercise, or uncontrolled hypertension (Fardy et al., 1980; Steinberg, 1983). When contraindications are not present, there are many benefits to exercise for the elderly. These are found in the "Maintenance of Wellness" section.

The common rule of thumb used in increasing the activity level for any post-myocardial infarction client is the heart rate. It should be kept initially to the resting heart rate plus 20 during activity (Fardy et al., 1980). This rule of thumb is the same, no matter the age of the client. The difference arises because complications and other pathological processes may make elderly persons reach this heart rate with a much lower level of activity, possibly simply by walking across the room.

The intent of consistent exercise is that it should result in what is called the "training effect," even in the elderly. This will make it possible for the clients to perform routine activities of daily living with less of an increase in heart rate and thus with less demand for oxygen by the heart (i.e., the double product is lowered).

Peripheral Vascular Disease

Peripheral vascular disease is a common problem in the elderly, so common that many of its symptoms are believed by the general population to be "simply a part of getting old." The etiology of the process is primarily a superimposition of atherosclerosis and arteriosclerosis upon the normal changes that occur with aging in the vascular system. These normal changes are discussed in the section on "Aging of the Cardiovascular System" in this chapter. For discussion of the disease process, peripheral vascular diseases are divided into arterial ischemia (chronic and acute) and venous diseases.

Chronic Peripheral Artery Disease. Chronic arterial ischemia is the most common of the peripheral vascular diseases. With chronic ischemia, there is a slow progressive narrowing of the arteries in the lower extremities. Symptoms develop when the size of the arteries narrows to the point of not being able to transport sufficient oxygen and nutrients to meet the needs of the muscles, skin, and nerves in the lower extremities. The body develops collaterals similar to those that develop in the myocardium, but with continuation of the process eventually these are unable to keep pace with the circulation needs of the lower extremities, especially upon exertion.

Assessment Parameters

The most characteristic and common symptom of chronic arterial ischemia is intermittent claudication. The client usually complains of pain and/or cramping with walking the same distance. This sensation disappears with rest. Some individuals will not have pain but describe a feeling of fatigue or weakness. As the arteries become narrower, the distance the client is able to walk without experiencing discomfort continually shortens until the client reaches the point of having pain even while at rest. This progression may take several months or years, and many clients never reach this point in the process.

Other signs and symptoms that occur in chronic arterial narrowing are the sensation of coldness and then paresthesia in the extremities, especially the feet, thinning of the skin, diminished growth of hair, thickened and misshapen toenails, color changes in the limb with changes in posture, atrophy of the muscle mass, and slowed healing of any injury that occurs. Upon examination, the pulses distal to the location of narrowing will be diminished or possibly absent. Pallor of the affected extremity or extremities can be elicited by elevating the leg. When the leg is put in a dependent position, the limb takes more than 20 seconds for color to return, and then it frequently becomes rubor or cyanotic (Futrell et al., 1980; Rowe & Besdine, 1982). Sensation and skin temperature should also be checked as part of regular nursing assessments, as should the integrity of the skin. Another assessment tool to use is evaluation of blood pressure in the lower extremities, comparing these readings to those of the upper extremities. This is done at the ankle with a doppler. Pressures below 80 mm Hg are considered to be abnormal (Reichel, 1983).

As the disease process progresses to the point of pain at rest, ischemic fissures and ulcerations become more frequent. At this stage, pain at rest is a particular problem if the leg is elevated while in bed at night. For many clients, it is not until they reach this stage that they seek medical assistance. Until then, they may have simply decreased their activity levels to the point that the pain is prevented. Intervention is imperative now if gangrene and resultant amputation are to be avoided. The individual should be eval-uated by a physician to determine whether re-vascularization is possible.

Nursing Care and Medical Management

Nursing care for chronic peripheral arterial disease is primarily in the form of assessment for potential problems and client education to avoid problems. By assessing the elderly client whenever possible for the initial symptoms of the process, the progression can be slowed or stopped. If the client smokes, it is important for him or her to stop smoking. This is the greatest of the risk factors for chronic peripheral artery disease. Smoking probably causes vasospasms of the arterioles and results in a further reduction of the flow of blood (Reichel, 1983). Tight and constricting clothes can increase the number and severity of problems for these clients and should be avoided. Heating pads to "warm up" the legs and feet should also be avoided. It is difficult to convince elderly individuals that heating pads are not only dangerous but also relatively ineffective. The individual should also be cautioned against taking hot baths and instructed to test the water with an elbow rather than fingers. The client should be cautioned to check the feet daily for reddened areas and places where the skin is broken. If such an area is found, it must be watched closely and kept clean; shoes that rub or put pressure on the area must be avoided. If the redness lingers, or increases in area, medical assistance should be sought immediately. The same is true for any injury to the limbs.

Another precaution is avoiding exposure to cold temperatures. If it is necessary to be outdoors during cold weather, long underwear should be worn. Many clients also find it helpful to wear warm socks to bed. Properly fitting shoes are essential to avoid trauma to the feet. Emollients can be used on the feet and legs to help prevent dryness and cracking. When the sensation in the feet is diminished, toenails should be clipped with great care, preferably by a health professional. The client should be instructed to change positions frequently and not to cross the legs. Exercise should be encouraged.

Walking short distances that do not cause pain can increase the distance the person can tolerate, increase the collateral circulation, and increase blood flow in extremities that have vascular occlusion (Reichel, 1983).

In the person who has received revascularization or amputation, adhering to the treatment is imperative, especially stopping smoking. Follow-up studies have shown the frequency of occlusion in grafts of clients that continued to smoke is threefold that of those that stopped (Reichel, 1983). Clients with amputations run the risk of losing circulation in the remaining portion of the limb.

Acute Peripheral Artery Disease. Acute peripheral artery disease is the acute onset of ischemia, most often due to an embolus. It can also result from acute thrombosis, especially if the artery is already compromised by narrowing. Individuals who have aneurysms, atrial fibrillation, myocardial infarction, or any atherosclerotic and arteriosclerotic disease are at greater risk to develop an embolus or acute occlusive thrombus. Because of the suddenness of this process, collateral circulation cannot be established to compensate for the occlusion.

Assessment Parameters
Diagnosis of the process is not usually difficult. The classic signs and symptoms are the "Five P's" (Reichel, 1983, p. 124) that occur with abrupt onset:

1. Pain
2. Pallor
3. Pulselessness
4. Paresthesias
5. Paralysis

Not every client exhibits all these signs and symptoms. The presence of a sign or symptom is dependent on the size and location of the artery that is occluded and on the previous status of the artery and the tissue distal to it. This means that if there is already sufficient narrowing to cause diminished pulse or decreased sensation in the limb, the client may not be acutely aware of any change in status. It also depends on the individual's mental status and ability to communicate a change.

Nursing Care and Medical Management
The best form of management for this disease process is prevention. Individuals who are at high risk should be cautioned against constriction of the vessels in the lower legs, as discussed in the section on "Chronic Peripheral Artery Disease," and to seek medical attention at the first onset of symptoms. If an acute occlusion occurs, time in seeking treatment is important to the successful outcome of the treatment. Medical treatments used may be an embolectomy, which has a high success rate, anticoagulants, which must be used with great caution and close nursing assessment in the aged to prevent bleeding, or revascularization of the limb. If these treatments are unsuccessful or occur too late, amputation to a level of good blood supply becomes necessary.

Peripheral Venous Disease. Varicose veins and thrombophlebitis occur with increased incidence in elderly persons.

VARICOSE VEINS. Varicose veins develop more easily in the elderly population because of a combination of the veins losing their elasticity with age and the leg muscles weakening so that the veins are not supported as well.

Assessment Parameters and Management
With the onset of varicose veins there is venous engorgement in the extremity. The client complains of the calf aching and a feeling of heaviness that is relieved by elevating the extremity. As the process progresses, dependent edema develops and venous stasis may appear with a change in skin pigmentation. Management primarily consists of using support stockings to counteract stasis and swelling of the veins. The client should be encouraged to walk on a regular basis, if possible, and to elevate the legs peri-

odically during the day. This should help prevent venous stasis. The nurse practitioner should teach the client the signs and symptoms of thrombus formation and stasis ulceration. The nurse practitioner should also be vigilant for signs of severe venous dysfunction, as this would predispose to thrombus formation and/or stasis ulceration (Giorella & Bevil, 1985; Price & Wilson, 1986).

THROMBOPHLEBITIS. Thrombophlebitis occurs more frequently among elderly clients who have been on bed rest or had a recent trauma to the lower extremities. This trauma could be a result of either surgery or a fracture.

Assessment Parameters and Management

Signs, symptoms, and treatment of thrombophlebitis depend on the location of the vessel involved. If the thrombophlebitis occurs in a superficial area, the area will usually be red, warm, and painful and tender to the touch. Treatment for the superficial thrombophlebitis usually involves heat, rest, elevation of the leg, and use of elastic stockings until the symptoms have disappeared. For deep thrombophlebitis, there may be edema present, as well as distended superficial veins, a reddish cyanotic color, pain, and tenderness (McMahan, 1987). Along with the treatment provided for superficial thrombophlebitis, anticoagulants are frequently used when deep vessels are involved (Steinberg, 1983).

Careful nursing assessment must accompany the administration of the anticoagulants. Nursing care must include avoidance of positions and situations that may cause strain to the client, provision of adequate fluids, and alertness to the signs and symptoms of pulmonary embolism (Eliopoulos, 1979).

Both severe varicose veins and deep thrombophlebitis can damage the veins, causing chronic venous insufficiency, unless adequate support stockings are used. These stockings should be removed only at night and periodically to determine if edema is still present and use of the stocking is still needed. The signs and symptoms of chronic venous insufficiency include chronic edema over the lower third or more of the leg. Frequently, the area will develop a brownish pigmentation. If the edema cannot be controlled by support stockings, the tissue in the area will become hardened and fibrotic, and chronic stasis cellulitis will result (Steinberg, 1983).

Cerebral Vascular Disease

Cerebral vascular accidents, or strokes, occur when there is a disruption in the cerebral blood flow. The incidence of cerebral vascular accidents increases with age. Although commonly associated with the aging process, cerebral vascular accidents are due to a pathological process in the cardiovascular system. The occurrence of strokes is closely related to the presence of the cardiovascular risk factors leading to the development of atherosclerosis. Hypertension is especially important in contributing to cerebral vascular accidents. There are three common causes of strokes—cerebral thrombosis, embolus, and hemorrhage.

Assessment Parameters

The most frequent cause of cerebral vascular accidents is a cerebral thrombosis that becomes large enough to cause ischemia to cerebral tissue. Cerebral thrombosis is considered a disease of the elderly because its peak incidence is in persons 60–69 years of age (Price & Wilson, 1986). A thrombosis usually occurs in a vessel that has already been narrowed by an atherosclerosis plaque. The plaque increases turbulence of blood in the vessel and provides a rough edge on which the thrombus can form. If the narrowing occurs slowly enough, collaterals can develop. This can either avoid or decrease the severity of the infarction when an occlusion occurs. This type of cerebral vascular accident usually gives the client a warning, in the form of transient ischemic attacks (TIAs).

Transient ischemic attacks are at times called angina of the brain because, like angina pectoris, the symptoms stem from ischemia to an area, but there is no residual effect. They are, however, a sign of advanced atherosclerotic disease in the cerebral vascular system, and one third of the individuals that experience them will develop a cerebral infarction (Lewis & Collier, 1983). The etiology of TIAs is believed to be a microembolus that separates from a complicated atherosclerotic plaque (Lewis & Collier, 1983). The symptoms from TIAs last anywhere from a few minutes to a day. The symptoms can be any of those of a stroke, such as paresthesias, paresis, vision changes or loss, aphasia, or behavioral changes.

Cerebral vascular accidents due to thrombosis frequently have a progressive onset of symptoms, peaking in 1–2 days. They tend to begin during or immediately after sleep (Lewis & Collier, 1983; Price & Wilson, 1986). This is thought to be due to the lowering of blood pressure during sleep and the decrease in sympathetic activity. Sedation can also precipitate the stroke in these clients (Price & Wilson, 1986).

The second most common cause of stroke is an embolus. These clients are generally younger than the cerebral thrombosis client. A cerebral embolus usually originates in the heart or the carotid arteries. The amount of damage depends on where the embolus occludes an artery and what that artery feeds. A cerebral vascular accident from a cerebral embolus is usually sudden and completed at the start, rather than progressive, although progression can occur, and some clients will receive warnings from TIAs. The prognosis is usually not as good as the cerebral thrombosis.

The third and least common cause of a cerebral vascular accident is hemorrhage of a cerebral artery. When this occurs in the elderly individual, hypertension is usually present. Cerebral hemorrhage has an abrupt onset and rapid evolution. Severe headache and vomiting are frequent. When there is a hemorrhage of the brain or the subarachnoid space, there is compression and displacement of the surrounding brain tissue. If the hemorrhage is large, herniation of the brain may occur. When this happens, coma and death usually result. Prognosis of cerebral hemorrhage is extremely poor; approximately half of the clients do not survive (Lewis & Collier, 1983).

Nursing Care and Medical Management

The most successful part of the management of a cerebral vascular accident falls within the realm of prevention, i.e., getting the person to decrease risk factors. For detailed information on treatment during the acute phase, a general medical–surgical text should be consulted. General nursing care is the same for all causes of cerebral vascular accidents. Nursing efforts should be directed toward four objectives (Eliopoulos, 1979):

1. To maintain a patent airway
2. To provide adequate nutrition and hydration
3. To monitor neurological signs and vital signs
4. To prevent complications due to immobility

The nurse practitioner must remember that the elderly client is particularly vulnerable to developing contractures and decubitus sores because of the aging process itself and as part of the complications of immobility. Because contractures develop more easily in limbs with impaired circulation, correct positioning and early physical and occupational therapy are essential (Steinberg, 1983). Care must be taken to make sure the eyes close completely, especially if the client is unconscious. If an eye does not close completely by itself, it should be irrigated with sterile saline and possibly with sterile mineral oil, depending on the physician's preference, and taped closed with the aid of an eye patch. This should be checked frequently to ensure the eye is staying closed and should be changed daily or as needed to keep it clean and dry (Eliopoulous, 1979).

The client should be encouraged to learn self-positioning and turning as soon as the condition allows. This not only helps him or her to exercise the usable muscles, but also promotes some independence. Early promotion of independence in any area possible may make the difference in the client being able to persevere through the long and tedious process of rehabilitation. Rehabilitation should be started as soon as the client is conscious and stable. In addition to improving motor and language (communication) skills, rehabilitation should also address social and vocational skills. This means the person's self-esteem should be increased by constant stimuli, increased independence wherever possible, and frequent praise—for even the smallest of accomplishments. If possible, the sensory stimuli the client is accustomed to at home should be used, i.e., familiar people, television, radio. Rehabilitation for the stroke client is a long, slow process. This, added to the problems of mobility and sensory loss associated with aging, creates an extremely frustrating situation for both the client and the family (Hahn, 1987). A common problem encountered when the client returns to the home environment is that the family tries to do too much for the client. This takes away client independence, and the family should be cautioned to avoid this. They must also be warned that they may see personality changes in their loved one, especially when the individual becomes frustrated.

For more detailed information on specific parts of rehabilitation of stroke victims, a rehabilitation text should be consulted.

Congestive Heart Failure

Congestive heart failure is another cardiovascular disease that is seen with greater frequency in the aging population. Its primary cause is the atherosclerotic disease process. The effects of this process are exacerbated by the effects of aging. As discussed in the section on "Physiological Changes in Aging," the aging heart responds more slowly and less frequently to stressors. This fact, coupled with loss of elasticity of the vessels, contributes to congestive heart failure. There are some noncardiovascular diseases that end in congestive heart failure in aging clients. These could be pneumonia, hyper-

thyroidism, fever, or anemia. In these situations, congestive heart failure is considered reversible, and the client is treated for both the failure and the precipitating problem until both are resolved. This section does not deal with these situations, but only with the type of congestive heart failure more frequently seen in the elderly client that comes from the irreversible disorders.

In order to understand the causal factors of congestive heart failure and the manner in which the heart responds, the heart should be thought of as two separate pumps. The left pump is responsible for providing the body tissue with oxygenated blood by pushing the blood from the left ventricle through the systemic circulation. The right pump is responsible for receiving the unoxygenated blood from the systemic circulation and pushing it through the lungs for reoxygenation. If one of these pumps fails, it means that either oxygen is not being carried to the body tissues or unoxygenated blood and waste products are not being removed from the tissues.

When the heart is confronted with failure, compensatory mechanisms attempt to continue providing the body with needed oxygen. The first compensatory mechanism to take effect is tachycardia. This increases cardiac output initially but is only effective in the short term. As the heart accelerates, it not only increases the number of beats per minute, but it also decreases the time for the ventricle to fill, so a point is reached when the cardiac output is diminished and failure is increased.

The second and third compensatory mechanisms occur more slowly. The muscle fibers of the myocardium lengthen and thicken in order to be able to contract more forcefully. The chambers also become enlarged as the volume of blood the chamber can hold is increased. These mechanisms are initially effective in compensating for the heart failure. Yet, there are problems associated with these mechanisms as well. One is that the heart can literally outgrow its blood supply in an attempt to increase the cardiac output. The other problem is that Starling's law is only effective to a point. This law states that the more myocardial fibers are stretched during diastole, the stronger the force of contraction. The increased stretch is accomplished by increasing the volume of blood in the ventricle during the diastole. The amount of stretch is called the preload. The myocardial fiber, as pictured in Starling's law, is frequently compared to the elasticity of a rubber band. The further it is stretched, the harder it bounces back. As is true of the rubber band, the myocardial fiber weakens with continual overstretching, and its elasticity lessens. This will lead to an increase in the volume of blood left in the chamber after the contraction, which again increases the severity of the failure. The volume of blood remaining in the left ventricle after a contraction is called the afterload.

Congestive heart failure develops when there is a failure of one or both sides of the heart. This happens when the myocardium is forced to beat against an area of higher pressure. The result is a backup of blood in the areas of higher pressure. For example, in hypertensive disease, the left pump is pushing blood into vessels with higher pressure. To deal with this, the heart uses its compensatory mechanism to override the pressure and continue to provide the body with the oxygen it needs. Eventually these compensatory mechanisms become ineffective, and the signs and symptoms of congestive heart failure appear.

Assessment Parameters of Left-Sided Congestive Heart Failure

Left-sided congestive failure can be due to hypertension, myocardial infarction in the left ventricle, or aortic or mitral valve disease. These situations result in decreased cardiac output, an insufficient amount of oxygenated blood being carried to the body tissues, and a pooling of blood in the left side of the heart. With pooling in the left side, the blood begins to back up in the system, first into the lungs. This results in the first signs of left-sided failure, dyspnea on exertion (DOE), dry hacking cough, and fatigue. The cough and the DOE are due directly to the blood pooling in the lungs. The fatigue is due to the body tissues failing to receive adequate levels of oxygen. As the failure progresses, the person becomes more and more fatigued, becomes dyspneic with less and less exertion, and the cough becomes increasingly productive—first with white or clear mucus and progressing to the pink frothy mucus of pulmonary edema, which is considered a medical emergency. When assessing the elderly person in failure, the nurse practitioner will find tachycardia, bounding pulses, S-3 on auscultation of the heart, and rales in the lungs. A medical history usually discloses that the client is sleeping on more than one pillow. At times the client may not even be aware they are doing this to relieve dyspnea. This suggests they may have paroxysmal nocturnal dyspnea (PND). The use of additional pillows is the client's way of keeping the fluid of congestive heart failure in the lower portion of the lungs. If the pillows are not used, the PND results from the fluid moving up in the lobes as the person sleeps, leaving less breathing space for the client.

Assessment Parameters of Right-Sided Congestive Heart Failure

Right-sided congestive heart failure can be due to a myocardial infarction in the right ventricle, although this is rare, disease of the pulmonic or tricuspid valves, pulmonary hypertension or, most commonly, progression of left-sided failure to where the right ventricle is pumping against high pressure. Whatever the cause, failure in the right side backs blood up into the systemic circulation. The individual will complain of swelling in the feet and ankles first. As the failure progresses, the edema in the lower extremities will become pitting and progress up the leg. Along with the dependent edema comes nocturia of one or two times per night. This is because the fluid that accumulated in the feet and legs during the day is reabsorbed from the tissue and excreted by the kidneys during the night. Initially this mechanism will be successful in reducing the swelling completely by morning. As the failure worsens, however, the edema will remain in the morning. Another symptom of progressive failure is anorexia. This is due to the blood pooling in the abdomen. On assessment, the nurse practitioner may find hepatomegaly and ascites. The congestion that results throughout the systemic circulation increases the pressure in the renal tubules as well. The result is an increased reabsorption of sodium by the tubules, further contributing to edema and the congestive heart failure. When anorexia is present, the client will be able to better satisfy nutritional needs with small, frequent meals throughout the day.

Nursing Care and Medical Management

The general goals of management of congestive heart failure are to correct the sodium and water retention and the elevated right- and/or left-sided filling pressures (Steinberg, 1983). The most common medical management used to achieve these goals is a combination of a diuretic and digitalis. In mild cases the diuretic may be successful alone by decreasing the circulation volume, thereby decreasing the overload. This decreases the work load of the heart and, in turn, the failure. Digitalis is used because it is effective in improving cardiac output in the face of heart failure. It does this by improving the force of the contraction. It also improves renal perfusion with the improved cardiac output. Another known effect of digitalis is decreased potassium levels through blockage of the sodium pump. The possible result of hypokalemia must be monitored closely, particularly if diuretics are also used, because hypokalemia can lead to lethal ventricular arrhythmia. Because of this, the client is usually given oral potassium to supplement dietary intake. Yet another effect of digitalis is on the junctional tissue, where it slows conduction through the tissue. This is helpful if the client has tachycardia or atrial fibrillation because it slows the ventricular rate to provide time for adequate filling.

The nurse practitioner must be vigilant for signs of digitalis toxicity, which can block stimulation and increase the irritability of the ventricle to the extent that lethal arrhythmias result

(Futrell et al., 1980). Elderly persons frequently develop digitalis toxicity because their renal filtration rate is decreased; this allows digitalis to accumulate in the system until toxic levels are reached. The first indications of toxicity are gastrointestinal symptoms. The individual may experience anorexia, nausea, vomiting, and/or diarrhea. The client usually has a heart rate below 60 beats per minute at this time. For this reason, it is important that the client learn how to count his or her pulse accurately, if at all possible. Some people will develop "colored" vision as another symptom of digitalis toxicity. If the toxicity is not reversed, the client can develop any number of lethal arrhythmias.

Nonmedical management of congestive heart failure consists of restricting the client's activity to the level the body can tolerate without stress. This means without shortness of breath, which is the first signal that the tissues are not receiving enough oxygen. Persons who experience shortness of breath at rest will need to keep their head elevated while in bed; the physician may also order oxygen therapy.

Clients with congestive heart failure need to be shown ways in which they can gain control of their health. This can also increase compliance with the management plan. The client should understand as much as possible about the disease and be given guidelines regarding when to seek medical assistance. The nurse practitioner can best do this by describing the progression of symptoms that are experienced and noting the point at which medical assistance should be sought. Significant others must be included in this teaching because they may be able to recognize changes before the client does. This is because as the failure progresses a decreased amount of oxygen is provided to the brain, so that the client's mental acuity decreases. This may be especially noticeable at night or after the client has been in a recumbent position for a while.

The client needs to reduce salt intake. As discussed in the "Maintenance of Wellness" section, this may be extremely difficult for the elderly person after years of high sodium intake, but is extremely important for controlling the congestive heart failure. The congestive heart failure client must also exercise. The initial level of exercise and the speed with which it is increased is usually more conservative than with other types of cardiac clients. The exercise program is usually governed more by the client's shortness of breath than heart rate, but both must be watched. Efforts to reduce the other risk factors given in the "Maintenance of Wellness" section should also be instituted to help keep the congestive heart failure under control:

1. No smoking
2. Decrease in weight if obese
3. Decrease in lipid intake
4. Control of hypertension and diabetes

The "Maintenance of Cardiovascular System Wellness" section provides discussion of how these are implemented in the nursing care of the congestive heart failure client.

Anemia

Anemia is a common problem among the elderly. Its presence in any age group is considered a sign of a disorder or deficiency, rather than a disorder in and of itself. The label of anemia is given whenever the erythrocyte, hemoglobin, or hematocrit level is below normal (Natow & Heslin, 1980).

The normal production of erythrocytes is dependent on a number of nutrients. Iron, vitamin B_{12}, folic acid, protein, pyridoxine, ascorbic acid, and copper are known to affect production. A deficiency in intake and body stores in any one of these can result in anemia (Natow & Heslin, 1980). When the hemoglobin level drops below normal there is a subsequent drop in the oxygen-carrying capacity of blood. This places the body in a compromised state when faced with a stressor. As discussed in the section on "The Normal Aging Process of the Car-

diovascular System," the elderly client is already in a slightly compromised position. Therefore, the development of anemia carries with it grave consequences.

The common manifestations of anemia in the elderly are likely to be dyspnea, angina pectoris, fatigue, and pallor. Dyspnea and angina are particularly common among individuals with coexisting coronary heart diesease. These and other general signs and symptoms of anemia are found in all anemic clients.

The two types of anemia seen most frequently in the elderly are iron-deficiency and megaloblastic anemia (Brocklehurst & Hanley, 1981; Natow & Heslin, 1980; Reichel, 1983).

Iron-Deficiency Anemia
Iron-deficiency anemia is the most frequent type of anemia in the elderly population. The most common cause of iron-deficiency anemia is blood loss. This blood loss is frequently slow, chronic, and intermittent, so its presence may not be known to the client. The common causes of such loss of blood resulting in anemia may be carcinoma of the right side of the colon, hiatus hernia, peptic ulcer, polyps, or hemorrhoids (Reichel, 1983). All of these have an increased frequency in the aging population. Chronic aspirin intake, frequently seen in clients with arthritis, can be another source of gastrointestinal blood loss that can cause iron-deficiency anemia.

Assessment Parameters
The client with iron-deficiency anemia will present the common manifestations of anemia: dyspnea, fatigue, pallor, and possibly angina. It is possible for iron-deficiency anemia to be due to dietary deficiencies, but this usually occurs only with highly restricted diets or in alcoholic clients. Therefore, a source of blood loss must be sought if iron-deficiency anemia is found.

Nursing Care and Medical Management
Management for iron-deficiency anemia is dependent on the source of the problem. If blood

loss is the cause, then the problem must be corrected. If dietary deficiency is the cause, then an iron supplement along with a higher intake of iron-rich foods is the treatment. At times blood loss is combined with a dietary deficiency, in which case correction of the problem underlying the blood loss and addition of a dietary supplement will hasten recovery.

When dietary changes and supplements are used to speed recovery after the site of blood loss is found and hopefully corrected, or in the few cases where the anemia is truly from a dietary deficiency, there are several factors to keep in mind. The first is that the iron in meat has a higher absorption rate than that of vegetables. This can also affect the absorption rate of iron supplements given, so the meat should be increased even when supplements are given. Another factor to remember is that delayed release preparations and enteric-coated iron supplements are not completely absorbed. Any supplement should be given with food in order to minimize the gastrointestinal irritability. This also increases compliance with the management plan.

Megaloblastic Anemia

Megaloblastic anemia is characterized by the presence of large nucleated red cell precursors in the bone marrow. In the elderly, this is from vitamin B_{12} or folic acid deficiency.

Vitamin B_{12} deficiency is usually caused by a lack of the intrinsic factor that results in a situation known as pernicious anemia. The intrinsic factor is necessary for vitamin B_{12} absorption. Nutritional deficiency of vitamin B_{12} is extremely rare (Natow & Heslin, 1980; Reichel, 1983).

Assessment Parameters

The symptoms peculiar to this type of anemia are neurological disturbances, including paresthesia, progressing to gross disturbance in gait (Reichel, 1983). Other common symptoms are anorexia and low-grade fever. The Schilling test is commonly used to diagnose pernicious ane-

mia. In this test, chromium-tagged vitamin B_{12} is administered and its recovery rate in the urine over a 24-hour period is determined. In pernicious anemia, the recovery rate is less than 2%. This demonstrates a probable lack of the intrinsic factor, resulting in the failure to absorb the vitamin B_{12}. To ensure that the diagnosis is accurate, the test is run again, administering the intrinsic factor along with the tagged vitamin B_{12}. If pernicious anemia is present, the recovery rate will then be greater than 10%. If the recovery rate is still low, other causes of vitamin B_{12} deficiency must be considered. These are usually malabsorption due to disease of the small intestines or a resection of the terminal ileum. Only rarely is the deficiency due to inadequate dietary intake (Reichel, 1983).

Nursing Care and Medical Management

Management of vitamin B_{12} deficiencies is through intramuscular administration of B_{12}. Unless the deficiency has been shown to result from dietary deficit, the treatment must be continued for life. Because dietary deficiency is so rare, for all practical purposes treatment is continued for life.

Folic acid deficiency, in contrast to the other anemias discussed, is often caused by nutritional deficiency. Other causes include disorders of the proximal portion of the small intestine where folic acid is absorbed, medications that interfere with folic acid utilization, and alcoholism (Reichel, 1983). Some of the medications that can interfere with folic acid utilization are barbiturates, glutethimide, or aspirin (Natow & Heslin, 1980). Folate deficiency is usually managed by oral administration of folic acid and institution of a balanced diet. If the client is an alcoholic and continues to drink, the utilization of the folic acid given will be inhibited.

When treating folate deficiency, the importance of careful diagnosis of this as the cause of megaloblastic anemia cannot be stressed enough. If an incorrect diagnosis is made and folic acid is given to the pernicious anemia client, the signs and symptoms will be corrected while the neurological complications continue to progress (Reichel, 1983).

SUMMARY

The aging process brings many changes in the cardiovascular system that are not directly related to a pathological process, but that set the stage for pathological processes to progress more quickly. In order to slow the development of pathological processes in the cardiovascular system, the elderly person must try to alter as many risk factors as possible. Altering these risk factors is also an important component of the treatment for each of the disorders discussed, with the exception of anemia.

Four main cardiovascular system disorders are discussed: (1) hypertension; (2) ischemic diseases, which include angina pectoris, myocardial infarction, peripheral vascular disease, and cerebral vascular accident; (3) congestive heart failure; and (4) anemia, which includes iron-deficiency and megaloblastic anemia.

Hypertension is a common problem in the elderly population. Although blood pressure generally rises somewhat during the natural aging process, current research shows that blood pressure should be treated when the systolic pressure is 160 mm Hg and above or when the diastolic pressure is 90 mm Hg and above. The key to successful treatment has been shown to be "go slow and start low." Whenever possible, the first step of treatment should be to alter the risk factors that are present. Treatment with medication can then be instituted, if necessary.

Ischemic disease is any disease process in the cardiovascular system that is caused by a decline in the blood's capacity for carrying oxygen and nutrients to a tissue. Included in this class of diseases are angina pectoris, myocardial infarction, cerebral vascular accidents, and peripheral vascular disease. All of these are primarily due to atherosclerotic disease. The vessels affected in angina pectoris and myocardial infarction are the coronary arteries. The vessels affected in cerebral vascular accidents are in the neck and brain. The peripheral vessels are the ones affected in peripheral vascular disease, especially those in the lower extremities. Treatments for these disorders include decreasing risk factors, the use of medication, and, in some situations, surgery.

Congestive heart failure is a disorder that results when either the left or right side of the heart fails to pump blood adequately and a back-up of blood results. The heart attempts to compensate for the failing state by tachycardia, increasing the size of the heart chambers, and increasing the size and strength of the myocardial fibers. These compensatory mechanisms are successful only up to a point, after which the client develops symptoms. Congestive heart failure is treated by decreasing the risk factors and with medications.

Anemia is a common problem in the elderly population and contributes to the symptoms of ischemic disease already present. Its presence is considered a sign of a disorder or deficiency, rather than a disorder in and of itself.

REFERENCES

American Heart Association. (1975). *Exercise testing and training of individuals with disease or at high risk for its development, a handbook for physicians.* (unpublished).

American Heart Association. (1980). *How you can help your doctor treat your high blood pressure.* Dallas, TX: Author.

American Heart Association. (1981). *An older person's guide to cardiovascular health.* Dallas, TX: Author.

American Heart Association Nutrition Committee. (1982, March/April). Rationale of the diet–heart statement of the American Heart Association. *Arteriosclerosis, 4,* 177–191.

Applegate, W. B., Zwaag. R. V., Dismuke, S. E., & Runyan, J. W., Jr. (1982). Control of systolic blood pressure in elderly black patients. *Journal of the American Geriatric Society, 30*(6), 391–396.

Baldini, J. (1981). Knowledge about hypertension in affected elderly persons. *Journal of Gerontological Nursing, 7*(9), 542–551.

Bemis, C. E. (1981). When is coronary arteriography indicated? *Geriatrics, 36*(9), 89–99.

Brocklehurst, J. C. (1985). *Textbook of geriatric medicine and gerontology* (3rd ed.). New York: Churchill Livingstone.

Brocklehurst, J. C., & Hanley, T. (1981). *Geriatric medicine for students* (2nd ed.). New York: Churchill Livingstone.

Bullock, B. L., & Rosendahl, P. P. (1984). *Pathophysiology adaptations and alterations in function.* Boston: Little, Brown.

Cape, R. D., Coe, R. M., & Rossman, I. (Eds.). (1983). *Fundamentals of geriatric medicine.* New York: Raven Press.

Cooper, K. H. (1981). *The new aerobics.* New York: Bantam Books.

Dawber, T. R. (1980). *The Framingham Study: The epidemiology of atherosclerotic disease.* Cambridge: Harvard University Press.

Denham, M. J. (1980). *The treatment of medical problems in the elderly.* Baltimore: University Park Press.

Ebersole, P. & Hess, P. (1981). *Toward healthy aging: Human needs and nursing response.* St. Louis: Mosby.

Eisdorfer, C. (Ed.). (1982). *Annual review of gerontology and geriatrics.* New York: Spring.

Eliopoulos, C. (1979). *Gerontological nursing.* New York: Harper & Row.

Fardy, P. S., Bennett, J. L., Reitz, N. L., & Williams, M. A. (1980). *Cardiac rehabilitation: Implications for the nurse and other health professionals.* St. Louis: Mosby.

Forbes, E. J., & Fitzsimons, V. M. (1981). *The older adult: A process for wellness.* St. Louis: Mosby.

Futrell, M., Brovender, S., McKinnon-Mullett. E., & Brower, H. T. (1980). *Primary health care of the older adult.* North Scituate, MA: Duxbury Press.

Giorella, E. C., & Bevil, C. W. (1985). *Nursing care of the aging client: Promoting healthy adaptation.* Norwalk, CT: Appleton-Century-Crofts.

Gresham, G. A. (1980). *Reversing atherosclerosis.* Springfield, IL: Thomas.

Harper, A. E. (1981). Dietary guidelines for the elderly. *Geriatrics, 36*(7), 34–40.

Hahn, K. (1987). Left vs right what a difference the side makes. *Nursing 87, 17*(9), 44–47.

Hill, M. N. (1987). Diuretics for mild hypertension: Still the best choice? *Nursing 87, 17*(9), 62–64.

Joint Committee on Detection, Evaluation and Treatment of High Blood Pressure. (1984, May). The 1984 report of the Joint National Committee on Detection, Evaluation and Treatment of High Blood Pressure: A cooperative study. *Archives of Internal Medicine, 144*(5), 1045–1057.

Lewis, S. M., & Collier, I. C. (1983). *Medical-surgical nursing: Assessment and management of clinical problems.* New York: McGraw-Hill.

Libow, L. S. & Butler, R. N. (1981). Treating mild diastolic hypertension in the elderly: Uncertain benefits and possible dangers. *Geriatrics, 36*(11), 55–59.

Lindeman, R. D. & Klinger, E. L., Jr. (1981). Combating sodium and potassium imbalance in older patients. *Geriatrics, 36*(8), 97–106.

Malasanos, L., Barhouskas, V., Moss, M., & Stoltenberg-Allen, K. (1981). *Health assessment.* St. Louis: Mosby.

McMahan, B. E. (1987). Why deep vein thrombosis is so dangerous. *RN, 50*(1), 20–23.

Moser, M., Guyther, J. R., Finnerty, F., Richardson, D. W., Langford, H., Perry, H. M., Wood, D. E., Krishan, I., Branche, G. C., & Smith, W. (1977, Jan. 17). Report of the Joint National Committee on detection, evaluation, and treatment of high blood pressure. *Journal of American Medical Association, 237*(3), 255–261.

Natow, A. B., & Heslin, J. A. (1980). *Geriatric nutrition.* Boston: CBI.

O'Brien, D. K., & Pattee, J. J. (1981). Hypertension in older patients: What drugs to use and when. *Geriatrics, 36*(8), 111–116.

Peitzman, S. J., Bodison, W., & Ellis, I. (1982). Care of elderly patients in a special hypertension clinic. *Journal of the American Geriatrics Society, 30*(1), 2–5.

Price, S. A., & Wilson, L. M. (1986). *Pathophysiology: Clinical concepts of disease processes* (3rd ed.). New York: McGraw-Hill.

Radin, A. M., & Black, H. R. (1981). Hypertension in the elderly: The time has come to treat. *Journal of the American Geriatrics Society, 24*(5), 193–200.

Reichel, W. (1983). *Clinical aspects of aging* (2nd ed.). Baltimore: Williams & Wilkins.

Rodman, M. J., & Smith, D. W. (1979). *Pharmacology and drug therapy in nursing* (2nd ed.). Philadelphia: Lippincott.

Rowe, J. W., & Besdine, R. W. (1982). *Health and disease in old age*. Boston: Little, Brown.

Saxon, S. V., & Etten, M. J. (1978). *Physical change and aging: A guide for helping professions*. New York: Tiresias Press.

Schrier, R. W. (1982). *Clinical internal medicine in the aged*. Philadelphia: Saunders.

Selzer, A. (1983). *Principles and practice of clinical cardiology*. Philadelphia: Saunders.

Smith, I. (1982). *Medical care for the elderly*. New York: SP Medical and Scientific Books.

Steinberg, F. U. (1983). *Care of the geriatric patient in the tradition of E. V. Cowdry* (6th ed.). St. Louis: Mosby.

Underhill, S. L., Woods, S. L., Sivarajan, E. S., & Halpenny, C. J. (1982). *Cardiac nursing*. Philadelphia: Lippincott.

Yurick, A. G., Robb, S. S., Spier, B. E., & Ebert, N. J. (1980). *The aged person and the nursing process*. New York: Appleton-Century-Crofts.

12

COMMUNICATING WITH THE AGED

This chapter (1) reviews the age-associated changes in cognitive processes, especially in the areas of intelligence, learning, memory, and motivation as they relate to the elderly, (2) discusses means of communicating with the elderly effectively, and (3) offers strategies useful in teaching the elderly and assessing learning needs.

"We're not getting older, we're getting better," is a phrase often heard in working with the elderly. How they are getting better and how best to help them become better need to be addressed by health care providers. One method is to build effective helping relationships through education and experience with the elderly. Gershowitz (1982) advocates that health care providers for the elderly build relationships based on trust and the elderly client's existing repertoire of responses. Perhaps the best place to begin is with a review of the cognitive changes generally found in the elderly.

EXPECTED CHANGES IN COGNITIVE PROCESSES

Cognitive changes are unique with each individual and are related to the onset, rate, and pattern of aging. In general, the psychological and mental changes of aging are more gradual and occur later than do the corresponding physical changes. However, some clients have reported becoming "old" all of a sudden, seemingly overnight. Weber (1980) noted that there is no single cause for aging. Some clients become aware of their aging almost instantaneously; however, the aging process begins at birth and proceeds at varying rates with each individual. Intelligence, learning, memory, and motivation are aspects of the cognitive process that should be considered when assessing and caring for the aged.

Intelligence

Intelligence and functions of the brain, providing there are adequate oxygen and nutrition and no diseases, do not undergo major changes with aging. Minute changes in the brain's functioning, with a resultant decline in intelligence does seem to occur in about the fiftieth year. This decline, according to Lieberman (1965), is so small that barring any physical or neurological problems, general intelligence, problem solving abilities, judgment, and creativity are maintained into old age. Mental deterioration does not occur until 6–12 months before death (Lieberman, 1965).

Learning

Learning is an ability that is retained well into old age. The older client learns more quickly than the young in situations that require redundant information. However, tasks requiring innovation, analogies, or new classification systems are more difficult for the older client (Murray & O'Driskoll, 1979). According to Lieberman (1965), elderly clients are capable of learning and maintaining the ability to learn until shortly before death.

Memory

Memory in the elderly client seems to be a problem, particularly in ordering the time sequences of more recent events and in immediate recall of recent events (Murray & O'Driskoll, 1979; Lawson, 1975). However, long-term memory, including such components as (1) vocabulary, (2) personal history, (3) past experiences, and (4) basic knowledge, is very resistant to the decrements normally caused by the aging process (Murray & O'Driskoll, 1979). Those aspects of learning that are less dependent on short-term memory, e.g., synthesis, analysis, comparison, and ability to organize content, do not decline with age. Memory will effect new learning when the client loses some elements of immediate information needed to process, code, or synthesize new information (Sterns & Sterns, 1981). Memory loss does not necessarily occur in later maturity.

Motivation

Motivation, according to Coleman, Butcher, and Carson (1980), both energizes and directs an individual's behavior. An individual's motivation is affected by the individual's perception of his or her situation and its potential to be either satisfying or frustrating. Coleman and colleagues (1980) indicate that there are no age limits to the motivation to (1) develop and use one's potentials, (2) enrich one's experiences and satisfactions, and (3) expand one's relationships.

Motivation for the elderly client is within oneself and can best be drawn out in a climate of respect and acceptance.

THE AGING PROCESS AND ITS EFFECT ON COMMUNICATION

The aging process often has profound effects on a person's ability to communicate. Neurological and sensory changes affect the ability both to receive information (e.g., read, hear conversations) and to transmit information (e.g., speak and write). Assessment of the client's neurological status has been previously discussed (see Chap. 4) but should be reconsidered when viewing a client's ability to communicate.

Good vision is needed for many purposes— to read, see the television, dial the telephone, or to lip-read, if one's hearing is impaired. Vision may be impaired by physiological problems, such as cataracts or glaucoma, or by environmental factors, such as poor lighting or dirty eyeglasses.

Hearing losses may lead to fear, anger, hostility, and psychological problems, such as paranoia and depression. The loss may be only slight, so that a hearing aid is helpful, or it may be so great that lip-reading or written communication is necessary in order to communicate effectively. The gerontological nurse practitioner must consider such possibilities when assessing or teaching an aged client.

Neurological changes, such as organic brain syndrome or aphasia, may lead to communication difficulties. Organic brain syndrome has often been too conveniently used as an umbrella diagnosis, but it is an indication of confusion and disorientation that disrupts the communication process. Obviously, a confused person cannot correctly perceive or disseminate information.

Either receptive or expressive aphasia, usually due to cerebrovascular accident, creates a communication barrier. The client may, indeed, be able to comprehend, but be unable to respond to, words spoken in their presence. On the other hand, clients may be able to make sounds that they believe to be appropriate responses to questions but that are actually unintelligible.

Thought processes may be slowed by neurological changes, and response patterns may be prolonged. Speech too may become slower. These changes result from degeneration of neurons and deterioration of synaptic transmission between neurons. Reduced vascular supply to the neurons, resulting in impaired functioning, is often the origin of the neuronal problem.

Diminished perception of touch can also be a communication barrier, especially if a person has decreased vision and hearing. Touch is an important means of communicating that another is present and cares. Individuals with poor vision may wish to use the sense of touch to ''read'' the time on a clock (without a crystal) or to learn Braille.

APPROACHES FOR COMMUNICATING WITH THE AGED

Biological changes that affect communication gradually occur with the aging process. There is usually a marked decrease of the senses involved with communication after the late mid-adult years, between the ages of 55 and 60 years. Because the onset of these changes is usually gradual, the individual is able to adapt to them and maintain communication. The gerontological nurse practitioner must be aware of the adaptations that might occur and be observant for them during the assessment process.

The structural and neurological changes (see Chap. 4) that occur within the ears interfere with the transmission of sound waves. The nurse practitioner can assess the degree of bone and air conduction by using a tuning fork. An otoscope is used to assess the ear canals for possible obstruction with cerumen and the tympanic membrane for intactness. Many times the client's ability to hear is enhanced when excessive

or impacted cerumen is removed. Many elderly clients have experienced multiple ear infections during childhood, resulting in perforation(s) of the tympanic membrane that prevent(s) conduction of the sound waves to the bony structures in the middle ear. Most likely these perforations have not been patched surgically; therefore, the nurse practitioner should plan care to prevent water from entering the ear and remain vigilant to the signs of infection.

The changes that occur in the ears usually result in misinterpretations or an inability to interpret the sound waves correctly. The client usually adapts to these changes by turning toward the source of sound; at times, the individual may be observed cupping the hand behind the ear lobe to assist in directing the sound waves into the ear canal. Many elderly persons experiencing hearing loss adapt to this loss by reading lips. Therefore, it is important to note this adaptation and inform those caring for the client to place themselves directly in front of the client when speaking. The nurse practitioner must also be aware that, with the neurological changes that occur with aging, one loses the ability to hear high-pitched tones, and responses to sound are slowed. This makes it imperative not only to stand directly in front of the client when speaking but also to speak slowly and in lower-pitched tones.

With the decrease in hearing ability of the aged, vision becomes one of the adaptive mechanisms to maintain effective communications. However, visual problems also occur as a result of the aging process, e.g., decreased peripheral vision, cataracts, and inability to accommodate for acuity. These visual problems interfere with effective communications; therefore, the nurse practitioner must make the appropriate assessment to determine the degree and existence of visual impairment(s). Once these impairments are identified, they must be considered when speaking to the client. It is important that the client visualize the person speaking in order to see lip movements, which augment the interpretation of the sound waves picked up by the ears. The aged client must be aware of the nurse practitioner's presence; therefore, it is essential that the nurse practitioner avoid speaking to the aged clients behind their backs or to their sides.

The nurse practitioner must continually assess the degree of visual impairment in order to plan for other means of communication, e.g., Braille or talking books. It is most advantageous to begin Braille instruction before total visual impairment occurs.

The aged person experiencing hearing loss may use mechanical means (a hearing aid) to magnify sound waves. It is important to note that hearing devices amplify *all* sound; this can cause problems for older clients until they learn to be selective of what they wish to hear. The nurse practitioner should be aware of the type of hearing aid used by the client. Understanding the operation of the hearing device will assist in determining how to direct one's speech in order for the device to effectively pick up the projected sound waves. For example, if the client carries the amplifying unit in the front shirt pocket, one should speak directly toward the unit in order for the microphone in the unit to pick up the projected sound waves. Most likely if the nurse would speak to the back or side of the client, the pocket style hearing device would be ineffective in picking up and transmitting the sound.

APPROACHES TO ESTABLISHING A RELATIONSHIP

Establishing a relationship of trust with elderly clients can help them to lead as full a life as possible. Research has shown the importance of effective communication and has provided a theory foundation in planning care.

Importance of Trust

Gibb (1964) suggests that trust between individuals is essential for an effective relationship in which sharing, planning, and organizing are desired. Trust, acceptance of oneself and others,

an open climate, and subsequent growth are described by Gibb as interrelated variables that facilitate effective individual and group growth. This growth, Gibb feels, occurs in a concurrent fashion among the four variables and is optimal when a sequential order is maintained. According to Gibb, trust is a vital element in effective communication and growth.

Friedlander (1970) tested Gibb's suggestion that trust is vital to group growth. He did so by comparing two sets of groups on the accomplishment of groups initially high or low in trust. Specifically, the question was: Does a group with higher initial trust accomplish more over time than groups with lower initial trust? The results indicate that trust increases the probability of effective relationships and promotes group effectiveness. Friedlander also noted that trust served as a catalyst in promoting group effectiveness and increasing individuals' perceptions of the value of the group, which lends support to the contentions of Gibb.

Egan (1975), speaking specifically in relation to working with individuals, said that the client must come to trust the helper. Trust, according to Egan, is vital. To the client, its ultimate meaning may be described as follows: (1) I am entrusting myself to you, (2) you will use your skills to care for me, (3) you will not hurt me, and (4) you will try to see that I do not hurt myself.

Carkhuff and Anthony (1973) have used the word *critical* to describe the importance of creating an atmosphere of true concern and interest in the client. This true concern and interest provides a climate that enhances the probability of a relationship of trust developing between the client and helper. Brammer (1981) and others (Hansen, Pound, & Warner, 1976) have noted a number of behaviors that nurse practitioners can employ in establishing a relationship of trust with a client.

Promoting Trust

Mutual trust between the client and the nurse is the key to open communications. The probability of establishing a relationship of trust can be enhanced by the nurse practitioner's use of (1) modeling behaviors, (2) physical arrangements of the office, and (3) nonverbal behaviors.

Modeling Behaviors

A client's first impression of the nurse practitioner may be of the nurse walking to the office or going to the parking lot at the end of the work day. This first impression is often formed without the nurse's awareness. It is, therefore, important that nurse practitioners be seen to practice the behaviors and life-style that they are attempting to promote (Argyle & Kendon, 1967). For example, what does the overweight nurse practitioner working with a client on weight control or the nurse practitioner who chain smokes working with a group of clients with respiratory problems tell these clients? Modeling is a tool or mode of influence that is often overlooked or misused.

Physical Arrangements

Clients' perceptions of the nurse practitioner are affected by the office setting. Argyle and Kendon (1967) have noted that when individuals talk to each other over the corner of a desk, a feeling of cooperation prevails. However, when two people face each other across the desk, they are far more inclined to see each other as competitors. Thus, the nurse practitioner can increase the probability of establishing a helping relationship with the client by arranging the office to remove or minimize the artificial barriers to communication that the desk can create.

Nonverbal Behaviors

Brammer (1981) has identified a number of nonverbal behaviors that have an important bearing on the type and depth of the interaction between two people. Brammer contends that the attending behaviors of the nurse practitioner will either help or hurt the relationship with the client. The nonverbal attending behaviors include (1) high frequency of eye contact, (2) maintaining a comfortable distance, (3) leaning forward, (4) main-

taining a comfortable body posture, (5) facing the client squarely, and (6) equal eye level.

Eye contact with the client is one of the more important nonverbal attending behaviors to be employed by the nurse practitioner (Rorden, 1987). Many cultures place a great deal of value on maintenance of eye contact during interpersonal interactions. Some cultures believe that a person's soul can be stolen through prolonged eye contact. Also, the nurse practitioner must realize that many clients become very uncomfortable when eye contact is maintained for a period of time. However, it becomes very important for the nurse practitioner to maintain a high frequency of eye contact to observe the client for other nonverbal cues as well as to indicate the nurse practitioner's interest and concern.

The distance between client and the nurse practitioner will influence the interaction. If a great distance, say 8–10 feet, is maintained, the probability of the client discussing anything personal or meaningful is greatly reduced. On the other hand, if the nurse practitioner is too close to the client avoidance and withdrawal behaviors frequently result. These avoidance behaviors include the client breaking eye contact, turning away from the nurse practitioner, dropping the head, or moving back in the chair. Although the distance between the nurse practitioner and the client will vary according to the client, 3–4 feet is generally a comfortable distance for most clients and will help promote confidence and trust.

Consider now the nonverbal attending behaviors of leaning toward or back from a client and the subtle effect it has on an interaction. Leaning back could be interpreted as an avoidance behavior, a rejection of the client, or a lack of interest in what was being discussed. Leaning back enhances the probability that the client will feel rejected. On the other hand, leaning forward enhances the probability of nonverbally communicating interest, concern, and attentiveness.

A comfortable body posture is difficult to describe because of the many variations it may take. A number of *do nots* perhaps will suffice to convey the idea: (1) do not sit with the arms crossed over the body—this posture may make one feel comfortable and secure but may make the client feel being shut out or that the nurse practitioner is guarded or uninterested in listening to the client; (2) do not sit on the edge of the chair—this position may be comfortable, but it may communicate to the client that the nurse practitioner is either in a hurry to get to some other place, ready to leave or, for whatever reason, eager to end the interaction with the client; and (3) do not sit with the legs crossed—not only can this posture be interpreted as closing the client out, but it may also be viewed as expressing a casual attitude toward the client's feelings, thus reducing the probability that the client will share any in-depth concerns. Generally, both feet on the floor combined with the other nonverbal attending behaviors will increase the probability that the client will interact in a meaningful and productive manner with the nurse practitioner.

Carkhuff (1973) and Brammer (1981) noted the importance of facing the client squarely. The nurse practitioner who keeps the shoulders parallel to the client's shoulders enhances the probability of helping the client to communicate more effectively. Often the client will see the slight turning away by the nurse practitioner as rejection or a lack of interest. Thus, the subtle difference between facing the client squarely and facing him or her at an angle may have a profound effect on the scope of the interaction between the client and the nurse practitioner.

One other nonverbal attending behavior that warrants attention is eye contact between the client and the nurse practitioner. The nurse practitioner should keep the eye level with the client as nearly equal as possible. If the client has to look up at the nurse practitioner, the client is placed in an inferior position and may become intimidated. If the client has to look down on the nurse practitioner, the client may perceive the nurse practitioner to be in an inferior position and unable to be of assistance with the client's problem(s).

Lastly, one nonverbal attending behavior that seems to be the most positive or devastating to a relationship is touch. Touching the client communicates the nurse practitioner's concern for and desire to relate in a helping way. However, the possibility exists, due to individual and cultural differences, that the client may infer some meaning to being touched other than the concern implied by the nurse practitioner. More often than not, if the nurse practitioner uses the other attending behaviors, the client will begin to relate concerns, and touch may not be needed. However, if with the use of the other attending behaviors the client does not begin to relate concerns, the nurse practitioner may find that touching the client in a nonthreatening manner may signal the assurance the client needs to begin relating personal concerns.

THE VERBAL PROCESS OF HELPING

The process of helping a client begins with the nurse practitioner attending to the client. As the attending is taking place, the client begins to explore with the nurse practitioner the situation and circumstances of the problem. Carkhuff (1973) outlined the Helping Process presented in Figure 12–1.

In the exploration phase of the interaction, the nurse practitioner continues to attend and respond to the client, as the client relates the situations and circumstances of the problem. During this phase, the nurse practitioner attempts to assess the client and the client's perception of the problem. The nurse practitioner assesses the client's status on the following dimensions: (1) physical, (2) intellectual, and (3) emotional, as the client relates to the problem.

On the physical dimension, the nurse assesses the client's condition by making tentative judgments about the client on the basis of (1) height–weight ratio, (2) posture, and (3) overall appearance. The tentative judgment of a client who, for instance, is grossly overweight would be quite different from the tentative judgment rendered about an extremely thin client. The

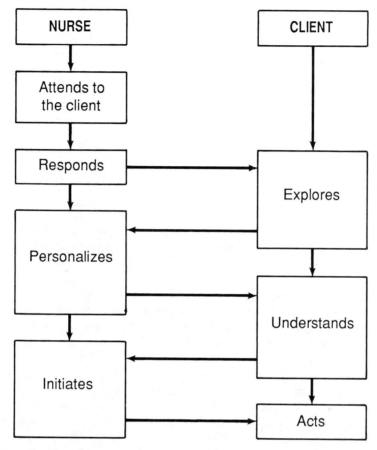

Figure 12-1. The Helping Process. (Adapted with permission from Carkhuff, Robert R., *The Art of Helping.* Amherst, MA: Human Resource Development Press, 1973, p. 21.)

posture the client maintains gives the nurse practitioner an indication of how the client views himself or herself, the problem, and the circumstances the client is experiencing. The client slumped in a chair may be expressing defeat or hopelessness, whereas the client sitting erect and well back in the chair may be indicating an attitude of anxiety or alertness in relation to the problem. The client's overall appearance offers some indications to the nurse practitioner about the current status: Is the client's clothing clean and neat, or is it rumpled and ragged? Are the shoes clean and in good condition, or are they scuffed and cracked? Is the client's hair combed and neat, or is it unkempt and matted?

The intellectual capabilities of the client are indicated to the nurse practitioner by the client's choice and use of words in relating the situation and circumstances of concern. Many times the client who is experiencing strong emotions will resort to very basic terminology to express experiences. The client who appears somewhat confused or perhaps uncertain about what is being experienced at the moment will often use nebulous terminology.

There are a number of indices the nurse practitioner can use to assess the client's emotional status: the rate of speech, the volume of speech, the nonverbal behaviors, and the frequency and types of eye contact employed by the

TABLE 12–1. INDICES FOR ASSESSMENT OF EMOTIONAL STATUS

Behavioral Indices	Clients' Emotional Status	
	Strong Emotional Involvement	Confused or Low Emotional Involvement
Rate of speech	Fast	Slow–hesitant
Volume of speech	Loud/very quiet–flat	Slow–few if any
Eye contact	Constant–piercing/total avoidance	Tentative/soft

client. For the purpose of clarity, Table 12–1 presents some general guidelines for the nurse practitioner to consider when assessing the emotional status of the client.

As the nurse practitioner assesses the physical, intellectual, and emotional dimensions of the client, the nurse practitioner prepares to respond. The nurse's response should confirm (1) an interest in what the client is experiencing and (2) the fact that the nurse practitioner has been listening. In order to be most effective, the nurse practitioner should say as few words as possible.

According to Carkhuff (1973) and Brammer (1981), an accurate response reflects two elements that have been communicated by the client: (1) the feeling and (2) meaning of the client's experience. In essence, the response to the client's initial exploration should correspond with or be a reflection of the client's experience in terms of feeling(s) the client is expressing and the reason(s) or meaning(s) of the experience.

Blake and Bichekas (1981) have noted that a skill that nurse practitioners can develop prior to working with clients is that of developing a vocabulary of feeling words. There are literally hundreds of feelings experienced and numerous words used to describe them, each of which has its own meaning to the individual who is using the word; it would thus seem to be impossible for the nurse practitioner to choose a word that would accurately reflect what the client is feeling. To further compound the problem, feelings

are often implied, hidden, or in some way disguised due to a cultural teaching that inhibits the direct expression of feelings.

One method that can be used to develop a feeling vocabulary is to begin by listing types of feelings. The list might consist of such types of feelings as anger, confusion, fear, happiness, and sadness. The next step in developing a feeling word vocabulary would be to classify the intensity of feelings into three degrees—strong, moderate, and mild.

The nurse practitioner can begin expanding and developing a feeling vocabulary, thus enhancing the probability that the client's expressions of feeling will be recognized and reflected accurately. With accurate reflection of the client's feelings, the nurse practitioner contributes to the client's experience of being attended to and listened to as an individual of worth and respect.

The next stage of the Helping Process outlined by Carkhuff (1973) is personalizing. A personalized statement consists of three elements: (1) the feelings expressed, (2) the meaning attached to the feelings, and (3) the assumption of responsibility for the problem by the client. The client usually indicates to the nurse practitioner when there is a readiness to move to this stage. The client's readiness is indicated by stating a lack of skill or inability to deal with his or her experience. The task of the nurse practitioner is to personalize the client's statement.

In this illustration, the nurse practitioner could personalize the problem expressed by the client as follows:

> Nurse: "You are really frightened because you might become sick and possibly helpless and you are not sure you can cope with it."

In the example, the nurse practitioner stated the feeling "frightened," the meaning or reason for the feeling, "might become sick and helpless," and placed the responsibility for the problem with the client: "You are not sure you can cope with it."

At this point in the Helping Process, after the first personalized statement by the nurse practitioner, the client makes a choice to accept or reject the responsibility for the problem.

The client may refuse to accept responsibility for the problem, for example:

> Client: "No, it's not that I don't know what to do; it's just that I'm scared. You know, I've really been feeling great, and besides that, no one in my family. . . . ."

The nurse practitioner should continue to explore the client's perception of the situation until the client again indicates a lack of skill or inability to deal with the experience(s). However, the client may accept the responsibility for the problem, for example:

> Client: "Yes, I am concerned. Losing my health would be terrible and I don't know if I can do anything to prevent it. It really scares me."

The nurse now needs to proceed with the client to the next phase of the Helping Process. The client's readiness to move is indicated by the client's expression of confirmation of: (1) feeling—"I am concerned," (2) meaning—"losing my health," and (3) acceptance of responsibility—"I don't know if I can do anything to prevent it."

The next phase of the Helping Process is for the nurse practitioner to initiate movement toward tentative goals or solutions with the client. The tentative goals or solutions are implied from the client's statements about the situation.

In the previous illustration, the client has stated fear and concern about "losing my health" and was not sure how to cope with the loss of health or how to prevent it. This is the clue from the client to the nurse practitioner to move on to the next phase of the Helping Process, the Initiation Stage.

The Initiation Stage entails that the nurse practitioner make a statement of a tentative goal or solution to the experience of the client in addition to the feeling, meaning, and responsibility of the problem of the client. In this instance, the nurse might say something like this:

> Nurse: "You are frightened because you may become sick and helpless. You are not sure if you could cope with being helpless. It sounds as if you would really be interested in knowing how to maintain your health and reduce your chances of getting sick."

In this statement, the nurse practitioner has summed up the client's situation as the client has shared thus far. The nurse practitioner stated the client's feeling ("You are frightened"), meaning ("you may become sick and helpless"), placed the responsibility with the client ("you are not sure if you could cope"), and offered a tentative goal or solution ("interest in knowing how to maintain your health and not get sick"). The client at this point in the Helping Process may choose to accept or reject the tentative goal or solution.

The client may reject the tentative goal or solution, perhaps with a statement like this:

> Client: "Yes, I am frightened about my health and becoming helpless. But I think I'll just keep on keeping on. I mean what is the use, I'm old. . . ."

With this statement the client confirms the feeling and meaning of the nurse practitioner's response but rejects the tentative goal ("I'll just keep on. . ."). When the client rejects a tentative goal or solution, the process reverts to the Exploration Stage to further clarify the client's experience.

On the other hand, the client may accept the nurse practitioner's initiating statement, with a statement something like this:

> Client: "Yes, I'm scared about becoming sick and helpless. I'm not sure what to do, but sure want to do all I can to stay healthy."

The nurse practitioner can then explore the client's present activities and practices and build on these practices to develop a plan or program with the client to enhance, maintain, and promote a state of well-being.

ASSESSMENT OF LEARNING NEEDS AND TEACHING STRATEGIES WITH THE ELDERLY

Bille (1980, p. 256) states "The elderly client can learn what the practitioner teaches if an appropriate philosophy of education and other teaching variables are customized to the individual." Meeting the educational needs of the client has become a legal responsibility with the advent of the "Patient Bill of Rights" (Roach, 1981). This responsibility of meeting educational needs includes instructing the client in continuing health needs and how to carry out the care measures after discharge (Roach, 1981).

Assessment

Rogers (1980) believes the quality of teaching can only be as good as the assessment on which it is based. In order to effectively assess the learning needs of the older client, Rogers advocates that the condescending attitude of "older people do not know what is best for them" be replaced with the attitude "older people can be taught to decide what is best" and that such teaching can begin in the assessment of the client. During the

assessment process the nurse practitioner should include the client as a collaborator in the planning of health care.

Collaborating with the clients in this way reinforces their sense of being independent, mature individuals capable of influencing their own health status. It also enhances the probability that clients will have a sense of power and control, therefore, increasing the likelihood that they will be motivated to participate in developing a greater sense of self-determination (Sterns & Sterns, 1981).

An effective assessment, according to Rogers (1980), begins with the nurse practitioner reviewing the client's health record. Making use of the available information allows the nurse practitioner to demonstrate respect for the client by having prepared for the assessment and thus relieved the client from having to repeat (possibly for the umpteenth time) his or her health history. It is important that the nurse practitioner establish rapport with the elderly client, as this will enhance not only the relationship but the learning activity as well.

In an effective assessment, the client should be informed of the nurse practitioner's role and task as well as the role and responsibility of the client. The nurse practitioner's role is to assist the client to identify problems, goals, and options; the client's responsibility is to choose among the options available and take action to implement the chosen option to achieve the goal. Research indicates that although elderly clients tend to avoid taking risks, they will take action to deal with a problem when perceived as an unavoidable risk.

In an effective assessment, the task of the nurse practitioner and client is to turn the problems into goals, so that more time is devoted to goals than to problems. Goals describe what the client would like to have happen. Once the client's goals have been stated, the nurse practitioner can work with the client to evaluate their feasibility as well as the variables that may impede their attainment. By focusing on the client's goals, the nurse practitioner can emphasize the positive attributes and health factors of the client that may compensate for an illness or disability. Attention to goals rather than problems, to abilities rather than disabilities, is a key factor in effective assessment.

Teaching Strategies

Teaching is an ongoing process and is an ever-present opportunity in each interaction. A factor noted by Aspy and Roebuck (1972) is emphasized by the title, "Kids Don't Learn from Teachers They Don't Like." Egan (1975) believes that it is vitally important that the client trust the nurse practitioner. In essence, it seems that the relationship between the client and nurse is one of the more important "strategies" to be considered in teaching.

Teaching initially takes place during the assessment process (Taylor, 1987) when the nurse practitioner explores with the client alternatives and options for attaining goals. One particularly useful teaching strategy in assessing the aged is for the nurse practitioner to summarize, in writing, the options and alternatives for each problem identified, and the positive attributes of the client that contribute to the attainment of the goals. These notes can serve the client as reminders by providing important points that would be helpful in attaining goals.

In the Helping Process, it is important to keep communication within the client's frame of reference. Thus, the usage of jargon or medical/surgical terminology may convey little or no meaning to the client. The nurse practitioner's vocabulary should be monitored and may need to be modified to teach effectively. Technical terms or procedures should be defined in terms or phrases understandable to the client.

Repetition of important points will serve to reinforce learning. Repetition is especially important when the client is learning some new information or applying information to a new or novel situation. Occasionally, repetition of entire teaching sessions may be necessary, es-

pecially if a session was taught at a time when the client is either psychologically and/or physiologically distracted or if so much information was given at one time that the client was unable to assimilate it.

Attention must be constantly directed to the psychological and physiological status of the client before and during teaching. Effective teaching is difficult, if not impossible, when the client is experiencing a disruption from either a psychological or physiological source. Psychologically the disruption may be due to the nature of the topic, such as loss of sight or hearing or change of body image, or perhaps to feeling overwhelmed by more information than can be assimilated. The nurse practitioner using the attending behaviors with the client will be able to detect and possibly avoid these problems and work with the client in pacing the instruction to the client's needs.

The nurse practitioner working with the client to develop a flow chart or map as to how to achieve the goals the client has chosen is another teaching strategy. Assisting the client in drawing a map or path of the necessary steps and time frame to achieve the health goals gives the client a tangible plan that can promote feelings of self-determination and worth. Operationally defined behavioral steps, graphically displayed, are effective means for promoting and maintaining positive health practices and for the personal empowerment of the client (Stensrud & Stensrud, 1982).

As Bille (1980, p. 263) stated, "Perhaps the most important strategy in teaching the elderly client is letting the client be the individual human being that he is." The elderly need to be allowed to make decisions about their own life-style. In order to customize teaching, an effective assessment includes the client in making decisions and determining what is important to one's life-style. The nurse practitioner should identify the extent of the client's knowledge about the condition and/or situation (Rogers, 1983) before developing an individualized teaching plan.

SUMMARY

Research indicates that barring any physiological problems, an elderly client in the areas of intelligence, learning, memory, and motivation does not differ markedly from younger clients. Changes in these cognitive elements as one matures occur idiosyncratically and on an individual basis. Assessment of the client by the gerontological nurse practitioner on these cognitive elements serves as a basis for development of a holistic care plan for the client.

The ears and eyes must also be assessed by the nurse practitioner to determine the existence of any impairments. Determination of visual and hearing problems will assist the nurse practitioner in planning for more effective communications. The nurse practitioner should be cognizant of the usual biological changes that occur with hearing and sight. Knowledge of these expected changes will guide the nurse practitioner to speak slowly in low-pitched tones directly in front of the aged client.

Development of a trusting relationship with the client is extremely important. The nurse practitioner can enhance the probability of helping and establishing a relationship of trust with clients by (1) being aware and acting on the effect of behaviors that represent positive modeling of healthy living, (2) arranging the office or positioning to promote a positive interaction with the client, (3) assessing the nonverbal attending behaviors in an interaction, (4) developing and using a feeling vocabulary, and (5) working with the client through the Helping Process to identify a problem(s) or develop a plan of action for the client to deal more effectively with the situation.

A number of factors must be considered by the gerontological nurse practitioner in assessing the client, and a number of strategies are useful in teaching the elderly client. The challenge for the nurse practitioner is to determine how the client views himself or herself and the ideas the client has for adapting to the condition. Effective assessment and teaching of the elderly client are enhanced by working with the client to identify goals and helping the client to attain the skills needed to reach those goals. Each client is an individual and bears ultimate responsibility for his or her health status. The nurse practitioner can assist the individual to identify goals and teach the skills necessary to achieve these goals, but the client has control, not only over the choice of goals, but over whether those goals are achieved.

REFERENCES

Argyle, M., & Kendon, A. (1967). The experimental analysis of social performance. In L. Berkowitz (Ed.), *Advance of experimental social psychology* (Vol. 3). New York: Academic Press.

Aspy, D. N., & Roebuck, F. (1977). *Kids don't learn from teachers they don't like.* Amherst, MA: Human Resource Development Press.

Belderston, T. W. (1981). Rental concept proposed for middle-income elderly. *Contemporary Administrator, 6*(2), 10–14.

Bengtson, V. L. (1973). *The social psychology of aging.* Indianapolis: Bobbs-Merrill.

Bille, D. A. (1980). Educational strategies for teaching the elderly patient. *Nursing and Health Care, 2,* 256–263.

Blake, R. H., & Bichekas, G. (1981). In J. E. Meyers and M. L. Ganikos (Eds.), *Counseling older persons* (Vol. II). Falls Church, VA: American Personnel and Guidance Association.

Botwinick, J. (1969). Disinclination to venture response versus cautiousness in responding: Age differences. *Journal of Genetic Psychology, 115,* 55–62.

Brammer, L. M. (1981). In J. E. Meyers and M. L. Ganikos (Eds.), *Counseling older persons* (Vol. II). Falls Church, VA: American Personnel and Guidance Association.

Capuzzi, D. (Ed.). (1982). The school counselor, aging education. *American Personnel and Guidance Association, 29*(4), 259–322.

Carkhuff, R. R. (1973). *The Art of Helping.* Amherst, MA: Human Resource Development Press.

Carkhuff, R. R., & Anthony, W. A. (1973). *The skills of helping.* Amherst, MA: Human Resource Development Press.

Carter, C. (1976). Community mental health programs and the elderly. *Nursing Clinics of North America, 11*(1), 125–133.

Coleman, J. C., Butcher, J. N., & Carson, R. C. (1980). *Abnormal psychology and modern life.* Dallas, TX: Scott-Foresman.

Egan, G. (1975). *The skilled helper.* Monterey, CA: Brooks-Cole.

Friedlander, F. (1970). The primacy of trust as a facilitator of further group accomplishment. *The Journal of Applied Behavioral Science, 6*(4), 382–400.

Gershowitz, S. Z. (1982). Adding years to life: Remotivating the elderly people in institutions. *Nursing and Health Care, 3,* 141–145.

Gibb, J. R. (1964). *Climate for trust formation in T-group theory and laboratory method.* New York: Wiley.

Hansen, J. C., Pound, R. E., & Warner, R. W. (1976). Use of modeling procedures. *Personnel and Guidance Journal, 65,* 242–245.

Kirchner, W. (1958). Age differences in short-term retention of rapid changing information. *Journal of Experimental Psychology, 55,* 352–358.

Lawson, J. S. (1975). Changes in immediate memory with age. *British Journal of Psychology, 56,* 69–69–75.

Looney, D S. (1975). Senility is also a state of mind. *Nursing Digest, 14,* 13.

Lieberman, M. (1965). Psychological correlates of impending death. *Journal of Gerontology, 20,* 181–190.

Murray, R. B., & O'Driskoll, D. L. (1979). *The nursing process in later maturity.* Englewood Cliffs, NJ: Prentice-Hall.

Murray, R. B., & Zentner, J. P. (1979). *Nursing assessment and health promotion through the life span.* Englewood Cliffs, NJ: Prentice-Hall.

Myers, J. E., Fried-Finnerty, P., & Graves, C. H. (Eds.). (1981). *Counseling Older Persons* (Vol. I). Falls Church, VA: American Personnel and Guidance Association.

Myers, J. E., & Ganikos, M. L. (1981). *Counseling Older Persons* (Vol. II). Falls Church, VA: American Personnel and Guidance Association.

Pine, G. J. (Ed.). (1980). Counseling and values. *American Personnel and Guidance Association, 24*(2), 66–135.

Roach, W. (1981). The patient's right to know. In D. Bille (Ed.), *Practical approaches to patient teaching.* Boston: Little, Brown.

Rogers, J. C. (1980). Advocacy: The key to assessing the older client. *Journal of Gerontological Nursing, 6,* 33–36.

Rogers, C. (1983). *Freedom to learn.* Columbus, OH: Charles E. Merrill.

Rorden, J. W. (1987). *Nurses and health teachers: A practical guide.* Philadelphia: Saunders.

Selye, H. (1974). *Stress without distress.* Philadelphia: Lippincott.

Smith, S. P., Jepson, V., & Perloff, E. (1982). Attitudes of nursing care providers toward elderly patients. *Nursing and Health Care, 3,* 93–98.

Stensrud, R. H., & Stensrud, K. (1982). Counseling for health empowerment. *Personnel and Guidance Journal, 71,* 377–381.

Sterns, H. L., & Sterns, R. S. (1981). In J. E. Meyers and M. L. Ganikos (Eds.), *Counseling older persons* (Vol. II). Falls Church, VA: American Personnel and Guidance Association.

Taylor, R. A. (1987). Making the most of your time for patient teaching. *RN, 50*(12), 20–21.

Weber, H. (1980). *Nursing care of the elderly.* Reston, VA: Reston Publishing.

13

VARIATIONS IN MENTAL HEALTH OF THE AGED

Aging is inevitable, and the health care professional can assist elderly persons to do this within their capabilities. Being old does not necessarily mean that life stops. The personality traits and characteristics that one had as a young person are still with the elderly person. Coping strategies may change because of sensory deficits, multiple losses, or diminished physical strength and energy; nevertheless the elderly experience feelings like any other age group. By identifying sensory deprivation, body image, territoriality, and loss/separation as concepts, gerontological nurse practitioners can operationalize the plan of care without losing sight of the fact that each concept is unlikely to occur as a single entity, and yet the nursing intervention will require different approaches for each concept.

STEREOTYPING

Rokeach (1968) defines stereotypes as beliefs or opinions that have no implicit direction. They are used to minimize ambiguity, to bolster self-esteem, or as a means of social control. The media have done little to promote a positive image of the elderly, but rather have perpetuated the idea that the elderly suffer from cognitive decrements, depression, confusion, and physical impairment. Hess and Markson (1980) supported the findings that rarely did the media provide a positive image of the elderly.

Some attempts are being made to correct this situation, however. The American Association of Retired Persons, an advocacy group for the aged, has directed efforts toward increasing acceptance of the aged by society. Eyde and Rich (1983) suggest that aging should be viewed as a developmental phase of the life-span, with more recognition of the diversification and lack of homogeneity within the group. More public education would help to remove the myths as well as the misunderstandings of the aging process.

Age prejudices do exist. A review of the literature reveals multiple prejudices that result in negative stereotypes by the population in general as well as the aged themselves. The elderly have difficulty receiving appropriate physical and mental health care because societal prejudices, myths, and stereotypes characterize their infirmities as incurable and their very existence as noncontributory to society. Health care providers have been heard to say, "What can Mrs. Jones expect? She is seventy-five years old." Because nurses are influenced by personal prejudices, one may be in error to ascribe a symptom and/or behavior to the aged personality when in essence a physical problem may be influencing the behavior of the aged. If these same behaviors/symptoms were observed in a younger person, such stereotyping would not occur. Consider the following example: Over a period of several months, Jane had observed that when her mother was in a group, she was quiet, withdrawn, and did not participate verbally or nonverbally with the group. She appeared to be in her own world, exhibiting depressive behaviors, apathy, and disinterest in the surroundings. Jane's assessment included the social withdrawal behaviors exhibited by her mother, but she felt social validation was necessary. After exploring these observations with her mother, Jane learned that her mother could not hear when multiple conversations were going on in a large group; therefore, rather than continually ask people to repeat their comments, which was embarrassing and in her own mind was a stereotype of the aging process, she preferred to remain quiet and alone. This situation illustrates the stereotyping that often takes place with the elderly. This was a physical problem (hearing loss) which was initially attributed to stereotypical behaviors "expected" of the elderly, namely withdrawal, depression, and lack of interest. Fortunately, the physical problem had a solution. Often the evaluation is much more complex, requiring in-depth exploration of the behaviors in order to institute the appropriate treatment.

As one examines the employment field choices of nurses, it is alarming to note how very few recent graduates choose the field of gerontological nursing. Caring for the aged is unpopular with nurses. Studies have shown that nurses least prefer working with the aged; as a result, there are more than 1 million elderly needing nursing care and only approximately 40,000 registered nurses employed full time in gerontological care.

Why is gerontological nursing not a desired field of employment for nurses? Why are nursing students not interested in working with aged cli-

ents? Among the reasons might be the values of the industrialized United States and the stereotypes regarding aging and the aged. Our children are taught early to value youth. The media are full of talk about youthful beauty. Billions of dollars are spent annually on cosmetics, beauty aids, and clothes designed to help people appear young. We live in a society that values economic productivity and work and ignores aging and the closure of life. Older citizens are a reminder of reality, a reality with which we are not comfortable. The aged remind us that our bodies will change, that our physical and mental health will decline, that our family and friends will leave us, and that each of us must face and work through the denial and fears of our own mortality. The aged are also devalued because they are seen as being nonprogressive and no longer productive, maintaining old values and resisting new ideas, and getting sick and dying.

If the elderly person in the nursing home is stereotyped as senile, incontinent, and dying, then gerontological nursing is not likely to interest too many future nurses; however, nurse educators must recognize the stereotypes that nursing students have toward the elderly and influence these attitudes. Hart, Freal, and Crowell (1976) reported that when students had positive experiences with the "healthy" elderly and when students had guided learning experiences with the "sick" elderly, the positive attitude continued. The research of Wilhite and Johnson (1976) suggests that changes in student attitudes are functionally related to the attitudes of the faculty toward the aged.

Stereotypes about the aged do exist in today's society; unfortunately, aged persons know this and tend to share these beliefs. Although much has been written about the nuclear family and the holistic functioning person, society denies that the elderly form a heterogeneous population, with individual personalities and lifestyles. Service agencies provide programs into which all the aged are supposed to fit simply because they are old.

SENSORY DEPRIVATION

Sensory deprivation in the aged has been recognized as a deficit, but reduction in the capability of the senses does not necessarily cause maladaptive behavior. The number of taste and smell receptors may be decreased, but the significance of the loss will not have the same meaning to the individual as the loss of hearing or vision (Weber, 1980).

Hearing loss occurs in 30% of the older population, affecting men more frequently than women (Pfeiffer, 1980); it causes a greater social isolation than blindness (Butler & Lewis, 1982). Eighty percent of the elderly have fair to adequate vision, and most need glasses for reading (Pfeiffer, 1980; Butler & Lewis, 1982).

It is important to consider the adaptive capabilities of the individual. Human beings have the ability to survive but are dependent upon the reception and integration of information from the eyes, ears, skin, muscles, and joints. The human organism can tolerate decreased sensations without manifesting behavior changes. Reduction of sensations may be the result of disease or injury as well as advancing age (Schwab, 1973).

Individuals may deny or compensate for sensory deficits, particularly if the changes are gradual. If the change is rapid, it is often accompanied by emotional reactions and denial. Declines in the sensory function of the elderly may contribute to isolation and reductions in the amount of incoming stimuli. This, then, can cause difficulties in the processing of information. The capacity of the central nervous system to integrate stimuli may be limited or distorted. Failing eyesight, decreased hearing ability, and decreased location and position sense can cause further difficulty in handling complex stimuli (Thomas, 1979).

Sensory deprivation is a stress that can cause behavioral changes. Individual differences come into play in determining when and how stress is handled. Culture, education, personality structure, and genetic traits also influence behavior patterns. Controlling emotions and aggressive behavior has the potential for creating discord (Thomas, 1979) because of the challenges of the neuroendocrine and psychomotor impulses and physiological states. If the discord lasts long enough, the individual may have difficulty in handling stress (Giorella, 1980).

Old age is a period during which profound crises frequently occur. The psychological events leading to sensory deprivation may be seen in all ages, but it is more conspicuous in the aged because they are vulnerable to stress. The lifelong capacity to cope effectively with stress may diminish in the elderly when remaining strengths are unequal to the intense and frequent demands for adjustment (Thomas, 1979; Johnson, 1979).

Several generalizations can be made regarding stress (Butler & Lewis, 1982): (1) higher levels of stress cause unpleasant sensations; (2) stress is a consequence of personality variables and genetic factors; (3) when a critical level of somatic dysfunction is reached, variation in cognition occurs; and (4) psychological and social antecedents accompany the physiological manifestations of stress. When communication is not effective, the health care professional needs to intervene and assist the elderly to adjust to the environment. Being aware that sensory defects may result from losses in hearing, vision, or motor skills can help the elderly modify or enhance the quality of life.

SELF-IMAGE/SELF-ESTEEM

Old age is the phase of life during which the individual becomes more acutely aware of the biological, social, and psychological adaptive mechanisms that affect one's capacities to revise one's self-image. A person who has had rewarding life experiences (home, marriage, good health, intact family, meaningful interpersonal relationships, education, productive years, and a sense of autonomy) will be more likely to have a valued identity (Schwartz, 1975). Unrewarding life experiences (such as poverty, broken families, membership in deprived groups, minimal education, and little productive achievement) tend to diminish the individual's ability to adapt.

World, state, and local events also influence the individual's adaptive mechanisms. The television brings instant news to the listener (Busse & Pfeiffer, 1969). There are constant reminders that the Social Security system faces insolvency, that the economy is either in a state of growth or decline, and that gold and silver market prices somehow affect inflation and the stock market. The national and world scene is also unstable, with political pressures and potential arenas for violence and war. Negotiation processes are a constant reminder of the instability of the world around us. These situations cause major concern for the health and welfare of older members of our society. Will the aged have the same rights when our nation needs money or when our society needs more space? Even the person who planned for retirement might find it difficult to maintain an identity and self-worth during these troubled times.

One's self-esteem is also negatively affected by aging. Youth and productivity are valued in our society and this intimidation can be carried into the family. It is seen in role reversal as adult children assume responsibility for the management of their parents' affairs. The loss of memory, loss of friends, baldness, dentures, decreased hearing and visual acuity, and changes in physical attributes all contribute to the changes in self-image (Lee, 1976).

How one adapts depends upon a number of factors, one of which is the person's ability to accept the fact that he or she is no longer a young person but is rather in the final phase of life. Acceptance is based on a person's past experiences of success and capacity for accurately assessing himself or herself. A sense of self is an outgrowth of one's roles, values, and goals. It may become necessary to abandon one role and

substitute another (Spencer & Dore, 1975). Ways of using one's energies should be planned, and alternative ways of maintaining security and self-esteem should be developed.

SPACE/TERRITORIALITY

The elderly are often faced with moving from their homes into smaller dwellings because of financial, physical, or mental constraints. This move is usually traumatic, particularly if it is not desired by the individual; time is needed for grief resolution. All too frequently individuals are institutionalized and, where they once had privacy, they now have to deal with an unknown roommate and the institution's personnel (Giorella, 1980). Personal space, that is, the physical distance between the individual and others, is often limited. Individuals need to be able to define, control, and protect the space around them (Lewis, 1981). Each person needs personal space, although the amount needed may vary, as women are more likely to tolerate less space. More space is needed when the client approaches the nurse practitioner than when the nurse practitioner approaches the client (Murphy, 1981; Lewis, 1981).

Privacy is a basic human right, and one should have the freedom to decide what one wants others to know about oneself. Persons do need the opportunity for social interaction in order to develop effective ties; however, closeness and distance are essential if possible interaction continues (Edney, 1974). Institutional settings have limited space, and the decreased personal space can create an environment for adverse stimuli and interpersonal conflict. Regardless of the space requirement, territory is essential (Johnson, 1979; Allekian, 1973). Territorial boundaries aid the individual in maintaining identity and feelings of security. If territory cannot be established, anxiety, withdrawal, loss of identity, and loss of reality can occur. According to Johnson (1979) and Allekian (1973), the presence of others in the setting and their intrusion into the elderly person's territory often create anxiety; this anxiety increases in direct proportion to how strongly one identifies the territory as one's own. Females develop higher levels of anxiety than do males when territorial intrusion takes place.

LOSS/SEPARATION

Elderly persons have emotional needs similar to those of younger individuals. They have other universal needs: living as long as possible; obtaining release from tiring tasks; safeguarding skills, possessions, rights, and authority; remaining active participants in the affairs of life; and, as death nears, withdrawing from life in a timely, honorable, and comfortable fashion (Palmore, 1969).

Havighurst (1973) has identified ten developmental tasks of adulthood: worker, mate, parent, homemaker, son/daughter, citizen, friend, organization member, religious affiliate, and user of leisure time. As each task becomes more difficult to carry out, the aging individual has to cope with multiple losses at the same time that physical decrements, such as decreased strength/ energy, chronic illness, loss of hearing, and diminished sight are occurring. Losses occur more frequently with a cumulative effect, and one may neglect to appreciate the rapidity and the intrusive nature of the losses upon the elderly (Butler & Lewis, 1982). Each loss, whether the loss of a loved one, the loss of health, the loss of body function, the loss of a job, the loss of economic status, the loss of valued possessions (home, property, memorabilia), the loss of membership or status, or the loss of a pet, is a real threat; and change of status is irrevocable (Palmore, 1969).

Loss is inevitable; the extent of the grief reaction depends upon the value of the lost object to the person. It may last 3–12 months, after which interest in the environment is renewed and psychic energy is restored.

When part of the self is lost, the loss becomes more difficult and complex to manage. Loss usually initiates a disorganizing emotional reaction (McNulty, 1977). It is not unusual to see the grief reaction become prolonged and merge into depression. Other persons may become angry and seek a scapegoat to blame for their troubles. Still others will withdraw to avoid risks, thus increasing the momentum toward isolation and the avoidance of reality. Another reaction is the loss of one's sense of identity. Reactions of grief, shame, and hostility are generated, causing increased conflict which then can interfere with the person's reality orientation and rehabilitation efforts (Verwoerdt, 1980).

The elderly are aware that time does not necessarily cure all ills but know that living with losses is inevitable; how one copes is not always clearly defined. There are those who are involved in the network of interpersonal activity, but there are those who find little that is inspiring or rewarding. As with all ills, loss can be denied only a short while (McNulty, 1977).

COMMON DISORDERS

Loss and loneliness are present throughout the life cycle; however, their impact increases with advancing years. Older persons are more likely to be separated by death or distance from family and friends and to lose the ability or opportunity to be gainfully employed. The elderly may also be restricted in the type of activities they can perform because of poor health, e.g., failing eyesight or hearing. Lack of transportation may be another factor in further isolating the aged.

Grief

Grief, as defined by Freedman, Kaplan, and Sadock (1976), is an alteration in mood and affect consisting of sadness appropriate to a real loss. In the aged, a most significant human loss is the death of a marital partner. This loss results in grief and is particularly stressful for the aged person because similar relationships are unlikely in the future and the void is very difficult to fill. Bereavement is a highly traumatic experience for the elderly. The symptoms of grief are similar regardless of age—feelings of deep sadness and lessening of self-esteem, decline of interest in one's surroundings, general retardation of motor activities, aimless wandering, inability to concentrate, agitation, anorexia, and insomnia. Also typical are self-accusations, feelings of guilt, regrets about the past, and wishes that more affection had been shown. These feelings are more prevalent if the bereaved person had experienced ambivalence toward the one who died.

It is important to note that the grieving person will turn continually to the lost object and tend to dwell on the memories of the past. This activity is a necessary part of mourning and should be encouraged. The grieving person should be encouraged to reminisce about the deceased person. The individual who is able to complete the grieving process promptly is more likely to return to a normal psychological state sooner and more completely than the person who attempts to avoid or delay the experience. Mourning is not accepted as healthy in our society, and in many cases it is not allowed. The person who is classified as being brave, who exhibits little sadness or grief, is recognized positively by society. However, denial may prolong the grief process, as mourning plays an essential part in making a healthy adjustment to loss. It will normally free the bereaved person from maintenance of tie-ups with the deceased (Fromm-Reichmann, 1950) and helps one to complete the grief process so that one's energies can be redirected to new interests.

All individuals, including the aged, need to work through the grief process by continuing with routine tasks, by support from significant others, and by reduction in the feelings of abandonment and loss. The individuals providing support should be aware that grief is expressed in numerous ways.

Anger is a stage of the grief process and may be directed at the loved one for leaving or at the health care providers for not preventing the death. This anger needs to be expressed and explored with a person who can provide understanding and empathy.

The profound effects of loss of a spouse are exemplified in the following case study: Mr. and Mrs. Thompson had been married for 51 years and had three children. They had been in reasonably good health, each had retired from gainful employment, and were enjoying activities with other senior citizens. While on a trip sponsored by a senior citizen organization, Mrs. Thompson became ill and died.

Following the death of his wife, Mr. Thompson lost all interest in his children and outside activities and experienced a loss of appetite, a loss of energy, and insomnia. Within a period of 6 weeks he had lost 20 pounds. He continued to live alone because he "did not want to be a burden to anyone." He would get up very early but would not get dressed. He ate very little, but insisted that he be responsible for preparing his meals. His continual comments were, "I have nothing to live for, why did she have to die? What am I going to do? I do not want to live without her."

This example serves to illustrate the severe feelings of loss, helplessness, and desperation experienced. The loss of a spouse or significant other is not the only cause for grief in the aged; it is, however, the most profound. Loss of health, forced retirement, decreased financial assets, loss of possessions (by burglary or fire), loss of social status, or mutilating surgeries are also unpleasant realities for the elderly person. These events can result in many of the previously discussed symptoms of grief.

Depression

Depression is a morbid state characterized by mood alterations such as sadness and loneliness, by low self-esteem associated with self-reproach, by psychomotor retardation and at times agitation, by withdrawal from interpersonal contact, and at times a desire to die (Freedman et al. 1976). Depression is the most common mental health disorder in the aged and, as indicated by the definition, is sometimes characterized by the desire to die; therefore, suicide is of major concern in the care of a depressed client. The suicide rate among the elderly is higher than in any other age group, and the suicide rate for men increases with every decade of life (Blazer, 1982).

The following case study illustrates the feelings of loneliness, helplessness, despair and grief experienced by a depressed aged person (Wilson, 1987). Mrs. Green is a 75-year-old widow who had been active in church and community activities until the death of her husband 1 year earlier. Immediately following his death, Mrs. Green returned to her usual activities, and friends commented as to "how well she was doing." However, within 3 months of Mr. Green's death, the activities had diminished. Mrs. Green's son, Paul, had spent a great deal of time with her immediately after his father's death; but, since she was "doing so well" and the family members were so busy, their visits became less and less frequent.

On one occasion, when the son came for a visit, he noticed that his mother had not combed her hair and was dressed in a very old skirt and a blouse that did not fit. This was uncharacteristic of Mrs. Green, as she had always been an immaculately groomed person. When Paul asked about Mrs. Green's well-being, she expressed feelings of fatigue and described a weight loss, and an inability to sleep. She would awaken about three o'clock in the morning, get up, and just sit in a chair until sunrise. Paul questioned Mrs. Green about involvement in community activities and found that his mother had not participated in some time. When questioned further, it was learned that Mrs. Green felt inadequate without her husband. He was the outgoing member of the family. The questions bothered Mrs. Green, and she began to cry uncontrollably, saying "I am so alone, I have nothing to live for, I'd rather be dead, I don't belong anywhere to anyone."

This illustration is an example of the feelings of loneliness and loss experienced by the aged depressed. Following the loss of her spouse, Mrs. Green experienced reduced self-esteem. Because her life had revolved around Mr. Green, she had difficulty seeing herself without him.

As nurses confront care situations such as this, how does one assess the client for depression? The nursing assessment needs to be comprehensive and should include behavioral manifestations, nursing history, and physical and mental status examinations (Tancredi, 1987).

The *Diagnostic and Statistical Manual of Mental Disorders* (American Psychiatric Association [APA], 1987) categorizes depression as an affective disorder. The pertinent behavior of a major depressive episode is a disturbance of mood, accompanied by a full or partial manic or depressive syndrome, that is not due to any other physical or mental disorder (APA, 1987). Major depression, a subclassification of the category, is pertinent to this discussion.

Mrs. Green was admitted to a community hospital with a plan of nursing care that included rest and directed activity. Essential to this care was a primary nurse who could give the client individualized care and warmth and provide an environment conducive to a feeling of protection and security without making undue demands. Additionally, the plan called for the family to provide support and convey to Mrs. Green that she was both cared for and thought to be worthwhile. Friends were also included in the plan and were encouraged to visit and to talk with Mrs. Green about happenings in the community.

This example illustrates one possible cause of depression in the aged; however, there are other causes such as disease, drug usage, disappointments, and threats of physical harm or abuse. These situations may be real or imagined and need investigation. Depression in the aged is complex and many times multicausal in origin. Butler and Lewis (1982) point out that the increased incidence of depression with age, in both men and women, suggests a relationship to the emotion-laden life events in middle and later life—the children leaving home, the culmination of career possibilities, the first signs of physical aging, and the sense of time passing more quickly. The impact of these events depends on the individual's personality, previous life experience, and contemporary circumstances.

Loneliness

Loneliness, according to Williams (1978), is a feeling that there is no one who cares what happens. This feeling is expressed as self-pity, thus making that person think only of himself or herself and the things expected from others. The effects of this feeling of loneliness can be very distressing, as it often causes feelings of deprivation, helplessness, and low self-esteem.

Loneliness is a common and very serious problem in the aged. It occurs frequently in the elderly because they often experience the loss of a significant relationship, particularly the loss of a spouse. This loved one may have provided a real sense of interpersonal intimacy. Frieda Fromm-Reichmann (1950) addresses the disintegrative effect of feeling alone, unappreciated, and unloved, which she considers to be a particularly difficult stress in our group-conscious culture. The aged person who has previously been shy and dependent on the marital relationship to meet the need for belonging may, upon the loss of the marital partner, become extremely withdrawn and isolated and experience a painful sense of being all alone in the world.

Thurmott (1977) explains that the degree of loneliness felt by the aged may depend in part on the life-style that the individual or family had in the past as well as personality. Those persons who are outgoing and have enjoyed the companionship of family and friends will continue to do so in later life, thus minimizing the feelings of loneliness and self-pity.

Everyone experiences loneliness at some stage of life (Williams, 1978). The precipitating

factors may vary; however, the aged are called upon to make numerous changes, such as adapting to new means of transportation, different living quarters, and the (frequently rapid) physical problems affecting themselves and their friends. Adaptation to change may have been uneventful in the past; with increasing age, however, these changes constitute major stressors.

Williams (1978) found, when working with a group of aged women, that loneliness was mentioned by each member of the group. When each member was asked to discuss some problems associated with compliant behavior related to health care, the subject of loneliness was predominant. The group members asserted that a lack of understanding on the part of others is a cause of their loneliness; however, there was a note of sadness, depression, and hopelessness.

In order to provide quality nursing care for the lonely elderly person, it is essential that the gerontological nurse practitioner develop a trusting relationship and exhibit a willingness to listen. The elderly can be assisted in dealing with feelings of loneliness by establishing relationships with others—the nurse, family and friends. Essential to the plan of care for the aged is the inclusion of family and friends. Many older people have extensive support systems to help them deal with isolation and loneliness; others were not as fortunate. This latter group is a symbol of society's prophecy that being old means being senile and nonvalued. With the elderly comprising a steadily increasing percentage of our society, it is essential that this negative image of the aged be challenged; otherwise society will fail in its mission of providing for all its members (Eyde & Rich, 1983).

Guilt

Each person has inhibitions or fears that have been a hindrance in the past; with the incapacities of old age, anxiety and anger may reoccur. Individuals who have been minimally self-reliant, goal directed, and involved in problem solving suffer from feelings of failure when they are faced with functional losses. As these feelings increase, so do feelings of helplessness and fear. Fear and the feeling of worthlessness continue to feed upon one another to the point where the individual is no longer able to achieve personal gratification. A sense of frustration is present; anger takes over, followed by a fear of retaliation. This behavior is repetitious, and guilt feelings reappear. As the emotional disorganization state appears, the individual takes on a culturally accepted dependency role (Butler, 1978).

Grief is a concept related to guilt. The grief process begins with an awareness of loss followed by shock and disbelief. The feelings of loss may be followed by a period of denial and later by the mourning stage. This is the period when a person feels hurt. Often guilt and self-blame arise, particularly if there was an ambivalent relationship with the object of the guilt. Following the grief, anger, hostility, and rejection are often projected; as time passes, psychic energy is renewed and life begins to take on new meaning (Gramlich, 1978).

Elderly persons frequently need help to work through the grief process. Sometimes denial helps the person to live in a state of unreality. Others need to be helped to work out the grief process by remembering and talking about the pain, guilt, and anger that is continually present. Feelings of intolerable guilt can lead to suicide. Sharing of guilt feelings can be therapeutic and can also provide the grieving person time to work through feelings of anger and hostility. When depression follows the loss of a person or object that has been held ambivalently by the individual, there is an introjection of the lost object. The hostile impulses toward the object take on the form of self-accusation, self-blame, and guilt. The attention to the loss with the encouragement to participate in activities that have meaning to the individual will help in renewing feelings of self-worth (Busse & Pfeiffer, 1969).

The aged person has time to reflect, and the life review is often filled with unresolved conflicts and regrets. Guilt arising from deeds of omission or commission is real, and the individual needs to seek ways to resolve the problem. It may be in prayer, increased religious activity, repayment of a debt, or a request for forgiveness. This is a serious concern and should not be treated lightly. It is an act of relieving one's conscience in preparation for another life after death (Falk, 1971).

Anxiety

Anxiety is considered to be a result of conflict and is viewed as a threat. It may be real, anticipated, or imaginary, and may be related to the self-concept, self-esteem, or the environment; however, the threat is not clearly perceived. Anxiety levels may range from mild to panic stages, where the perception changes from heightened awareness to almost nonfunctioning cerebral integration (Travelbee, 1971). Anxiety is a state of tension that is produced originally by external causes. If anxiety occurs over a long period of time, physiological manifestations come into play and psychosomatic illnesses may result. However, if psychological manifestations are more predominant, neurotic or psychotic behavior may be seen (Wilson & Knerse, 1979; Gregg, 1952). Adaptive processes need careful study, as the boundary between psychological and physiological illness is not clear-cut, and many health care professionals have a tendency to stereotype the behavior of the elderly (Busse & Pfeiffer, 1969).

The elderly are often faced with changes, and the individual's capacity to deal with stress and to resolve crises is quite different at various points of the life cycle. The decreased physical capacities of aging place a heavy burden on psychological resources. For example, the media continually refer to the insolvency of the Social Security system. This can add to the buildup of anxiety in the aged, particularly as this may be their only source of income. The threat is real and external; and the anxiety may be manifested as rigid thinking, psychosomatic illness, or a paranoid state.

Another area that needs to be explored is the

prevention of sexual expression by the elderly. Sexual behavior is frequently repressed, and many elderly persons do not lose their sexual desire, whether they are in nursing homes, in their own homes or in mental institutions. They are prevented from expressing normal sexual feelings, and it is not unusual to see elderly persons in a nursing home taking off their clothes, grasping at a member of the opposite sex, babbling, and constantly searching for something. Many of these individuals are heavily tranquilized. Nursing home personnel have value systems that direct them to view sexual intimacy as an object for ridicule, and the majority of nursing homes try to prevent sexual expression. This denies an older person who has always been sexually active the opportunity to obtain sexual release. Pervasive anxiety is, therefore, experienced by many elderly persons, and the therapeutic environment that would allow for greater sexual freedom and expression is practically nonexistent. The dehumanizing practices by uninformed professionals in the treatment and care of the elderly only foster dependency and mental illness.

A study of institutionalized aged in a state mental institution indicated that 94% did not belong there, and less than 5% required some degree of custodial care (Kassel, 1976; Busse & Pfeiffer, 1969). In order for an individual's needs to be gratified, the dynamics of personality require contact or transaction with the external world; the elderly should be viewed as any other group. They have the same basic needs as others in our society. The degree of attainment may change, but the desire for love, security, health, housing, and safety are always present.

Confusion

Confusional behavior is more common in the aged than any other segment of the society. This behavior is characterized by deficits in the following areas: memory, concentration, attention, orientation, comprehension, compliance, mood, and interpretation of the environment.

Confusional states always have an underlying cause; this might be physical or emotional in nature. Examples of disorders that might cause confused behavior in the aged are infection, vascular diseases, severe anemia, endocrine disorder, hyperthyroidism or hypothyroidism, heart and kidney disease, sensory impairment (loss of hearing and loss of sight), side effects of drugs, hypothermia, dehydration, disruption in activities of daily living, and distortion of time and space cues. Organic brain syndromes are common disorders of aging resulting in a state of confusion and disorientation. Severe anxiety and/or a bipolar personality disorder (manic depressive state) may also result in confusion. Because there are numerous causes of confusion in the aged and a variety of symptoms characterized in the behavior, the person may be erroneously diagnosed and thus deprived of appropriate health care; therefore, if adequate care is to be provided for the confused client, it is essential that the physical and mental status be properly assessed. Once the cause of the confused state has been diagnosed, treatment can be started.

Specifics related to the nursing care of a confused client should focus on consistency and routine. The plan of care should provide for consistency of nursing personnel assigned to the client; orientation questions and reorientation to day, time, and place, with corrections when errors are made by the confused client; routines related to activities of daily living, with decisions being made by the client and assistance when necessary by the care-giver and consistency of expectations by all personnel. If the client receives mixed messages or there is lack of consistency, the confusion may be intensified. The client should be treated with dignity, kindness, and courtesy at all times; the nurse practitioner will need to be extremely patient (Montgomery, 1987).

Another cause of confusion in the elderly is a move to unfamiliar surroundings—either a change of residence (such as moving in with or close to relatives) or admission to a hospital or long-term care facility. This change may cause the elderly person to become extremely frightened or aggressive. The family or nurse practitioner, whichever the case might be, needs to be prepared to deal with this reaction with kindness and reassurance. It is helpful to try to maintain as many constants in this transition as possible, such as moving familiar furniture into the new place of residence. If the client is in the hospital, having familiar pictures in sight, a calendar and clock visible, and fluids always available and encouraged, allowing ambulation when possible, ensuring that the room is well lighted, allowing clients to wear their own night clothes when possible, and allowing for continuation of their routine activities of daily living all serve to provide reality orientation.

Hypochondriasis

Hypochondriasis, as described by Butler and Lewis (1982), is a somatoform disorder. It usually involves an excessive concern with one's physical and emotional health, accompanied by various bodily complaints for which there is no physical basis.

Individuals labeled as hypochondriacs are usually characterized by multiple complaints about their physical health and sometimes display a particular preoccupation with digestive and excretory functions. These complaints are not necessarily imaginary but are emotional in nature and need to be treated as such. The aged person may be experiencing feelings of loneliness, loss, guilt, and despair and he or she needs understanding, acceptance, and care. The cry for help may be communicated through the sick role. This role usually results in increased attention from family and care-givers, and this may help the client feel important, cared about, in control, and less isolated. By using these symptoms, the clients can manage to have their needs met by controlling persons around them. For example, Sam noticed that, following the death of his father, each time he planned an out of town trip his mother became ill and made such

statements as "I feel so bad," "I really don't think I can take care of myself if you leave," "You wouldn't leave with me being sick, would you?"

Many hypochondriacs develop a pattern of going from physician to physician, or they may be consulting one physician for minor conditions which have been highly exaggerated. Health care providers and families find the hypochondriac very frustrating and may even develop feelings of resentment; therefore, activities of avoidance may come into place.

The gerontological nurse practitioner should be aware that the aged person with hypochondriacal symptoms is best cared for by a person who is able to develop an understanding, supportive relationship and listen in an empathetic manner. The family and significant other(s) should be included in the plan of care so that they can be assisted in providing a supportive relationship. Additionally, the family may need assistance in understanding the disorder and their feelings about the aged relative. The goal of care can best be met through an accepting, supportive, caring relationship to assist the aged person to cope with the feelings that precipitated the somatic complaints.

Suicide

Suicide is among the ten leading causes of death in the aged. Males over 65 years of age commit suicide three times more often than 20–24-year-old males. White females over 65 years of age commit suicide twice as often as their youthful counterparts. The rate is highest in the 45–54-year-old age group for women and it increases among men 85 years and older. Nonwhite and white suicide rate ratios are similar until the age of 35 years, at which point the rate for the white population increases. Persons with professional backgrounds, such as dentists, physicians, and lawyers, and the unskilled have the highest suicide rate; however, after age 65 years, the unskilled and the lower class have the higher rate of suicide. Income loss and rising costs for housing, food, and clothing may provoke feelings of desperation and anxiety, thus contributing to the increased number of persons committing suicide (Pelizza, 1979; Resnik & Cantor, 1978).

The national figures may not represent the total number of elderly persons who commit suicide. Because they have the time and opportunity to contemplate and plan their deaths, some individuals starve themselves to death, others fail to comply with medication routines, and still others delay seeking needed treatment or care or deliberately undertake dangerous activities.

The breakup of a symbiotic relationship caused by the death of a spouse can cause the surviving partner to contemplate and carry out suicide in the hopes of being reunited with the dead spouse. Regaining control is seen as another rationale for committing suicide. Abandonment, whether real or imaginary, is a factor in self-alienation. This form of suicide has previously been categorized as anionic. It is seen when there is a loss or absence of group rules or presence of societal regulations that are unacceptable for an individual to feel good and safe. The term *anionic* has been renamed *social disorganization*, and it is the pattern most frequently seen in the elderly (Resnik & Cantor, 1978; Pelizza, 1979).

A number of contributing factors for social disorganization are inherent in the life of the elderly. When a person retires, numerous social advantages cease: there is a loss of status, a loss of close associations with former colleagues/workers, and a loss of income; in some instances, the move to retirement communities or other housing arrangements can disrupt interaction with family and friends. The problem is compounded when physical or mental disability occurs, especially if the threat is severe enough to decrease the individual's mobility and ability to maintain self-care. Decisions relative to health and welfare begin to be made by others. The loss of independence and self-esteem continues to exacerbate the already present problems (Schneidman, 1965). Death of a spouse and friends are inevitable. Changes resulting from

death do not necessarily occur as a single event and may be compounded by more than one loss. Elderly persons experiencing these losses often display suicide threats, and these should be considered as more than a casual statement (Butler & Lewis, 1982).

Butler (1978) considers suicide accidents as preventable in the older population. Most of the suicides are the result of depression; the public, including the health care professionals, should be alert to the signs and symptoms of depression. Old age is often accompanied by loss, grief, and despair. Even individuals with cerebroarteriosclerotic disorders experience lucid moments and need help in coping. All elderly persons may need help, but the degree of assistance depends on their being able to adapt and integrate values appropriate to their life-styles. There is no period in life that is subject to as many negative forces as old age. These may occur with suddenness, in numbers that are overwhelming, and with extreme intensity. Life review goes on simultaneously and is shaped by contemporary experiences; its failures and outcomes are affected by the individual's own outlook on life (Busse & Pfeiffer, 1969).

Drug Dependence

The pharmacodynamics of drug therapy should be carefully considered in the drug regimes of the aged. Drugs must pass across several membranes; with age, there is less likelihood that complete absorption will take place (Hayes, 1982; Williamson, 1980; Peterson, Whittington, & Payre, 1979). Alteration of drug distribution in the elderly is also affected by a decrease in body mass, a decrease in total body water, a reduction in intracellular and extracellular space, and an increase in fat deposits. Many of the active functional tissues are replaced by fat; highly lipid-soluble drugs, such as phenobarbital and diazepam, have a more pronounced and longer duration of effect (Hayes, 1982). There is also a possibility that some elderly persons have lower plasma albumin levels, which makes unbound protein fractions higher. This can have significance with warfarin and phenytoin levels because less of the drug will be protein-bound (Williamson, 1980).

Drugs are excreted through the kidneys either by passive filtration at the glomerulus or by active secretion into the filtrate. There is an approximate 30% reduction in the glomerular filtration rate and decreased blood flow in the kidney as well as shrinkage of the parenchyma (Gotz & Gotz, 1978). These physiological changes result in more readily attained higher plasma levels in the elderly than in the younger person. This has significance in the use of oral medications and especially intramuscular injections (Hayes, 1982; Allen, 1980). Drug metabolism takes place primarily in the liver. The microsomal enzymes are responsible for drug metabolism; however, there is decreased enzyme activity in the aged, which intensifies drug sensitivity and response (Allen, 1980; Hayes, 1982).

Drugs interact at a receptor site, but, with age, there is a decrease in the number of viable and active cells. The pharmacological action of the drug may be greater because the dose per milligram of active tissue is increased (Allen, 1980).

The homeostatic response to the internal environment is important for the body's vital functioning. When it is impaired, a number of deficiencies may result: an inability to adjust to high or low temperature; limited regulatory mechanisms for maintaining blood sugar levels; a decreased ability to restore acid base equilibrium; and a decreased response to orthostatic stress (Gotz & Gotz, 1978).

Personal characteristics including psychological and physiological variables contribute to compliant and noncompliant behavior. The involutional changes that take place during the aging process, such as a loss of body mass, decreased transport across cellular membranes, diminished renal function, and reduced cardiac reserve and output, are known; however, a major parameter in drug research, namely safety and efficacy, has only been minimally explored in the elderly population (Williamson, 1980).

There is evidence that older individuals use more drugs than younger persons. The population over age 65 years constitute 10% of the United States population and they use 22% of the prescribed and over-the-counter drugs (Hollister, 1977). In a study by Benson (1977), it was found that each nursing home resident used two to seven drugs a day and was the person most likely to have a drug-induced illness. Forty percent of the drugs used in nursing homes were central nervous system drugs such as pain killers, sedatives, and tranquilizers. Tranquilizers represented 20% of the total drugs administered in a nursing home. The elderly used three times as many medications and spent three times as much for drugs as did their younger counterparts (Peterson, Whittington, & Payre, 1979). The high usage of tranquilizers, antidepressants, sedatives, and hypnotics reflects the anxiety, depression, and insomnia experienced by the aged (Butler & Lewis, 1980).

A National Institute for Drug Abuse (1977) study revealed that 50% of elderly persons using psychotropic drugs indicated that they could not perform their daily activities without the agent. Thirty-nine percent of this group indicated they took several kinds of drugs, both prescriptive and over-the-counter, increasing the potential for adverse drug reactions. In skilled nursing centers, 10% of all drugs were tranquilizers, 35% were sedative hypnotic agents, and 8.5% were antidepressants; 25% of clients were taking more than one tranquilizer, and 6% were taking more than one sedative.

Data on narcotic addiction among the elderly are lacking; however, Copel and Stewart (1971) found a number of addicts between the ages of 45 and 75 years, many of them were not in treatment programs, and had camouflaged their habits. There is little information regarding the extent of the addiction. Any drug can be habit forming in a person disposed to become dependent on drugs. These are people with dependent personalities who are constitutional leaners. They lean on members of their families, they draw on social agencies, rituals, alcohol, or on drugs (Poe & Halloway, 1980). There are indications that younger people and people who are now middle-aged are more tolerant and more conditioned to the use of drugs than are those who are now elderly. Use of illicit drugs (heroin, marijuana, or cocaine) by the aged is not significant. Heroin use is less than 1% (Benson, 1977).

There are two distinct groups who become alcoholics, those who do so after 60 years of age and those who have had a long history of alcoholism. Depression, social isolation, and feelings of hopelessness were seen in elderly individuals with a drinking problem. They are, however, able to give up alcohol more quickly than their younger counterparts. Stress factors, such as loss of loved ones, retirement, loneliness, and physical illnesses, may be contributors to the development of alcoholism (Zimberg, 1979). It is difficult to determine the cause of alcoholism, but it does exacerbate mental illness. Suicide is higher among alcoholics (Forni, 1978). How the factors of retirement, poverty, minority status, urbanization, and poor health contribute to the development and persistence of alcoholism is not fully known, but there does appear to be an association (Kola & Kosberg, 1981).

Drug misuse and abuse and clinical abuse of the aged are so interwoven with physical illness that the abuse patterns are not clearly definable. Early identification of the ''at risk'' client could facilitate the relieving of the symptomatology of underuse, misuse, and abuse (Blackwell, 1972; Ellor & Kurz, 1982).

NURSING CARE

The aged population is the one group that the health care professional will come in contact with, either in an institution, in the community, or in the family setting. The majority of aged persons are physically and mentally competent, are goal directed, are secure, and have satisfying personal and interpersonal relationships. Unfortunately, this is not the group that the health professional sees most frequently, and the nurse practitioner is the person most likely to have the responsibility for planning and implementing the care for the aged individuals who have physical and mental health impairments. In order to provide more individualized care, Gordon (1982) suggests the use of functional health patterns in making the assessment and in determining the signs and symptoms of dysfunctional patterns. Gordon further suggests that this typology of functional health patterns contains a set of health-related areas quite familiar to nurses. These following eleven items serve as a guide for assessment and lead nurses to a nursing diagnosis (Gordon, 1982):

1. *Health-perception–health-management pattern:* Describes client's perceived pattern of health and well-being and how health is managed
2. *Nutritional–metabolic pattern:* Describes pattern of food and fluid consumption relative to metabolic need and pattern indicators of local nutrient supply
3. *Elimination pattern:* Describes patterns of excretory function (bowel, bladder, and skin)
4. *Activity–exercise pattern:* Describes pattern of exercise, activity, leisure, and recreation
5. *Cognitive–perceptual pattern:* Describes sensory–perceptual and cognitive pattern
6. *Sleep–rest pattern:* Describes patterns of sleep, rest, and relaxation
7. *Self-perception–self-concept pattern:* Describes self-concept pattern and perceptions of self (e.g., body comfort, body image, feeling state)
8. *Role–relationship pattern:* Describes pattern of role-engagements and relationships
9. *Sexuality–reproductive pattern:* Describes clients' patterns of satisfaction and dissatisfaction with sexuality pattern; describes reproductive patterns
10. *Coping–stress–tolerance pattern:* Describes general coping pattern and effective-

ness of the pattern in terms of stress tolerance

11. *Value–belief pattern:* Describes patterns of values, beliefs (including spiritual), or goals that guide choices or decisions

The nursing diagnoses should be stated to include outcome, predictions, and nursing interventions. The evaluation should include the outcome in the process.

When first seen by the health care professional, the aged person often presents multiple health problems. The assessment should include a review of the body systems and a psychosocial evaluation including the appraisal of cognitive, affective, and psychomotor functioning. A family history should be included to provide clues regarding family relationships and communication patterns. Information about the use of leisure time and frequency of social contact needs to be elicited, including church affiliation and religious practices.

The place of residence is often an important assessment factor because neighborhoods change. If a person has lived in a house for 35 years or more, chances are, if it is a single-family residential area, the majority of the neighbors are elderly or the residences may have changed from single ownership occupancy to rental property. When this occurs, the property is usually occupied by transient renters. Deterioration of the neighborhood may occur and be followed by poverty and crime. The aged person is in a very vulnerable position. By understanding their fears, frustrations, and stresses, the health care professional can help further the quality of the aged person's life (Carp, 1975).

Case Presentation

Mrs. Massey was a 75-year-old woman who lived alone. She was brought to the hospital by ambulance. A neighbor saw Mrs. Massey fall as she went out her back door and, as she tried to get up, fell again. Mrs. Thomas, the neighbor, had just moved into the house next door and did not know Mrs. Massey's name. When she got to Mrs. Massey, she saw that her leg was in a funny position and that she couldn't get up. Mrs. Thomas called for the ambulance.

Mrs. Massey was still in her nightgown and robe when she arrived in the emergency room. She was not wearing glasses, and a partial plate was missing. She was extremely upset and kept saying, "Please find Cleo" or "I couldn't find Cleo." The more the staff questioned her, the more upset she became. Mrs. Massey's concern for Cleo made it impossible to obtain needed information. Her physical condition required treatment. They were told by the ambulance driver that Mrs. Thomas, the neighbor, was trying to locate someone who knew something about Mrs. Massey and that she would call the emergency room.

The preceding example is not an unusual occurrence in a large city emergency room. Knowledge about the person was needed in order to initiate the treatment process. Each system of health care providers has a specificity that often borders on depersonalizing the individual, and it requires that identifying cards and numbers be provided. Without them, an individual loses his or her identity. When this is compounded with a communication problem, an individual can be lost in the system. The professional nurse is the major link between the person requiring health care and the other health care providers. The level of care the nurse provides is based on health-related information; using several concepts from this chapter, such as confusion, sensory deprivation, loss/separation, and anxiety, tentative inferences can be made. The physical injury is beyond the scope of this chapter, but it has the need for immediate care. The nursing assessment should consider the physical and emotional behaviors of the client in planning care.

Older persons when aroused and exposed to a different environment may, because of diminished sensory activity and decreased speed in integrating information, demonstrate a defective orientation to time and space. This state of confusion results in incoherent statements, motor agitation, anguish, and fear. Sensory deprivation may appear when the individual is separated from familiar objects or surroundings, and this is further compounded if the structural components of the sensory organs receive little information.

This can be precipitated by loss/separation, anxiety, or injury. In this situation, the elderly individual may have decreased ability to organize information.

Mrs. Massey presents evidence that she has an emergency situation; certain problems need to be resolved, with the assessment occurring simultaneously with the treatment plan. The clinical cues are relevant: (1) Mrs. Massey is obviously upset and agitated, and (2) she has a physical dysfunction. The cues may be clustered using Gordon's typology. It is noted that the patterns of cognitive–perceptual and coping–stress-tolerance are present. Consideration should also be given to determine the degree of threat that is being internalized by Mrs. Massey (Gordon, 1982).

Using the nursing diagnoses, the following may be identified: (1) alteration in comfort, (2) impaired communication, (3) ineffective coping, (4) potential for trauma, (5) knowledge deficit, (6) impaired mobility, (7) disturbance in body image, (8) alteration of auditory perception, and (9) moderate anxiety (Kim & Moritz, 1982). Even though these may be tentative, the nurse needs to consider the desired outcomes, the plan of care to reach the outcomes, and the implementation of nursing care and evaluation (Gordon, 1982).

Mrs. Thomas learned, after knocking on several doors, that Mrs. Massey attended the First Methodist Church, and the ensuing events took place:

1. Reverend Smith went to Mrs. Massey's house, picked up her very large black bag, locked up the house and told Mrs. Thomas that he would be back to pick up Cleo, Mrs. Massey's cat, who was now safely in the house
2. The minister and his wife went to the hospital and found Mrs. Massey in the emergency department
3. He gave Mrs. Massey her black bag, and she proceeded to take out her hearing aids, glasses, and partial dental plate
4. Mrs. Massey also appeared relieved to see Reverend and Mrs. Smith
5. The emergency department staff was able to collect the required information from Mrs. Massey
6. The minister assured Mrs. Massey that the cat would be taken to the veterinarian
7. Mrs. Smith continued to stay with Mrs. Massey

Several areas need further explanation. Reverend Smith said that the black bag held a duplicate of every important paper owned by Mrs. Massey. Additionally, he had copies. The bag was also used to store Mrs. Massey's partial plate, eyeglasses, and hearing aids at night. When Mr. Massey died, she had the responsibility of settling his estate. He had not kept her informed about his business, income, or debts, and she had to find out this information from a number of sources. This was time-consuming as well as frightening for someone who had never had any financial responsibility during their 60 years of marriage. She kept the bag near her at all times. Even the placement of her glasses, hearing aids, and teeth were significant actions. It represented the need to control her environment in order to feel safe. Cleo, the cat, was symbolic of a loved one, and leaving her was a loss/separation from a significant other.

Not all aged persons are as well organized as Mrs. Massey. The health care professional should encourage the aged to interact more openly with someone who can help them in their estate planning. Although many will see this as a means to say "you want me to die," others will understand the importance of lessening the burden for others regardless of the income.

One week later, there were several changes in Mrs. Massey's appearance. Her hair remained uncombed, she had on one hearing aid, and her teeth were in a denture cup on the bedside table. She had not touched her breakfast. Physically, Mrs. Massey was progressing, her hip pinning was successful, and all physical signs were within normal limits. When asked if she wanted to comb her hair and complete her morning hygiene, her response was, "I don't think I'm going to live; I have no one to look after Cleo and me,'' and she turned her head away from the nurse. Mrs. Massey was experiencing feelings of worthlessness that were caused by her feelings of helplessness and loss of self-esteem. Illness often precipitates those feelings, and it is accentuated when there is little emotional support (Pfeiffer, 1980). Depression often follows loss, and suicide is not uncommon. The feelings of worthlessness use energies that might be channeled in other directions. The aged need to be in an environment where dignity and self-respect are preserved.

There are a number of universal guidelines/principles that can be used in planning and nursing care. The most important principle is to foster the individual's own potential. If the person values independence, encourage independence; if the person values religion, the plan of care should be to encourage participation at religious services. The nurse practitioner should also consider the vocational interests or the leisure time interests in planning care.

An example of fostering an older person's potential was that of an 85-year-old school teacher whom we will call Miss Murphy. Miss Murphy decided that she would move into a nursing home after experiencing several blackout spells. Miss Murphy was viewed as a difficult client because she complained about everything. She saw the elderly as being complacent about their care, and every day she had a list of complaints that she took to the management. An astute nurse recognized that Miss Murphy needed something to do with her time and suggested to the speech therapist that Miss Murphy, because of her background in special education and teaching reading skills, might help her with the rehabilitation program in progress for the stroke clients. Miss Murphy was elated, and she remained busy most of the day. She also enlisted a male resident, Mr. Caldwell, who was a retired speech teacher, to help in the program. She noted that the male clients responded more readily to her and suggested that Mr. Caldwell help with the women. The speech therapist enjoyed working with her co-therapists, as she called

them. Miss Murphy stopped complaining and stated, ''I feel like I'm doing something that is badly needed.'' Linn and Gurel (1969) noted an increased mortality during the first 3 months following the move to a nursing home.

Elderly persons often experience grief, and they need help and encouragement in discussing their loss, pain, guilt, and anger. The nurse practitioner can help the individual to remember the loved one and remain nonjudgmental when anger, hostility, and blame surface. Mrs. Massey may not have had the time to complete the grief process following the death of her husband, or she may have been using denial; however, when the physical injury occurred, she became more reaction-sensitive to past losses. Grief may be delayed, and Mrs. Massey needed help in expressing her feelings of abandonment and anger.

Institutionalization, whether in a hospital or nursing home, can precipitate emotional changes, and individuals may need help in focusing on their physical location. Environmental deprivation or sensory overload may produce disorientation and hallucinations. Staff should promote reality orientation. Increased efforts should be made to involve persons in activities that have meaning for the individual. For example, consider an instance where all the clients had to make potholders. Not everyone wanted to participate in this activity and for many persons it became busy work; for some individuals it had meaning and purpose, however, and for them it was an acceptable pastime. The potholder can serve as a gift or be sold.

Dress, makeup, and activities of daily living are necessary accessories to further self-image. Clothing, shoes, and the opportunity to view oneself for critical appraisal can enhance the process. Health care personnel need to encourage cleanliness, neatness, and appropriateness in dress. Kind evaluation and helpful hints can provide the elderly with the sense that they ''look good.'' Successful adaptation leads to an increase in self-confidence and mental well-being (Byrne & Thompson, 1973).

Older people have their individual differences, too, and the life experiences, intelligence, interests, or background are much the same as in the general population. In order for society to change, more significance needs to be placed on the positive aspects and the value of the aged person's contribution to society. Lessons from other cultures, in which the elderly are venerated, may not exist in our society, but the health care professional has the responsibility to see that the aged receive care in a noncritical atmosphere in which the needs are identified. Creative planning may include anticipatory nursing intervention; it may also include changing the system in which one finds the elderly, such as encouraging the use of pets (Francis, 1981) or an advocacy program where the aged and youth participate (Strumpf & Mezey, 1980) in concrete activities such as gardening or cooking. Families will often share in their parents' accomplishments; and, regardless of any diminished increments in the physical or emotional state, positive reinforcement is more apt to bring desired results. Staff and families need to be realistic and not impose their values on the aged individual, but encourage the health role.

SUMMARY

Growing old is inevitable, and the health care professional can assist the aged person to grow old within his or her capabilities. The goal is to provide care, concern, and understanding toward the elderly by improving the knowledge components of care. The health care professional must be able to plan and provide care, act as an advocate, and provide a positive environment for the elderly. By identifying and being knowledgeable about the variations in the mental health of the aged, such as sensory deprivation, body image/self-esteem, space/territoriality, and loss/separation, the nurse can develop a plan of care that allows for these variations. This plan needs to be realistic and not value laden.

Positive feelings of joy, happiness, and accomplishment require less expenditure of energy than do feelings of guilt, frustration, and anger. By accentuating the successes, the health care professional is more likely to be able to assist the aged to maintain healthy mental attitudes.

REFERENCES

Aguilera, D. C. (1980). Stressors in late adulthood. *Family and Community Health, 2*(4), 61–69.

Allekian, C. I. (1973). Intrusions of territory and personal space, *Nursing Research, 22*(3), 236–241.

Allen, M. D. (1980). Drug therapy in the elderly. *American Journal of Nursing, 80*(8), 1474–1475.

American Psychiatric Association. (1987). *Diagnostic and statistical manual of mental disorders* Washington, DC: Author.

Benson, M. (1977). The elderly and drugs—Problem overview and program strategy. *Public Health Reports, 92*, 43–48.

Blackwell, B. (1972). The drug defaulter. *Clinical Pharmacology and Therapeutics, 13*, 841–847.

Blazer, D. (1982). *Depression in late life.* St. Louis: Mosby.

Brock, A. M., & Madison, A. S. (1977). The challenge in gerontological nursing. *Nursing Forum, 16*(1), 95–108.

Burnside, I. M. (1973). *Psychosocial nursing care of the aged.* New York: McGraw-Hill.

Busse, E. W., & Pfeiffer, E. (Eds.). (1969). *Behavior and adaptation in late life.* Boston: Little, Brown.

Butler, R. N. (Ed.). (1978). Overview on aging. *Aging: The process and the people.* New York: Brunner/Mazel.

Butler, R. N., & Lewis, M. I. (1982). *Aging and mental health* (3rd ed.). St. Louis: Mosby, pp. 74–75.

Byrne, M. L., & Thompson, L. F. (1972). *Key concepts for the study and practice of nursing.* St. Louis: Mosby.

Carp, F. M. (1975). Life style and location within the city. *The Gerontologist, 15*, 27–34.

Chenitz, W. (1979). Primary depression in older women. *Journal of Psychiatric Nursing and Mental Health Services, 17*, 20–23.

Coleman, J. C. (1972). *Abnormal psychology and modern life* (4th ed.). Glenview, IL: Scott, Foresman.

Copel, W. C., Goldsmith, B. M., Waddell, K. J., &

Stewart, G. T. (1972). The agency narcotic addict: An increasing problem for the next decade. *Journal of Gerontology, 27,* 102–106.

Copel, W. C., & Stewart, G. T. (1971). The management of drug abuse in agency populations: New Orleans findings. *Journal of Drug Issues, 1,* 114–121.

Durkheim, E. (1951). *Suicide.* New York: The Free Press.

Eddy, D. N. (1986). Before and after attitudes toward aging in a BSN program. *Journal of Gerontological Nursing, 12*(5), 30–34.

Edney, J. J. (1974). Human territoriality. *Psychological Bulletin, 81,* 959–975.

Ellor, J. R., & Kurz, D. J. (1982). Misuse and abuse of prescription and non-prescription drugs by the elderly. *Nursing Clinics of North America, 17,* 319–329.

Epstein, C. (1977). *Learning to care for the aged.* Reston, VA: Reston Publishing, pp. 43–67.

Eyde, D. R., & Rich, J. A. (1983). *Psychological distress in aging.* Rockville, MD: Aspen Systems Corporation.

Falk, M. A. (1971). Psychosocial aspects of aging. *Illinois Medical Journal, 140,* 447–479.

Forni, P. J. (1978). Alcohol and the elderly. In R. C. Kayane (Ed.), *Drugs and the elderly.* Los Angeles: University of Southern California, Ethel Percy Andrus Gerontology Center, pp. 75–82.

Francis, G. (1981). The therapeutic use of pets. *Nursing Outlook, 29*(6), 369–370.

Freedman, A. M., Kaplan, H. I., & Sadock, B. J. (Eds.). (1976). *Modern synopsis of comprehensive textbook of psychiatry II* (2nd ed.). Baltimore: Williams & Wilkins.

Freedman, J. (1976). Under the surface of American's nursing home scandal. *Journal of Psychiatric Nursing and Mental Health Services, 14,* 41–42.

Fromm-Reichmann, F. (1950). *Principles of intensive psychotherapy.* Chicago: The University of Chicago Press.

Gallegher, D., & Frankil, A. S. (1980). Depression in (an) older adult(s): A moderate structuralist viewpoint. *Psychotherapy: Theory, Research, and Practice, 17,* 101–104.

Giorella, E. C. (1980). Give the older person space. *American Journal of Nursing, 80*(5), 898–899.

Goodstein, R. K. (1980). The diagnosis and treatment of elderly patients: Some practical guidelines. *Hospital and Community Psychiatry, 31*(1), 19–24.

Gordon, M. (1982). *Nursing diagnosis process and application.* New York: McGraw-Hill.

Gotz, B. & Gotz, V. P. (1978). Drugs and the elderly. *American Journal of Nursing, 78*(8), 1347–1351.

Gramlich, E. P. (1978). Recognition and management of grief in elderly patients. In M. Brown (Ed.), *Readings in gerontology.* St. Louis: Mosby.

Gregg, D. (1952). Anxiety—A factor in nursing care. *American Journal of Nursing, 52*(11), 1363–1365.

Hart, L. K., Freal, M. I., & Crowell, C. M. (1976). Changing attitudes toward the aged and interest in caring for the aged. *Journal of Gerontological Nursing, 2*(4), 10–16.

Havighurst, R. (1973). *Developmental tasks and education.* New York: David McKay.

Hayes, J. E. (1982). Normal changes in aging and nursing implications of drug therapy. *Nursing Clinics of North America, 7,* 253–261.

Hess, B. B., & Markson, E. W. (1980). *Aging and old age: An introduction to social gerontology.* New York: Macmillan.

Hofling, C. K., Leininger, M. M., & Bregg, E. (1967). *Basic psychiatric concepts in nursing.* Philadelphia: Lippincott.

Hollister, L. E., (1977). Prescribing drugs for the elderly. *Geriatrics, 32,* 71–73.

Hunt, P. (1977). The elderly: A challenge to nursing. Confusion in the elderly. *Nursing Times, 73*(49), 1928–1929.

Johnson, F. L. P. (1979). Response to territorial intrusion by nursing home residents. *Advances in Nursing Science, 1,* 21–34.

Kassel, V. (1976). Sexism in nursing homes. *Medical Aspects of Human Sexuality, 10*(3), 126–131.

Kayser, J. S., & Minnegerode, F. A. (1975). Increasing nursing students' interest in working with aged patients. *Nursing Research, 24*(1), 23–26.

Kim, M., & Morita, D. A. (Eds.). (1982). *Classification of Nursing Diagnosis.* New York: McGraw-Hill.

Kola, L. A., & Kosberg, J. I. (1981). Model to assess community services for the elderly alchoholic. *Public Health Reports, 96,* 458–464.

Lee, R. J. (1976). Self-images of the elderly. *Nursing Clinics of North America, 11*(1), 119–124.

Lewis, M. (1981). Personal space boundary needs of elderly persons: An empirical study. *Journal of Gerontological Nursing, 7,* 395–400.

Linn, M., & Gurel, L. (1969). Initial reactions to

nursing home placement. *Journal of the American Geriatrics Society, 17,* 219–222.

Marshall, C., & Wallenstein, E. (1973). Beyond Marcus Welby, Cable TV for the health of the elderly. *Geriatrics, 28,* 182–186.

McNulty, B. (1977). The elderly: A challenge to nursing. *Nursing Times, 73*(50), 1967–1968.

Montgomery, C. (1987). What you can do for the confused elderly. *Nursing 87, 17*(4), 55–56.

Murphy, K. E. (1981). Use of territoriality in psychotherapy. *Journal of Mental Health Services, 19,* 13–15.

Nagley, S. J. (1986). Predicting and preventing confusion in your patients. *Journal of Gerontological Nursing, 12*(3), 27–31.

National Institute of Drug Abuse Services. (1977). *Research report: A study of legal drug use by older Americans.* Washington, DC: United States Department of Health, Education and Welfare Publications.

Palmore, E. (1969). Sociological aspects of aging. In E. W. Busse & E. Pfeiffer (Eds.), *Behavior and adaptation in late life.* Boston: Little, Brown.

Pelizza, J. J. (1979). Suicide in the elderly: Can it be prevented? *Long Term Care and Health Services Administration, 3,* 85–91.

Peterson, D. M., Whittington, F. J., & Payre, B. P. (Eds.). (1979). *Drugs and the elderly: Social and pharmacological issues.* Springfield, IL: Thomas.

Pfeiffer, E. (1980). The psychosocial evaluation of the elderly patient. In E. W. Busse & D. G. Blazer (Eds.), *Handbook of geriatric psychiatry.* New York: Van Nostrand Reinhold.

Poe, W. D., & Halloway, D. A. (1980). *Drugs and the aged.* New York: McGraw-Hill.

Resnik, H. L. P., & Cantor, J. M. (1978). Suicide in aging. In M. Brown (Ed.), *Readings in gerontology.* St. Louis: Mosby.

Rokeach, M. (1968). *Beliefs, attitudes and values: A theory of organization and change.* San Francisco: Josey-Bass.

Schneidman, E. S. (1965). Preventing suicide. reprint from *American Journal of Nursing, 65*(5), 1–5.

Schwab, Sr. M. (1973). Caring for the aged. *American Journal of Nursing, 73*(12), 2049–2053.

Schwartz, A. N. (1975). An observation in self-esteem as the linchpin of quality of life for the aged—An essay. *The Gerontologist, 15,* 470–472.

Simon, A., Epstein, L. J., & Reynolds, L. (1968). Alcoholism in the geriatric mentally ill. *Geriatrics, 23,* 125–131.

Spencer, M. G., & Dore, C. J. (1975). *Understanding aging: A multidisciplinary approach.* New York: Appleton-Century-Crofts.

St. Pierre, J., Craven, M. F., & Bruno, P. (1986). Late life depression: A guide for assessment. *Journal of Gerontological Nursing, 12*(7), 5–10.

Strumpf, N., & Mezey, M. D. (1980). A developmental approach to the teaching of aging. *Nursing Outlook, 28*(12), 730–739.

Tancredi, L. R. (1987). The mental status examination. *Generations, 11*(4), 24–31.

Thomas, E. G. (1979). Application of stress factors in gerontologic nursing. *Nursing Clinics of North America, 14* 607–620.

Thomas, W. C. (1981). The expectation gap and stereotype of the stereotype: Images of old people. *The Gerontologist, 21*(4), 402–407.

Thurmott, P. (1977). The elderly: A challenge in nursing—Isolation and loneliness. *Nursing Times, 73*(48), 1884–1886.

Travelbee, J. (1971). *Interpersonal aspects of nursing.* Philadelphia: Davis.

Verwoerdt, A. (1980). Anxiety, dissociative and personality disorders in the elderly. In E. W. Busse (Ed.), *Handbook of geriatric psychiatry.* New York: Van Nostrand Reinhold.

Weber, H. I. (1980). *Nursing care of the elderly.* Reston, VA: Reston Publishing.

Whitehead, T. (1978). Confusing causes of confusion. *Nursing Mirror, 147*(12), 29–30.

Wilhite, M. J., & Johnson, D. M. (1976). Changes in nursing students' stereotypic attitudes toward old people. *Nursing Research, 25*(6), 432.

Williams, L. M. (1978). A concept of loneliness in the elderly. *Journal of the American Geriatrics Society, 26*(4), 183–187.

Williamson, J. (1980). Paving the way to safe prescribing for the elderly. *Geriatrics, 35*(9), 32–39.

Wilson, H., & Knerse, C. R. (1979). *Psychiatric Nursing.* Menlo Park, CA: Addison-Wesley.

Wilson, J. S. (1987). Unmasking depression. *NursingLife, 7*(6), 58–63.

Zimberg, S. (1979). Alcohol and the elderly. In D. M. Peterson, F. J. Whittington, & B. P. Payne (Eds.), *Drugs and the elderly: Social and pharmacological issues.* Springfield, IL: Thomas.

14

TREATMENT MODALITIES

Considerable concern has been expressed about the lack and underutilization of available mental health services by elderly adults (Birren & Renner, 1979; Gatz, Smyer & Lawton, 1980; Knight, 1978–79; Smyer & Gatz, 1979; Sparacino, 1978–79; Storandt, Siegler, & Elias, 1978). Presumably, those services that did exist were implicitly based on a model that stressed the irreversible decrements of aging, a model that until recently has dominated gerontological research and practice (Birren & Sloane, 1980; Kastenbaum, 1978; Storandt et al., 1978). Moreover, on the basis of evidence reviewed by Garfield (1978) and by Smith and Glass (1977) age per se does not emerge as a predictor of psychotherapeutic success. Although Luborsky, Chandler, Auerbach, Cohen, and Bachrach (1971, p. 151), for example, conclude that "older patients tend to have a slightly poorer prognosis," the studies reviewed did not imply that the samples were older patients and many lacked controls against which to assess the effects of therapy.

Why is there such a dearth of interest in the treatment of elderly adults? In part it is due to the feelings and attitudes of therapists regarding a variety of issues perceived to be relevant in treating the aged patient, again based on a lack of professional experience with elders and personal contact with aged persons (e.g., death, parental conflicts, fears of aging). A number of persons [notably Butler (1963) and Butler & Lewis (1981)] have discussed the professional "ageism" that pervades treatment of the aged in this regard, often resulting in the absence of care, or at best poor quality of care. Another factor behind the substandard care elderly patients sometimes receive is manifest in "countertransference" (Blum & Tallmer, 1977). As Hayslip and Kooken (1982, p. 183) note, this attitude "prevents many counselors from seeing their clients as real people—in terms other than those of physical decline, pain, disengagement from others, lessened intelligence, and rigidity." As Davis and Kopfer (1977) and Ford and Sbordone (1980) have noted, this negative attitude definitely interferes with treatment, unnecessarily complicates diagnosis, and generally disrupts both the lives of the older person and the therapist. Such biases are more likely if the therapist is younger, or has had limited contact with a wide range of elderly persons.

Another factor responsible for the lack of knowledge in this area is the attitude of potential clients toward receiving professional help. Suspicion, distrust, and ignorance are all factors that lead many to try to help themselves (Butler, Gertman, Overlander, & Shindler, 1979–80) rather than turn to others for such assistance.

Although there is some debate (see Lawton, 1978; Lawton & Gottesman, 1974; Smyer & Gatz, 1979) regarding both how to structure such training and utilize current personnel, it seems clear that future elderly (whose demand for therapeutic services seems likely to exceed the demand of the current elderly) will require services that are accessible and staffed by individuals with training in several areas, in order to maximize both the quantity *and* quality of professional therapeutic services to the elderly. Paying for emotional care (e.g., outpatient services) remains a problem for many whose insurance plans do not cover such treatment.

On the basis of the above work, indications are that according to current surveys, "between 6 percent and 16 percent of elderly asked indicated a need for counseling services, but that substantial differences are found in what service providers are offering versus what older adults themselves want" (Hayslip & Kooken, 1982, p. 285). Sensitivity to individual differences as well as "a recognition of the fact that mental health/mental illness is best conceived and treated when the interplay between physical health, stresses/supports in the environment, and the life experiences of the elderly person is emphasized, will heighten both today's aged and future cohorts' awareness and use of mental health services" (Hayslip & Kooken 1982, p. 285).

Rather than define treatment narrowly, the present review suggests that it may take on a variety of forms, each with its own goals. Such a view has been expressed by Levy, Derogatis, and Gatz (1980), who alternatively see therapy (or more properly, intervention) as focusing on the person *and* the environment, to facilitate a match between the two. A similar "model" has been advanced by Gottesman, Quarterman, and Cohn (1973) and is discussed more specifically below.

Treatment Modalities for the Aged

In addition to the above generic concerns regarding treatment of the aged, serious consideration must obviously be given to the therapeutic options open to the aged person in distress. Unfortunately, given that the area of gerontology is relatively new, interest in discussion of specific treatment modalities with the aged person has, in most cases, preceded an evaluation of the effec-

tiveness. Consequently, in the discussion to follow, the reader must be exceedingly *cautious* regarding the use of a particular mode of treatment. Regardless of how popular a given technique is, its effectiveness must be first defined in terms of the goals one has in mind, as well as in terms of the desires/needs of the elderly client.

At the present time, a number of approaches to treatment exist for the elderly person in need of help (both in the community and within the institutional setting). Although a specific model for the choice of treatment has been proposed by Gottesman, Quarterman, and Cohn (1973) (in spite of the fact that there are no established criteria allowing one to match therapies and disorders), these authors state that the factors governing one's choice of treatment should *always* involve (1) the *capacities* (physical, emotional, cognitive) of the elderly individual; (2) the *societal demands* regarding "appropriate" behavior for the aged; (3) the *expectations* of *significant others;* and (4) the expectations that the elderly person has for himself or herself. If, for example, as discussed by Gottesman and colleagues, an aged person wants to drive the car, but is not physically able (e.g., has had a stroke), the helper would encourage the individual to be more aware of physical limitations or would recommend that other arrangements be made (e.g., ask a friend or a family member for a ride, or take a bus). Alternatively, the source of the problem might be societal (age limitations on driver's permits) or rest with family members (they may demand that an older member continue to be independent because the respective member was always independent). Intervention might in these cases be directed at changing laws allowing older persons to drive or focus on altering the family's expectations of an older member.

Alternatively, Gotestam (1980) suggests that the primary concern should be with improving the *quality* and not necessarily only the quantity of life. More specific goals of therapy noted by Gotestam include (1) insight into one's behavior, (2) symptom relief, (3) relief to relatives, (4) delayed deterioration, (5) adaptation to a present situation, (6) improvement in self-care skills, (7) heightened activity, and (8) greater independence. Each goal is more or less important depending upon a number of factors, e.g., health or degree of support available to the client. Thus, "whether to opt for a long-term or a short-term approach, or whether outpatient (community-based) or institutional care is desired are *individual* decisions. Some types of therapy (individual, group, family) work better for some individuals (and for some therapists as well!) than for others. Some are more acceptable to older persons than others; some (individual therapy) are typically more costly than others (group therapy)" (Hayslip & Kooken, 1982, p. 289). Thus, there is *no single best* approach to/technique with older persons that will succeed in all situations or for all types of clients. In fact, it is likely (Eisdorfer and Stotsky, 1977) that a reliance on a single approach, to the exclusion of all others, virtually guarantees a less than mutually satisfying helping experience for both the counselor and the client.

As Hayslip and Kooken (1982) have noted, there are a large variety of forms of psychotherapy, and thus this review is by no means intended to be exhaustive. At the very least, one should keep in mind that the number of experimental investigations that have been done with elderly clients is small compared to those studies done with other age groups. Thus, in some cases, it is impossible to say with any certainty how effective a particular approach will be. In this light, discussions of some treatment approaches must be seen as descriptively valuable, in that they are, as yet, untested or rest upon a very thin knowledge base.

LIFE REVIEW THERAPY

One of the more popular approaches to the treatment of the aged person involves the use of the life review (Butler, 1963, Butler & Lewis, 1981). As Butler and Lewis (1981) point out, life review therapy is more extensive than a simple recall of the past, although reminiscence is a central component in this approach. They also point out that obtaining an extensive autobiography from elderly persons is important (relying on a variety of sources, e.g., family albums, genealogies), permitting them to put their life in order. Thus, conflicts of an intrapsychic nature, family relationships, decisions about success and failure, resolution of guilt, and a clarification of the elderly person's own values are potential benefits to be gained through the life review, which may be conducted individually, or in a group setting. However, the life review can be a frustrating, painful experience for many aged, who may require emotional support from a counselor for an extended period of time in order to deal with the by-products of this process (e.g., despair, guilt, hostility). Sherwood and Mor (1980, p. 867) indicate that reminiscence (life review) therapy is best utilized within a supportive setting to re-establish the elderly person's identity "in order to recover from a state of dissonance brought on by the realization that advanced age made it impossible to live up to past expectations of self." Sherwood and Mor (1980) note that reminiscence may not be appropriate for those elderly with a history of "social and psychological dysfunction." It may also be of limited use for those aged with few interpersonal resources (e.g., children, spouse, friends, grandchildren) or for those whose need to deny painful experiences (and for whom denial is a lifelong approach to one's problems) is greater than the benefits of a life review process (Peterson, 1980). One should also realize that reminiscing about one's past may occur at *many* points during the life cycle, and thus a life review process (as a preparation for death) is not characteristic of older persons in general (Hayslip & Martin, 1985).

OTHER MISCELLANEOUS APPROACHES

In addition to life review therapy, a number of rather esoteric approaches to treatment of the aged exist, including music therapy, remotivation, reality orientation, occupational therapy, exercise (dance) therapy, art therapy, and dramatics/role playing.

Music therapy relies upon playing instruments, singing, or listening to recordings to facilitate movement, enhance activity level, and increase one's sense of satisfaction and involvement with life. As noted by Hartford (1980), the few studies evaluating music therapy suggest that it does accomplish these goals. It is more properly thought of as a "technique," or an adjunct, in that it may be used within the context of a group situation, or life review therapy. Much the same can be said of art therapy, occupational therapy, exercise (dance therapy), and dramatics. To the extent that one is involved in art (either creatively or art as appreciation), participates in the writing, direction, or role playing of theatre/plays, or the joining of an aerobics group, interpretive dance, or a craft/skills group has many potential benefits. In addition to building self-confidence and a satisfaction with one's capabilities, these techniques allow one to build interpersonal skills, thereby lessening isolation. Most importantly, these treatment modalities, because they stress an involvement in something (an activity or interest) or someone, lessen the person's own rumination over past or present losses or unresolved conflicts. These activities keep one occupied physically as well as mentally, further reducing the possibility that one will devote time to persevering activities (e.g., mulling over the past) of a self-defeating nature.

REALITY ORIENTATION

Reality orientation (RO) stresses the reduction of confusion/disorientation (primarily within the institution), and may be highly structured, stressing orientation to time, place, and person, or be of an intensive 24-hour variety. The fact that it involves an environmental change (involving staff and family) makes it similar to milieu treatment (Folsom, 1968). Studies dealing with RO tend to be primarily descriptive, with generalized improvement or discharge from the

institution being the goals of choice (Sherwood & Mor, 1980); this research is methodologically flawed in many respects (e.g., not controlling for staff expectancy of improvement). Research by Zeplin, Wolfe, and Kleinplatz (1981) suggests that RO is effective in reducing disorientation (relative to controls), but that this effectiveness is limited to those elderly who are not severely disoriented or who are younger. The authors conclude that "The limited effectiveness of RO notwithstanding, it is useful as a vehicle to organize attention to the disoriented, thereby guarding against unjustified custodial policies" (Zeplin et al., 1981, p. 77). Zeplin and colleagues (1981) and Storandt (1978) both point out that adherence to a rigid treatment regimen often limits the effectiveness of RO. Given that it can be employed by nonprofessional staff (nursing aides), its use should be flexible, and possibly limited to those aged who are not profoundly deteriorated (Storandt, 1978). On the other hand, Storandt notes that the less disoriented patient may become hostile if exposed to RO indiscriminantly, requiring additional staff time and effort to deal with this anger.

As Hayslip and Kooken (1982, p. 295) note, "such participation may well prevent withdrawal and social isolation, as well as preventing cognitive deficits that may result from a lack of stimulation. The important principle to keep in mind is that of exposure to a demand for processing and retrieving information, or in simplistic terms, thought practice. Thinking skills cannot go unused for long periods of time without some deterioration taking place, whether such losses are experiential or organic in nature. Keeping the mind of the elderly person active is a prime objective of the therapist, and unlike psychotherapy with other age groups, may require daily or twice-daily sessions, if no other source of stimulation for the client exists or can be cultivated."

REMOTIVATION

Remotivation, which can also be employed by nursing aides, assumes that the "healthy" portions of the person's personality can be activated (Storandt, 1978). Acceptance by the therapist and other (structured) group members, "bridging" the client with reality, reinforcement of group interactions, and a "rediscovery" of previous satisfying activities are the central components of remotivation therapy. Increased social competence, self-care skills, and activity levels are the goals of this approach. Reviews of this technique (Storandt, 1978; Gotestam, 1980; Sherwood & Mor, 1980) offer a good deal of evidence that various forms of remotivation are successful in meeting the above goals for the institutionalized aged (it is to be noted that remotivation has been used with community living elderly as well), although (as with other therapies) there is some indication that the efficacy of this approach varies with patient status (favoring the more severely deteriorated). Storandt (1978, p. 286) feels that it "should not be seen as a panacea and deserves more detailed research in order to determine what aspects of the procedure lead to the greatest benefits for which types of patients and which components may be unnecessary or detrimental." It was also noted that remotivation may have its greatest impact initially, when interest in, and enthusiasm for, remotivation groups is highest in the staff and patients.

MILIEU THERAPY/
ENVIRONMENTAL MANIPULATION

Closely aligned with remotivation therapy is what has been termed "milieu therapy." Milieu therapy involves the creation of a *therapeutic community,* where all phases of the elderly patient's interactions with the staff are redesigned to benefit the patient and where increased social skills, greater responsibility for one's own actions, deeper involvement in structured activities, and increased self-esteem are the therapeutic goals. Milieu therapy also relies on peer pressure to achieve such goals. Sherwood and Mor (1980) feel that milieu therapy, whose descriptions vary from one "environment" to

the other and that is often used in combination with other (e.g., behavioral, group) methods, makes three assumptions: (1) that patient care shall be humane and noncustodial, (2) that its use will enhance ward management, and (3) that it will rely upon the immediate interpersonal resources of the environment in which it is utilized. Storandt's review also indicates that milieu therapy may work best with the older patient who is emotionally (psychotic) symptomatic but whose cognitive skills are still intact. Thus, the hostile, acting-out elderly patient who is very difficult to manage may not be a candidate for milieu therapy. Storandt (1978) notes that, although this approach has several potential drawbacks (e.g., minimal responsiblity being placed on patients per se for change, patient–staff discrepancies in goals), it may nevertheless benefit those elderly who have become very apathetic and unresponsive as a consequence of institutionalization. In addition to the above approaches, a number of what may be termed "environmental manipulations" may be appropriate and helpful in some situations. As Fozard and Popkin (1978) point out, simply clarifying or highlighting (making more discriminative) aspects of the environment may lessen anxiety, disorientation, and confusion in the elderly person. Such changes are numerous—speaking louder and more distinctly, lowering the tone but raising the volume of sounds (telephone, door bells), enhancing visual cues via color coding, avoiding glare by the use of flat paints and adequate, controllable ambient lighting, the design of "private" areas, encouraging the use of concrete (versus abstract) signs/symbols while enhancing memory function (Fozard & Popkin, 1978; Fozard, 1980; Kahn & Miller, 1978; Treat, Poon, Fozard, & Popkin, 1978) are only a few of the ways in which environmental demands/requirements might be eased to permit greater functioning in the aged. Additionally, Rodin and Langer (1977) and Langer and Rodin (1976) have noted the positive benefits in terms of improved physical health, morale, and enhanced self-esteem when older persons are given control over certain aspects of their everyday environment (e.g., visiting hours, being able to have plants in one's room, being able to choose from a variety of foods for one's dinner). Although these approaches would certainly not seem to be ''therapy'' in a traditional sense, they do possess a great deal of promise in this regard as ''environmental'' approaches to treatment. Gotestam (1980) refers to such approaches as ''prosthetic'' in that they compensate for the deficits an older person may have (e.g., self-care, locomotive, social). Further evidence of the efficacy of ''supportive'' environmental therapy with the aged involves increasing cues and rewards (prizes, snacks, money) for activity, increasing the availability of certain types of equipment (games, puzzles) or recreational activities, and permitting alterations in mealtimes and furniture arrangements (Gotestam, 1980). Target behaviors affected by these means are self-care skills, overall activity level, involvement in specific (e.g., recreational) activities, and social interaction (communication) with others.

Perhaps the most widespread approaches to treatment with the aged involve individual psychotherapy, group/family therapy, behavioral therapy, and psychopharmacological treatment. These therapeutic options should also be considered when determining an approach for treatment.

PSYCHOANALYSIS

Perhaps the best known and most misunderstood form of individual psychotherapeutic intervention is Freud's (1924) psychoanalysis. It is based on the assumption that, through insight (aided by the guidance of a therapist), one may come to grips with troublesome emotions that have been repressed via unconscious defense mechanisms. Although such defenses ordinarily operate very efficiently, a departure from this operation leads to the expression of anxiety, a sign that the control exercised by the ego (being reality-oriented) over the id (composed of instincts, wishes,

drives) and/or the superego (referring to one's morals, ideals) is weakening. Through free association, such conflicts between the ego, id, and superego, normally unconscious, are made conscious, and their meaning interpreted to the client by the therapist. Unfortunately, Freud saw very few older clients and himself was skeptical about his techniques' success with elderly persons, under the assumption that the effort required to change a personality whose defenses had been overused for years was not worth the limited time left to the elderly. Thus, because they were older, he assumed that, for them, change/growth was difficult if not impossible. Gotestam (1980) notes that other Freudian therapists, e.g., Abraham (1949) and Goldfarb (1953), were instrumental in pioneering changes in psychoanalytic therapy with the aged (e.g., regarding therapist supportiveness, the creative/therapeutic use of defenses, making use of the aged person's dependency needs, and permitting and utilizing transference to the therapist, who is perceived as a child substitute). There are, however, few reports dealing with insight-oriented, psycholanalytic treatment with the aged. Most are poorly designed and rely only on clinical judgment, making it difficult to reach conclusions regarding treatment efficacy. Gotestam (1980, p. 788) states that ''it is also important to consider the effects of transference and countertransference, which may play a more important role in therapy with older people than in more traditional therapy.'' Based on what is known at present, however, it is unfair to conclude that older clients are not capable of achieving insight.

GROUP THERAPY

Group therapy is a widespread alternative treatment for the aged, and is used quite often in both community and institutional settings. As noted by Hayslip and Kooken (1982, p. 295), ''the distinguishing feature of group therapy with the aged is that dependency needs can be used to their best advantage. This approach can take many forms, ranging from issue-oriented discussion groups, to groups designed to stimulate verbalization/interaction among group members, to groups specifically geared to promoting independence and a positive sense of self. They permit one to set realistic goals, while focusing on each client's strengths, thereby building group cohesiveness.'' Groups are typically short-term (when used within the institution) and informal in nature. Group therapy is often used in a variety of settings by those offering art therapy, dance therapy, or music therapy for elderly persons (see above).

Gotestam (1980) reviews the limited literature on group therapy with the aged and concludes that, despite its popularity in a variety of settings with the aged, its utility is largely undocumented. He attributes a great deal of the improvements in symptomatology to the attention given to the aged group members by the group leader.

Hartford (1980) comments on the variety of settings (largely linked to services offered to the elderly) within which group methods have been used with the aged over the past three decades: nursing homes, hospitals, private homes, day-care centers, retirement communities, senior centers. She notes many goals that might be effected through the use of group methods:

1. Individual growth/rehabilitation
2. Improved interpersonal relationships
3. Enhanced problem-solving/task achievement
4. Changes in the immediate surroundings
5. Changes in a social system/institution
6. Changes in attitudes and values of group members
7. Changes in society at large, regarding attitudes/treatment of the aged

She also notes, however, that group work (as is true of any treatment modality) can have negative, as well as positive, consequences, e.g., individual devaluation of self, socialization toward institutionalization, and increased loneliness or self-destructiveness. Although Hartford's treatment is largely descriptive and historical, she cites a great deal of observational evidence supporting the use of a variety of types of group therapy with the aged, e.g., the use of groups institutionally to lessen anxiety, isolation, and withdrawal and to enhance responsibility for self. Moreover, group work with community aged has been employed to deal with role loss/change (retirement, widowhood). Hartford (1980, p. 813) states that groups have many uses with the aged, e.g., ''for staying connected with the real world and with other people, for reconnecting after disengagement due to physical or emotional problems, for personal growth and enhancement, for new learning and survival, and for enrichment.'' In this light, reality orientation, remotivation, life review, art therapy, occupational therapy, dance therapy, and music therapy could be considered as specific instances of group treatment. In the role as group leader, the helper may facilitate discussion, provide structure, define goals, clarify what is being said, or simply be passively supportive. As Hartford (1980) notes, group therapy requires considerable expertise and may be used preventatively or in an ameliorative sense. Sadly, however, the use of group therapy with the aged has been relatively uncritical. The ''apparent lack of definitive research on group uses with the elderly, studies of groups where the elderly are subjects, textbooks in the methodology of group work practice with older adults, or example of work with the elderly in textbooks on group methods highlights the gap (between research and practice) that exists'' (Hartford, 1980, p. 822). A similar state of affairs exists regarding family therapy with the aged.

FAMILY THERAPY

Family therapy is another option available to the therapist who deals with older persons who are experiencing problems in communication (Butler & Lewis, 1981; Hayslip & Kooken, 1982; Peterson, 1973). As Hayslip and Kooken note (1982, p. 296) "changes in roles such as retirement or grandparenthood, problems accompanying chronic/acute illness, institutionalization of one's parent(s) or spouse, or conflicts arising when an older parent is being cared for at home by a middle aged child can be approached by bringing together all parties involved to set up clear expectations for behavior, improve communication, lessen distrust and guilt, or deal with hostility and anxiety."

Family therapy is also quite appropriate in dealing with parent–child conflicts centering around remarriage, struggles for power within the home, or restrictions on the aged person brought about by ill health, or by the divorce of an adult child. Family therapy allows each individual to express personal feelings, explore options, and increase sensitivity to another's point of view.

As Hartford (1980) notes, traditional family therapists have largely ignored the three-, four-, and five-generation families, although a great deal of information is available on family dynamics and mutual helping patterns in old age (see Sussman, 1976; Troll, Miller, & Atchley, 1979). Grauer, Betts, and Birnbom (1973) have successfully utilized family intervention to reunite a family who had placed a hostile elderly member in a day-care center. Dye and Erber (1981) report that the individual (residents only), group counseling, and resident-family group counseling were superior to a no-treatment control in facilitating the transition to a nursing home. In this case, a sharing of feelings and perceptions and focused problem solving characterized both treatment groups, who demonstrated lower self-reported anxiety and a greater feeling of internal control than did controls. Although such effects were evident immediately following the test, they did not carry over 6 months later.

Perhaps the most extensive discussion of family intervention has been provided by Herr and Weakland (1979), who have applied family

systems theory to work with the elderly. "Systems theory" in this sense treats the family as a system, the components of which are interconnected and mutually interactive. This approach then stresses the here-and-now nature of the interaction (handling of a problem versus the problem per se) involving family members. These authors see several primary problematic interactions involving elder family members: (1) scapegoating of the older person; (2) parent–child role reversal, where the adult child acts responsible for the older parent; (3) dyadic alliances, where pairs of family members (e.g. mother–daughter versus father) "team up" against one another; (4) symbiotic relationships, where the older parents cannot "let go" of their adult children (or vice versa); (5) incongruencies between what the older person expects and what the adult children expect from the parent; (6) role inversion, where, for example, due to the husband's illness, the wife assumes the husband's former duties; and (7) fearful withdrawal of the older person from those younger. Such communication difficulties may be elicited by age-graded events as illness, death, retirement, or institutionalization, or they may be of a long-standing nature. Herr and Weakland (1979) provide extensive, in-depth discussions of the family counseling process, and specific case examples dealing with issues such as confusion, hypochondriasis, intergenerational conflict, alternate living arrangements, independence/loneliness, and disability/death are provided. A general systems approach to gerontological counseling (within the framework of the older person–social system/culture interaction) has also been taken by Keller and Hughston (1981), who emphasize the "scheduling" of opportunities for communication/sharing, encouragement/support, "rational restructuring" by the older person, structured reminiscence, and "contracting" (defining and agreeing upon the consequences of a behavior pattern) as interventions aimed at several "levels" of unproductive behavior (attention-gaining, bossy, counter-hurting [striking back], and disablement [not taking responsibility]). Numerous case examples are also provided. Again, despite its popularity, family therapy has received little critical evaluation.

BEHAVIORAL APPROACHES TO TREATMENT

As Hoyer (1973) has noted, behavioral approaches to treatment are most consistent with a "person–environment interactive model" of development and aging. As opposed to psychodynamic notions of change, behaviorally oriented therapy focuses on the immediate, observable consequences of stimulus–response contingencies in the environment. Furthermore, although the principles that govern the formation, maintenance, and extinction (dropping out) of behavior are thought to be universal, behavior–consequence contingencies are specific to the individual. The application of a behavioral strategy involves (1) a definition and assessment prior to intervention of the desired target behavior, (2) a reinforcer (defined as a stimulus whose impact makes the desired behavior more frequent or of longer duration) whose effects on behavioral change must be identified and that may be self-administered, or administered by the therapist, and (3) the establishment of specific behavior–reinforcer contingencies. Positive (leading to pleasurable events and/or providing relief from aversive events) and negative (decreasing the frequency of a behavior by providing unpleasant consequences) reinforcing stimuli may be used for this purpose. A variation upon this theme is the *token economy,* where patients can earn tokens for desired behaviors, which can be later exchanged for appropriate rewards. Of course, ethical problems can be encountered if the therapist has too much control over the client's environment. Collaboration with family members and other professionals can help to avoid violations of the clients' rights (Hayslip & Kooken, 1982). Hayslip and Kooken (1982) also note that punishment appropriate for

such behaviors is generally severe and thus involves considerable risk to the client. They point out, however, "milder forms of punishment can be effectively utilized in programs to eliminate problem behaviors in the elderly. This risk can be minimized if the client is allowed to *participate* in making decisions about the behavior to be modified and agrees to the positive reinforcers and punishments in the program and when they should be administered" (Hayslip & Kooken, 1982, p. 293).

Another technique that can be utilized by the behavior modifier involves positively reinforcing a behavior that competes with the unwanted target behavior. "Contracting" is a form of behavior modification worthy of mention, where the client and therapist arrive at a clearly specified goal and agree upon a behavioral contract that the client should adhere to. Other behavioral intervention techniques can involve goal setting, modeling, or rehearsal (Rosenstein & Swenson, 1980).

Extensive discussions of the use of behavioral techniques with the aged are available (Levy et al., 1980; Rosenstein & Swenson, 1980; Hussian, 1981). In addition, there is ample well-designed research to support its efficacy in dealing with the modification of problem behaviors such as social interaction, incontinence, participation in a variety of activities, assertive behavior, walking, withdrawal, oral hygiene, orientation (to time, place, and person), self-stimulatory/inappropriate sexual behavior, wandering, speech behaviors, situational anxiety, pain-related behaviors, self-care, response speed, self-injurious behavior, and even grief. Moreover, behavioral methodologies have been utilized to successfully modify staff attitudes/expectations of elderly patients (Richards & Thorpe, 1978), which may indirectly have positive consequences for those aged persons. Behavioral technology with the aged possesses a number of conceptual and practical advantages: (1) it can be readily measured and its effects easily assessed, (2) goals can be readily defined, (3) it can be carried out and understood by staff at all levels of training, (4) it can be tailored to the individual patient (regardless of age), (5) procedures are relatively brief/economical, and (6) it can be adapted to the natural environment. Its use, however, demands a great deal of expertise, and it raises several ethical issues underlying treatment. As a number of gerontologists (Hoyer, 1973; Levy et al., 1980) have pointed out, the use of such techniques raises questions regarding (1) the long-term (versus the positive short-term) effects of such interventions (which may be harmful when such techniques are discontinued), (2) whether the reinforced behavior is actually within the person's capacities and/or will be supported by the immediate environment/staff (e.g., withdrawal of control), and (3) the need for careful selection of the behavior itself (e.g., reinforcing a prohibition against ingestion of foreign objects may be generalized by the patient to include the eating of food, leading to serious illness or death). Levy and colleagues (1980) also advocate a thorough investigation of the meaning of the environment as well as the unintended (versus the obvious) consequences of intervention. In short, "intervention for intervention's sake" is not always in the older person's best interests, depending upon his or her cognitive, health-related, and social/interpersonal resources and interpretation of the environment (e.g., "If I am not assertive? He was never that way before—is there something wrong?"). In many cases, it may be more feasible to change the enviornment per se or to leave things as they are, if one is unsure of the consequences of a given change.

In addition, cognitive–behavioral approaches to therapy and biofeedback training are options. Cognitive behavior therapy, an extension of behavioral therapy (Ellis, 1962; Meichenbaum, 1974; Beck, 1976) has recently been investigated with elderly persons (Kooken & Hayslip, 1984) in reducing test anxiety among older students.

"Cognitive behavior therapists believe that the way a person *thinks* largely determines the way he or she feels. In other words, thought causes emotional response. Cognitive behavior therapy is an attempt to help the client change his or her maladaptive thinking habits to relieve emotional disturbances such as depression, anger, and anxiety" (Kooken & Hayslip, 1982, p. 294).

Elderly persons, perhaps lacking feedback about themselves from others, often make "thinking errors" that in reality are quite inaccurate. Irrational assumptions relating one's age, or loss of skills once possessed, to feelings of self-depreciation may account for much anger, guilt, and depression in the aged. A competent cognitive behavior therapist, however, could instruct the elderly in substituting more rational thoughts in their place. Cognitive behavioral approaches to therapy have been successfully utilized to treat a variety of cognitive and emotional problems in the aged, e.g., depression, cautiousness, test anxiety, performance on intellectual tasks, and response speed (Labouvie-Vief & Gonda, 1976; Richards & Thorpe, 1978; Reidl, 1981).

Reidl (1981, p. 184) defines biofeedback as consisting of "measuring the electrical changes that accompany the body's physiologic processes, amplifying them, and feeding them back to the individual in either a visual or auditory signal . . . it involves control and alteration of response and stimulus by arranging contingencies . . . the reinforcement is the signal indicating success in attaining the physiologic state desired." In this case one might be interested in altering the individual's muscular tension, sweat gland activity, blood pressure, heart rate, or brain wave activity. Although biofeedback training, relative to control conditions (no biofeedback training, hypnosis, or relaxation training), has yielded mixed results, in many cases these data were based on studies of short duration and limited to the focus upon a single response. It does appear, however, to possess a great deal of potential in treating such problems as dermatitis, tension/stress responses, incontinence, migraine headaches, and pain, although it is expensive and time-consuming. An extensive discussion of biofeedback training in the aged has been provided by Woodruff (1980), who comments on the paucity of research on this modality for treatment of the aged. She cites several studies demonstrating biofeedback-related changes in electroencephalograph (EEG) activity, leading to changes in behavioral performance.

PSYCHOPHARMACOLOGICAL TREATMENT

With regard to psychopharmacological treatment (see Chap. 3), several major categories of drugs have been utilized with the aged. They include (1) antipsychotic agents and "antiparkinsonian" drugs (chlorpromazine), (2) antidepressants (tricyclics, monamine oxidase [MAO] inhibitors, lithium carbonate, estrogens), (3) antimanics (antipsychotics, lithium carbonate), (4) antianxiety agents/hypnotics (barbiturates, chloral hydrate, meprobamate, benzodiazepines, chlordiazepoxide, propranolol), and (5) cognitive-acting drugs (cerebral vasodilators, CNS stimulants, gerovital, anabolic substances, cholinomimetic agents [see Kapnick, 1978; Hicks, Funkenstein, Davis, & Kysken, 1980; Eisdorfer, 1975]).

Antipsychotic drugs are commonly used to treat agitation, violent behavior, irrational behavior, and perceptual disturbances (hallucinations) accompanying paranoid state/late life schizophrenia. Predictable side affects include extrapyramidal motor signs (tremors). Antiparkinson (anticholinergic) medication is often incorrectly prescribed to control tardive dyskinesia (involuntary facial, mandibular, and finger movements that may involve the limbs or trunk). Prolonged use of the antipsychotic drugs can lead to akathisia (uncontrolled restlessness/agitation) and sometimes glaucoma, constipation, and/or retention of urine. Major tranquilizers used to treat psychosis produce similar side effects. Most commonly, reduced dosage levels and/or "drug holidays" are recommended in these cases. Monoamine oxidase (MAO) inhibitors (antidepressant drugs) interact with foods having a high tyramine content (e.g., cheese, wine, bananas, meat tenderizers, and chocolate), causing hypertensive crises. Also, foods (e.g., chocolate) and beverages (e.g., coffee, tea, and soft drinks) containing caffeine will interact with MAO inhibitors, resulting in hypertension. Tricyclics can create many problems (arrhythmia, strokes, myocardial infarction, tachycardia) for those aged with cardiovascular disorders. Doxepin, amitriptyline, and imipramine are the recommended antidepressant compounds for use with the aged. Antimanics (lithium) often produce side effects of nausea, central nervous system (CNS) toxicity, and confusion. Antianxiety drugs (barbiturates) often produce "paradoxical" symptoms (excitement) and negatively affect enzyme action. Other minor tranquilizers (benzodiazepine) can be both physiologically and psychologically addictive. A variety of "cognitive-acting" drugs (e.g., hydergine) are used to supposedly reverse cognitive impairment, though their use in this regard has been questioned (Hicks et al., 1980). Electroconvulsive therapy (ECT) represents a viable approach to dealing with depressive symptomatology; it is contraindicated when a brain tumor is present and today not usually a treatment of choice. Many elderly fear it as well as its aftereffects.

It is probably accurate to say that drug treatment of the aged has historically been too often relied upon when other alternatives might have been of equal or greater efficacy. Extreme caution should be exercised when prescribing drugs for use with elderly clients. Older persons are particularly sensitive to drug effects; great individual differences exist regarding response to psychopharmacological agents. Polypharmacy is a pervasive problem with the aged. Furthermore, older persons are not as capable of metabolizing and excreting drugs as are the young (e.g., lithium carbonate). Most drugs (prescription or otherwise) have a longer half-life in older persons; they build up in concentration when fixed dosage intervals are used (due to age-related changes in fat to muscle tissue). Those that do so are not being used by the body and are thus ineffective. Moreover, this increases the likelihood of their interactions with other drugs (see Hicks et al., 1980) (e.g., particularly antipsychotics, antidepressants, antimanics, antiparkinson agents), medicines (anticongulants, antacids), and foods, which can result in a variety of side effects that may not only be harmful and exacerbate previous health problems (e.g. impairment of renal, liver, cardiovascular functioning) but may also be misdiagnosed as irreversible organic brain syndrome (OBS) (e.g., confusions, loss of memory, agitation, depression, paranoid delusions, hallucinations) and deemed to be untreatable by the unsuspecting diagnostician. Drugs may also produce a variety of symptoms that cause management problems in themselves. Such side effects can range from mild confusion, depression, and urinary or cardiac dysfunction to hallucinations or seizures. Ironically, such symptoms can lead to the administration of *more* drugs to alleviate the condition (which is seen as worsening) for which the drugs were originally prescribed, leading to more drug toxicity.

Hicks and colleagues (1980) also note that alcohol (see Woods, 1978) and analgesic (opiate) abuse may cause a variety of problems (i.e., behavioral/physical side effects) for the aged, complicating diagnoses. Also problematic are iatrogenic illnesses caused by direct and indirect drug action, making the differentiation of genuine somatic disorders difficult. Eisdorfer (1975, p. 57) comments that, although drugs should always be rationally and knowledgeably administered, their advantages in patient management/care should never be overlooked "given in appropriate degrees and in a carefully developed program."

RECOMMENDATIONS AND FUTURE DIRECTIONS

In light of the current state of the art regarding treatment approaches with the aged, it is safe to conclude that the literature is not complete enough at present to provide us with clear, consistent answers to many of the questions implicit in our discussion, e.g., Is one type of therapy more effective than another? Which approach is most effective for older versus younger clients? Are particular therapies more appropriate for certain disorders? What types of older persons respond best to what types of therapy under what conditions? Just as we might say with regard to potential clients who are younger, some persons certainly are motivated for, capable of, and can benefit from both professional and paraprofessional help. Therapy with the aged should always be oriented toward problem-solving (see Gotestam, 1980) and be geared to the individual. As pointed out by Hayslip and Kooken (1982, p. 298), "whether life review (reminiscence), insight, alleviation of symptoms, resolution of conflict, increasing social skills or self care behaviors is the goal, it seems clear that the elderly person should be the ultimate concern of the therapist."

The alleviation of distress may also require intervention at a societal level (Beattie, 1976; Lowy, 1980). As Beattie (1976) and Lowy (1980) have pointed out, altering attitudes toward the aged, effective use of community, family, and friends, and use of a variety of services (home-based care, outreach, hospice care, foster grandparent program, widow-to-widow programs, enhanced control over institutional regulations, routines and procedures) may prove to be as effective as intervention at the individual level. In fact, in some cases, the practicing clinician will often utilize various treatments in combination (e.g., pharmacological treatment and individual psychotherapy, individual and group therapy) to achieve a more effective state of affairs for the patient and family/staff.

One's own beliefs about aging, death, pain,

and illness, as well as feelings about one's own parents' aging, will bear on the choice of intervention as well as its success or failure with a particular client (Hayslip & Kooken, 1982). Views about development across the life-span (based upon implicit comparisons between the young and the older/personal recollections of youth) and about how personality as such functions (see Kastenbaum, 1978; Costa & McCrae, 1980) are likely to have an important bearing on whether one chooses to work with older clients at all, and which approach(es) is (are) selected for use with a particular client. Although many feel that existing personality theory has little to offer the gerontological counselor (Kastenbaum, 1978), views about aging and intervention with the aged and family development continue to be topics for discussing and research (see Baltes and Danish, 1980; Danish, 1981). Lawton (1976) also notes the importance of a variety of factors: discussing abstract ideas (i.e., dependency, conflict) in terms older persons can understand (using the older person's own words if possible), creating a supportive, trusting atmosphere to minimize anxiety, proceeding at a slow enough pace to allow the older client to become comfortable, encouraging the client to verbalize feelings that one would otherwise not choose to share for fear of being criticized, and being sensitive to sensory (visual, auditory, tactual) impairments. Hayslip and Kooken (1982, p. 287) emphasize the importance of being *real* with older clients. "Simply being able to express sadness, pain, anger, depression or loneliness is an invaluable service to aged persons who have no one else in whom they can confide. It may be particularly important to emphasize that it is all right to give up goals which are simply beyond their resources, such as maintaining power over grown children, or being totally independent."

In spite of the diversity of approaches to intervention reviewed here, it remains clear that older persons must be humanistically counseled on an individual basis, to avoid harmful generalizations about the ability of older persons to respond to treatment. Furthermore, choice of treatment must also be geared to each older individual. Clearly, such a recognition of client differences will enhance the chances of the older individual's responding positively to, and being satisfied with, each intervention, regardless of its nature.

SUMMARY

Until recently, the aged have largely been neglected as viable therapeutic possibilities, based upon a number of factors, e.g., notions of decline with age, unresolved feelings about older persons, as well as older persons' attitudes toward receiving professional help. Such neglect exists in spite of evidence suggesting that older persons are equally responsive to helping efforts as are younger persons.

A variety of potentially valuable interventions are available to older persons, e.g., psychoanalysis, behavioral-cognitive therapy, group and family intervention, and psychopharmalogical treatment. Moreover, a number of more specific techniques exist, e.g., remotivation, reality orientation, milieu therapies, life review, and biofeedback, that have been utilized with the aged. Regardless of the specific technique used, it must be one that is consistent with both the therapist's and the older client's goals and life circumstances. Available evidence largely fails to support (or deny) the efficacy of various therapies with the aged, although some findings indicate that certain types of techniques (e.g., life review, remotivation, reality orientation) are more effective with some types of older clients than with others.

Ultimately, the older person's welfare must be the primary concern of the therapist; knowing when not to intervene is as important as being skilled at various interventive techniques. Every older client must be considered as a unique individual, in order to maximize each individual's response to and satisfaction with both the help and the helper.

REFERENCES

Abraham, I. (1949). The applicability of psycho-analytic treatment to patients of advanced aged. In K. Abraham (Ed.), *Selected papers of psychoanalysis*. London: Hogarth Press.

Baltes, P., & Danish, S. (1980). Intervention and life-span development and aging: Issues and concepts. In R. Turner & H. Reese (Eds.), *Life-span developmental psychology: Intervention*. New York: Academic Press.

Baltes, P., Reese, H., & Lipsitt, L. (1980). Life-span development psychology. *Annual Review of Psychology, 31*, 65–100.

Beattie, W. (1976). Aging and the social services. In R. Binstock & E. Shanas (Eds.), *Handbook of aging and the social sciences*. New York: Van Nostrand Reinhold.

Beck, A. (1976). *Cognitive therapy and the emotional disorders*. New York: International Universities Press.

Birren, J., & Renner, V. J. (1979). A brief history of mental health and aging. In *Issues in mental health and aging*. Washington, DC: National Institute of Mental Health.

Birren, J., & Sloane, R. B. (1980). *Handbook of mental health and aging*. Englewood Cliffs, N.J.: Prentice-Hall.

Blum, J., & Tallmer, M. (1977). The therapist vis-a-vis the older patient. *Psychotherapy: Theory, Research and Practice, 14*, 361–367.

Butler, R. (1963). The life review: An interpretation of reminiscence in the aged. *Geriatrics, 26*, 65–76.

Butler, R., German, J., Overlander, D., & Shindler, L. (1979–80). Self-care, self-help, and the elderly. *International Journal of Aging and Human Development, 10*, 95–117.

Butler, R., & Lewis, M. (1981). *Aging and mental health*. St. Louis: Mosby.

Costa, P., & McCrae, R. (1980). Still stable after all these years: Personality as a key to some issues in adulthood and old age. In P. Baltes & O. Brim (Eds.), *Life-span development and behavior*. New York: Academic Press.

Danish, S. (1981). Life-span development and intervention: A necessary link. *Counseling Psychologist, 9*, 40–43.

Davis, R., & Klopfer, W. (1977). Issues in psychotherapy with the aged. *Psychotherapy: Theory, Research and Practice, 14*, 343–348.

Dye, C., & Erber, J. (1981). Two group procedures for the treatment of nursing home patients. *Gerontologist, 21*, 539–544.

Eisdorfer, C. (1975). Observations on the psychopharmacology of the aged. *Journal of the American Geriatrics Society, 23*, 53–57.

Eisdorfer, C., & Stotsky, B. (1977). Intervention, treatment, and rehabilitation of psychiatric disorders. In J. Birren & K. W. Schaie (Eds.), *Handbook of the psychology of aging*. New York: Van Nostrand Reinhold.

Eillis, A. (1962). *Reason and emotion in psychotherapy*. New York: Lyle Stuart.

Folsom, J. (1968). Reality orientation for the elderly mental patient. *Journal of Geriatric Psychiatry, 1*, 291–307.

Ford, C., & Sbordone, R. (1980). Attitudes of psychiatrists toward elderly patients. *American Journal of Psychiatry, 137*, 571–577.

Fozard, J. (1980). A time for remembering. In L. Poon (Ed.), *Aging in the 1980's: Psychological issues*. Washington, DC: American Psychological Association.

Fozard, J., & Popkin, S. (1978). Optimizing adult development: Ends and means of an applied psychology of aging. *American Psychologist, 33*, 975–989.

Freud, S. (1924). On psychotherapy. In S. Freud (Ed.), *Collected papers* (Vol. 1). London: Hogarth Press.

Garfield, S. (1978). Research on client variables in psychotherapy. In S. Garfield & A. Bergin (Eds.), *Handbook of psychotherapy and behavior change*. New York: Wiley.

Gatz, M., Smyer, M., & Lawton, M. P. (1980). The mental health system and the older adult. In L. Poon (Ed.), *Aging in the 1980's: Psychological perspectives*. Washington, DC: American Psychological Association.

Goldfarb, A. (1953). Recommendations for psychiatric treatment in a home for the aged. *Journal of Gerontology, 8*, 343–347.

Gotestam, K. G. (1980). Behavioral and dynamic psychotherapy with the elderly. In J. Birren & R. Sloane (Eds.), *Handbook of mental health and aging*. Englewood Cliffs, N.J.: Prentice-Hall.

Gottesman, L., Quarterman, C., & Cohn, G. (1973). Psychosocial treatment of the aged. In C. Eisdorfer & M. P. Lawton (Eds.), *The psychology of adult development and aging*. Washington, DC: American Psychological Association.

Grauer, H., Betts, D., & Birnbom, F. (1973). Welfare emotions and family therapy in geriatrics. *Journal of the American Geriatrics Society, 21,* 21–24.

Hartford, M. (1980). The use of group methods for work with the aged. In J. Birren & R. Sloane (Eds.), *Handbook of mental health and aging.* Englewood Cliffs, N.J.: Prentice-Hall.

Hayslip, B., & Kooken, R. (1982). Therapeutic interventions—Mental health. In N. Ernst & H. Glazer-Waldman (Eds.), *The aged patient: A sourcebook for the allied health professional.* Chicago: Year Book.

Hayslip, B., & Martin, C. (1988). Approaching death. In K. Esberger & S. Hughes (Eds.), *Nursing care of the aged.* E. Norwalk, CT: Appleton & Lange.

Herr, J., & Weakland, J. (1979). *Counseling elders and their families: Practical techniques for applied gerontology.* New York: Springer.

Hicks, R., Funkenstein, H., Davis, J., & Kysken, M. (1980). Geriatric psychopharmacology. In J. Birren & R. Sloane (Eds.), *Handbook of mental health and aging.* Englewood Cliffs, NJ: Prentice-Hall.

Hoyer, W. (1973). Application of operant techniques to the modifications of elderly behavior. *Gerontologist, 13,* 18–22.

Hussian, R. (1981). *Geriatric psychology: A behavioral perspective.* New York: Van Nostrand Reinhold.

Kahn, R., & Miller, N. (1978). Adaptational factors in memory function in the aged. *Experimental Aging Research, 4,* 273–290.

Kapnick, P. L. (1978). Organic treatment of the elderly. In M. Storandt, I. C. Siegler, & N. F. Elias (Eds.), *The Clinical Psychology of Aging.* New York: Plenum.

Kastenbaum, R. (1978). Personality theory, therapeutic approaches and the elderly client. In M. Storandt, I. Siegler, & M. Elias (Eds.), *The clinical psychology of aging.* New York: Plenum.

Keller, J., & Hughston, G. (1981). *Counseling the elderly: A systems approach.* New York: Harper & Row.

Knight, R. (1978–79). Psychotherapy and behavior change with the noninstitutionalized aged. *International Journal of Aging and Human Development, 9,* 221–236.

Kooken, R., & Hayslip, B. (1984). The use of stress inoculation in the treatment of test anxiety in older students. *Educational Gerontology, 10,* 39–58.

Labouvie-Vief, G., & Gonda, J. (1976). Cognitive strategy training and intellectual performance in the elderly. *Journal of Gerontology, 31,* 327–332.

Langer, L., & Rodin, J. (1976). The effects of choices and enhanced personal responsibility for the aged: A field experiment in an institutional setting. *Journal of Personality and Social Psychology, 34,* 314–350.

Lawton, M. P. (1978). Clinical geropsychology: Problems and prospects. In D. Nygaard (Ed.), *Master lectures on the psychology of aging.* Washington, DC: American Psychological Association.

Lawton, M. P., & Gottesman, L. (1974). Psychological services to the elderly. *American Psychologist, 29,* 689–693.

Levy, S., Derogatis, L., & Gatz, M. (1980). Intervention with older adults and the evaluation of outcome. In L. Poon (Ed.), *Aging in the 1980's: Psychological Issues.* Washington, D.C.: American Psychological Association.

Lowy, L. (1980). Mental health services in the community. In J. Birren & R. Sloane (Eds.), *Handbook of mental health and aging.* Englewood Cliffs, N.J.: Prentice-Hall.

Luborsky, L., Chandler, M., Auerbach, A., Cohen, J., & Bachrach, H. (1971). Factors influencing the outcome of psychotherapy: A review of quantitative research. *Psychological Bulletin, 75,* 145–185.

Meichenbaum, D. (1974). Self-instructional strategy training: A cognitive prosthesis for the aged. *Human Development, 17,* 273–280.

Peterson, J. (1973). Marital and family therapy involving the aged. *Gerontologist, 13,* 27–31.

Peterson, J. (1980). Social–psychological aspects of death and dying and mental health. In J. Birren & R. Sloane (Eds.), *Handbook of mental health and aging.* Englewood Cliffs, N.J.: Prentice-Hall.

Reidl, R. (1981). Behavior therapies. In C. Eisdorfer, (Ed.), *Annual review of gerontology and geriatrics.* New York: Springer.

Richards, W., & Thorpe, G. (1978). Behavioral approaches to the problems of later life. In M. Storandt, I. Siegler, & M. Elias (Eds.), *The clinical psychology of aging.* New York: Plenum.

Rodin, J., & Langer, E. (1977). Long-term effects of a control-relevant intervention with the institutionalized aged. *Journal of Personality and Social Psychology, 35,* 897–903.

Rosenstein, J., & Swenson, E. (1980). Behavioral

approaches to therapy with the elderly. In S. Sargent (Ed.), *Nontraditional therapy and counseling with the aging*. New York: Springer.

Sherwood, S., & Mor, V. (1980). Mental health institutions and the elderly. In J. Birren & R. Sloane (Eds.), *Handbook of mental health and aging*. Englewood Cliffs, N.J.: Prentice-Hall.

Smith, M., & Glass, G. (1977). Meta-analysis of psychotherapy outcome studies. *American Psychologist, 32*, 752–760.

Smyer, M., & Gatz, M. (1979). Aging and mental health: Business as usual? *American Psychologist, 34*, 240–246.

Sparacino, J. (1978–79). Individual psychotherapy with the aged: A selective review. *International Journal of Aging and Human Development, 9*, 197–220.

Storandt, M. (1978). Other approaches to therapy. In M. Storandt, I. Siegler, & M. Elias (Eds.), *The clinical psychology of aging*. New York: Plenum.

Storandt, M., Siegler, I., & Elias, M. (1978). *The clinical psychology of aging*. New York: Plenum.

Sussman, M. (1976). The family life of old people. In R. Binstock & E. Shanas (Eds.), *Handbook of aging and the social sciences*. New York: Van Nostrand Reinhold.

Treat, N., Poon, L., Fozard, J., & Popkin, S. (1978). Toward applying cognitive skill training to memory problems. *Experimental Aging Research, 4*, 305–320.

Troll, L., Miller, S., & Atchley, R. (1979). *Families in later life*. Belmont, CA: Wadsworth.

Wood, W. G. (1978). The elderly alcoholic: Some diagnostic problems and considerations. In M. Storandt, I. Siegler, & M. Elias (Eds.), *The clinical psychology of aging*. New York: Plenum.

Woodruff, D. (1980). Intervention in the psychophysiology of aging: Pitfalls, progress, and potention. In R. Turner & H. Reese (Eds.), *Life-developmental psychology: Intervention*. New York: Academic Press.

Zeplin, H., Wolfe, C., & Kleinplatz, F. (1981). Evaluation of a year-long reality orientation program. *Journal of Gerontology, 36*, 70–77.

15

APPROACHING DEATH

This chapter deals with the relevance that issues surrounding death and dying have for older persons, their families, and professional care-givers. Aging is often seen as a period in one's life that is associated with a variety of "negatives." Ill health, isolation and loneliness, uselessness, institutionalization, and ultimately death are associations that many people make when they consider old age—not only their own, but also that of others. Perhaps the most important of the above reasons for the resulting devaluation of the elderly is the association between death and old age. Kastenbaum (1978) notes that, "Together they have posed for many a classic ambivalence: one does not want to die, yet one does not want to grow old." It is the very belief that death is "more appropriate" for the elderly than for the young that has resulted, until recently, in the neglect of issues regarding death and dying in older persons. As Peterson (1980) has noted, although indications of a great deal of both popular and professional interest have emerged in the area of death and dying, substantive, empirically based research has lagged far behind.

In spite of the objective reasons for considering the worth of an older person's life to be no less than that of a young person, myths about aging abound, with the end result being that the life of an older person may literally be perceived as less worthy of saving than that of someone who is young and/or affluent. Perhaps the most poignant indication of such a view is described by Sundow (1967), who found emergency room staff to make a greater effort to save the life of a young person than an old person. He found that emergency care given to the elderly was similar to that afforded the alcoholic, the prostitute, or the vagrant.

Morever, Blauner (1966, p. 391) has written of the lessened impact of the death of an aged person on society, reflecting the lack of importance attached to the lives of the old. "The aged not only have become disengaged from significant family, economic and community responsibilities in the present, but their future status (politely referred to in our humane culture) is among the company of the powerless, anonymous, and virtually ignored dead."

More recently (see Kalish, 1985; Kastenbaum, 1985; Neugarten, 1977; Thomae, 1980), researchers and practitioners in the field of aging have come to reject the notion of older persons as necessarily disengaged from others. Thus, although some professionals undoubtedly see older persons in this very negative light, the prevailing view regarding aging is to see disengagement as one of *many* ways in which older persons cope with the aging process. Although some elderly do pull away from responsibilities, others remain involved in both family and community activities. Rosenmayr (1985), for example, has redefined the role of the aged in Western culture in terms of fulfillment and creativity.

This more balanced and more positive view

of the aged suggests that we now view death in very different terms, namely, seeing death as an opportunity for growth rather than as loss, thus investing death with more meaning and less negative connotations, whether we are young adults or elderly persons.

Several issues regarding death and dying as it pertains to the aged are salient for our purposes. These issues relates to (1) older persons' feelings and attitudes toward death, (2) the impact of loss on the elderly, (3) manifestations of death concerns among the aged, and (4) concerns the helping professional should keep in mind when dealing with older persons, where death is an ever-present consideration.

THEORETICAL VIEWS ON DEATH AND THE AGED

As noted above, both laypersons and professionals have a tendency to link older persons and death, sometimes with tragic consequences. It is frequently thought that, given the closeness of the aged to death, they are more fearful of death than are younger persons. This can lead caregivers to an avoidance of the topic with those older persons who genuinely need to air their feelings, or alternatively result in their focusing on death to the exclusion of other concerns that the older person may have. At the very worst, such a linkage may elicit feelings toward the aged ranging from passive dislike/avoidance to overt hostility and abuse and may lead to sub-quality care.

Erikson (1963) asserts that the final psychosocial crisis characteristic of old age is that of integrity versus despair. Although integrity is difficult to define objectively, it seems to possess the quality of completeness, of wholeness, the awareness that one has come full circle, and is therefore preparing for acceptance of death. Integrity is achieved by means of the process of introspection. The older person who fails to achieve a sense of integrity (implying a reintegration of the successes, failures, frustrations, and disappointments of one's past, present and

future, and being satisfied with the outcome) is despairing, according to Erikson. In effect, this person may say, "I am not free to die, give me more time to relive my life, to correct past mistakes, to atone for past failures." The resulting devaluation of the self is manifest in a fear of death, for death is seen as an event that cuts life prematurely short. Regret, depression, and sadness thus characterize the old person who is not able to successfully resolve this last psychosocial crisis of integrity versus despair. Implicit in this resolution are the older person's feelings about his own impending death.

A similar notion to Erikson's concepts of integrity/despair is Butler's (1963) formulation of the salience of death in the process of life review (see also Chap. 14). The life review is characterized by Butler as a recalling of past experiences and a re-evaluation of them, presumably culminating in an understanding of how these events and experiences have shaped one's life. The necessity of a life review is brought about by an awareness that one's death is imminent. Butler and Lewis (1981, p. 59) suggest that the eminence of old age (thought to be universal), reflecting a life review process, can result in ". . . a righting of old wrongs, making up with enemies, coming to acceptance of mortal life, a sense of serenity, pride in accomplishment, and a feeling of having done one's best."

On the positive side it serves, as Adams (1979, p. 45) has said, "as a primary compass (to) measure (one's) position in life (for) only when we understand where we have been can we decide where we wish to go. And the pilgrimage continues to the moment of life's end." On the other hand, it can generate considerable guilt, anxiety, and anger, with the ultimate result, perhaps, a decision that one's life was worth nothing, leading to suicide.

A third idea that reinforces the linkage of aging and death is embodied in the disengagement theory proposed by Cumming and Henry (1961). This theory suggests that it is natural for older persons to withdraw from both activities and relationships with others as they progress through old age. This leads to an intense preoccupation with one's self, under the assumption that most elderly persons desire such withdrawal. Implicit herein is the idea that death is a central concern to most older persons, and that disengagement permits them to get their "house in order" in preparation for death. The other side of this theory proposes that society also withdraws from older people, in this way preparing for their loss to the social group. Thus, notions of integrity versus despair, life review/reminiscence, and disengagement link aging and death in the minds of many professionals and laypersons alike.

Perhaps the most damaging consequence of these theories is that they doom the older person to what Schulz (1978) has termed a social death. That is, the aged are treated as if they are already dead, when they are in fact very much alive. In many cases, this social death takes the form of simple avoidance of the old although it might involve physical/emotional abuse by others (e.g., family, care-givers, nursing home staff) or talking in the presence of the older person as if the individual were an object, not a person. Marshall (1979), Kastenbaum (1978), Chapell (1975), and Wass (1979) have pointed out that institutions such as nursing homes or hospitals, or environments such as retirement villages implicitly socialize older persons to their deaths. In many instances, a climate is created by staff, fellow residents, or family that "legitimizes" death, making it more acceptable to those who must face it. In other cases, however, the concern with a preparation for death has the effect of "dehumanizing" the care that is given, resulting in a loss of self-esteem, deprivation/isolation from others (see Watson & Maxwell [1977] for an extensive discussion of staff–patient avoidance) or simply a giving up on life.

Kastenbaum (1978, p. 4) cogently summarizes many of the prevalent attitudes toward aging and death:

1. The old person is thought to be "ready" if not actually "longing" to see the final curtain descend
2. On a more philosophical level, death is "natural" and "timely" for the old person. Biologists make this point, with emphasis on the preservation of the vigor of our species through the "necessary elimination" of weakened and impaired specimens
3. On the more pragmatic level, it is inappropriate to attempt to extend the life of a person who is conspicuously old and ailing; such an action is decried as "indignity" or "not cost-effective," depending on the speaker's preferred vocabulary
4. The "social loss" (Glaser & Strauss, 1965) when an old person dies is minimal and is not a factor that must be taken seriously
5. Memorializations and rituals associated with the death also are not of particular importance; they may even extend the "morbid" aura of death over the surviving elders—in any event, the death has been expected so long that there is little need to prolong the scene with rituals of mourning and memorialization
6. Little could be done to extend the life of a sick and imperiled elder
7. The limited amount of social and medical resources available should be applied to care of the young, who still have so much life ahead of them

Because a considerable portion of elderly (estimated at 20% of those who reach age 65) end their lives in institutions (Kastenbaum & Candy, 1973) a death-oriented situation is a comparatively common occurrence in old age. Kastenbaum (1978, p. 5) notes, "So long as we can believe that old people are ready for death and that it is high time for them to leave the scene, we can also hold our emotional responses and professional services within acceptable limits. . . . If we just know that death is appropriate for old people, then there is little need to explore precisely what this old man or woman is thinking or feeling."

Beyond creating the damaging assumption that death and aging "go together," the above theoretical views are objectionable from a scientific, empirical standpoint as well. Disengagement theory has been rejected as a universal, normal, highly desirable pattern of adjustment to aging (Wass, 1979; Neugarten, 1977), although a lifelong pattern of disengagement may prove to be highly life satisfying for some elderly, as noted by Thomae (1980) and others.

Butler (1963, p. 67) notes that, although the life review is not restricted to the aged, it is nevertheless "more commonly observed in the aged because of the actual nearness of life's termination. . . ." It has been easy for professionals and others to forget this caution and most commonly assume it to be characteristic, indeed nearly unique, to the aged.

The idea of reminiscence (see also Chap. 14) has been studied in some depth by Romaniuk (1981), who notes that reminiscence is a complex phenomenon, one that is not limited to any single period of the life cycle. In fact, his review of the literature suggests that there is no relationship between age and frequency of reminiscence of one's life. Older persons, in spite of common belief to the contrary, do not spend more time preoccupied with their past lives than do the young. Romaniuk (1981) suggests that reminiscence may be more personality/trait-related (e.g., introversion–extroversion) than age-related. Further, reminiscence exhibits a great deal of variation in which events trigger it. Romaniuk and Romaniuk (1981) feel that "triggering" events usually involve change (e.g., parenthood, divorce, illness, retirement, relocation). Death of one's friends, the anticipation of one's own death, or the loss of one's mate most certainly involve changes in life-style, habits, interests, and relationships; these changes are not unique to older persons, however. Notions such as integrity or despair have been criticized in that they in effect represent idealized end points along a continuum (Birren & Renner, 1977). As such, they are *generalizations* about older persons and they offer little guidance as to how specific individuals vary along this continuum. Because older persons are more heterogeneous than are the young (Botwinick, 1978; Maddox & Douglas, 1974) it seems more useful

for professionals to be aware of these substantial individual differences found among older persons. Consequently, in practice, theories such as Erikson's, attempting to fit all elderly into a "stage," are at best crude attempts to describe the role that death plays in the lives of *some* elderly *some* of the time. In fact, Clayton (1975) has challenged the notion that psychosocial crises are ever "resolved" at all. Clayton maintains that older persons have compromised their way through previous crises, making it more likely that a complete resolution of this last crisis is simply not possible. It may be that older persons effectively "compartmentalize" their feelings regarding success/failure, e.g., their career in one compartment and their marriage in another.

Aging itself is debatable as a cause of death. Available data suggest older persons die most frequently from cardiovascular disorders (e.g., heart disease, strokes, high blood pressure) and malignant neoplasms (cancer), in that order. As Kastenbaum (1978) points out, the mortality rate for the aged has actually declined over the past 50 years, in spite of the fact that there are greater numbers of elderly and thus more deaths in an absolute sense. Paradoxically, the latter fact enhances the aging-death link, whereas the former tends to weaken this association.

HOW THE AGED SEE DEATH

As noted above, a central question bearing on the discussion of death and aging is that of the older person's views/feelings about death. Unfortunately, this is not a question for which there is a straightforward answer. The qualifiers in this case principally bear on (1) how death is interpreted (i.e., what the term means to the individual) and (2) how responses to death are best conceived.

The term *death* means many things to many people. As Kalish and Reynolds (1976) note, what frightens many of us about death per se is the fact that it involves *loss*. That which is lost through death can refer to a multitude of factors, e.g., the following (see Kalish & Reynolds, 1976):

1. Loss of ability to have experiences
2. Loss of uncertainty about subsequent events (after death)
3. Loss of the body
4. Loss of the ability to care for dependents
5. Losses suffered by family and friends
6. Loss of the opportunity to complete plans and projects
7. Loss of being in a relatively painless state

Kalish and Reynolds (1976) go on to mention that the loss of control over one's life is a salient issue for many persons, particularly those who are dying. As discussed above, dying in an institution can be very depersonalizing, and one frequently finds oneself the object of a variety of procedures and decisions regarding what will or will not be done to one's body, with whom time will be spent, and what possessions one is permitted to keep. All these decisions are presumably made in one's best interests, but one has little or no chance for input.

Another dimension is that, although some aspects of loss are important to some, these same considerations (see above) might not be important to others. For example, a young person may fear death because it represents an interruption of valued goals, whereas an elderly person may feel sorrow over the loss of the ability to care for others, be concerned about the impact of the death on others, or fear the loss of one's body (or what may happen to one's body after death).

In addition to death as loss, Kalish and Reynolds (1976) also discuss death in terms of time, i.e., death as an organizer of time as well as something that alters the manner in which we use time. For the old, time itself may be redefined. Thus, living life on a day-to-day basis may become more important than organizing one's life around future goals/plans. Without ignoring the past or being heavily invested in the future, many aged (particularly the most competent) seem to strike a balance in this regard (Ste-

vens-Long, 1979). Available literature definitely rejects the notion that as one ages, time, supposedly representing a smaller portion of one's total life, passes more quickly (Stevens-Long, 1979). Peterson (1980) does suggest that a sense of time pressure creates a great deal of stress for many middle-aged persons, but notes that this is speculative. Bascue and Lawrence (1977) have found that older persons turn away from the future and they interpret this as a means of coping with death anxiety. Thus, although death per se is literally a single moment in time, the criteria for death have already been spelled out (Veatch, 1979), and the meaning of death to older persons (as opposed to the young, or to other elderly as well) is likely to vary considerably, depending on one's value systems, interpersonal relations, goals, health, and whether one is caring for others or being cared for by them.

Research on the meaning of death, as well as responses to death, suggests that both are multidimensional constructs. Thus, in popular literature, and in everyday conversation, "death" concerns must be separated from those relating to the process of dying. Furthermore, fears about one's own death may differ from those surrounding significant others' deaths per se and/or dying (Schulz, 1978; Kastenbaum & Costa, 1977; Simpson, 1979). These concerns may or may not become manifest at a conscious, overt level of awareness. Thus, as Kastenbaum and Costa (1977) have noted, the absence of a fear of death at a conscious level of awareness may simply reflect the person's efforts at denial, and the true anxieties may surface at a covert, unconscious level (e.g., in terms of physical complaints, difficulty in sleeping, changes in one's eating habits, difficulties in completing a task, or even an abnormal concern with the welfare of others).

Research reviewed by Wass (1979) and by Kastenbaum and Costa (1977) suggests that, in spite of the usual assumption to the contrary, elderly persons do not report fearing death per se. They do, however, report fears of the dying process, e.g., dying in pain, dying alone, losing control over bodily functions/events, and changes in body image. In cases where these factors are clearly salient, ending one's own life may be perceived as preferable to living with the by-products of a slow, painful, lonely death. Hayslip, Pinder, and Lumsden (1981), Fiefel and Branscomb (1973), and Pinder and Hayslip (1981) have found that, although older persons and younger persons did not differ in consciously expressed death fears, there were substantial age differences in covertly expressed death concerns (e.g., fears of losing others, pain/suffering, loss of goals/achievements, loss of control). In this case, the differences suggested that older persons expressed more covert death fear than did the young, but less overt fear. Rather than age per se, factors such as health status, reflected in distance from death (Riegel & Riegel, 1972), may play a more important role in explaining death concerns in the aged (Marshall, 1975). In research by Jeffers, Nichols, and Eisdorfer (1961), Rhudick and Dibner (1961), Roberts, Kimsey, Logan, and Shaw (1970), Swenson (1961), Fiefel and Branscomb (1973), and Templer, Ruff, and Franks (1971), an "accepting" attitude toward death (a lack of self-reported fear) was shown among the elderly.

Although a variety of other factors interact with the age–death anxiety relationship, findings do not always present a consistent picture. Being alone and/or institutionalized, living in an urban setting, being in poor physical or mental health, being a female, and being poorly educated are all positively correlated with self-reported death fears, as reported by Mullins and Lopez (1982), Wass and Sisler (1978), and Wass, Christian, Myers, and Murphy (1978–79). However, studies by Bell and Batterson (1979), Christ (1961), and Swenson (1961) generally indicate an absence of a relationship between such factors as retirement, life satisfaction, religiosity, socioeconomic status, sex, and death fears. Moreover, ethnic variations in death fears have been observed by Kalish and Reynolds (1976) and by Bengston, Cuellar, and Ragan (1977).

Overall, it seems safe to conclude that there is a great deal of variability among older persons in their feelings about death, so that generalizations about the elderly are difficult to make. Thus, every older person should be approached as an individual. Their responses may range from what Kastenbaum and Aisenberg (1976) have termed "overcoming" (seeing death as the enemy, as external, as failure) to participatory (seeing death as internal, as a reunion, as a natural consequence of having lived).

In addition to research dealing with older persons' views and responses to death and dying, many reports deal with the elderly person's views and beliefs about a variety of death-related topics, e.g., afterlife, euthanasia, the right to die, funeral practices.

In addition to concerns relevant to death per se and to the dying process, another set of factors to consider in understanding aging and death relates to the elderly person's perceptions of what happens after death. In this sense, Kalish and Reynolds' (1976) treatment of death as punishment for sins becomes an issue of interest. Reynolds and Kalish (1974) found that, although older persons generally equate moral goodness with a longer life-span, a *majority* of those surveyed (regardless of age) agreed with a statement about the fact that accidental deaths showed the hand of God working among men. Thus, accidental death tends to be seen as retribution, rather than long life being seen as a reward. Obviously, when the older person who is dying has suffered a great deal, death may be seen as a release. Predictably, older persons in this study desired sudden death over a long, painful one.

Reynolds and Kalish (1974) have found that older persons, relative to the young, expected and wanted to live longer, possibly indicating that their feelings about the afterlife were negative. Kalish and Reynolds' (1976) review of this literature, however, suggests that those elderly who are more religious have lower death anxiety. Similar findings are reported by Wass and colleagues (1978–79). Wass (1979) and Kastenbaum and Costa (1977) found that the relationships between religiosity and fear of death are likely to be complex, dependent upon how each construct is measured. If an aged person is highly religious, he or she may fear death as an anticipated punishment for sin, or see death as a reward for a good life (see above, however). Persons who are not religious presumably have nothing to fear in this sense; however, the literal "nothingness" beyond death may elicit a great deal of anxiety.

Wass (1977) and Mathieu and Peterson (1970) found that some older persons in their sample were opposed to keeping a person alive by artificial means. They favored natural death (passive euthanasia). Many felt that such a decision belonged to God and held out hope for recovery, but under unusual circumstances (e.g., certain terminality and, without treatment, extreme pain), life could be cut short. Preston and Williams (1971) found that half of their sample of older persons rejected death through passive euthanasia under any circumstances as well as active euthanasia. One quarter favored a passive, but not an active, approach to ending life; one third accepted both types of euthanasia. Like most people, older persons wanted to be told if they were dying, and saw funeral prices as too high (Wass, 1979). It must be pointed out that such feelings may reflect an over-response to financial and/or emotional pressure from family. Most aged disapproved of lying in state, and although highly educated urban aged favored cremation, poorly educated rural elderly preferred burial (Wass, 1979). Kalish and Reynolds (1976) and Wass (1979) conclude that most elderly think about death at least "occasionally." This may reflect their experience with the deaths of others, but in addition can have positive benefits in facilitating funeral planning and the writing of a will, and encourage the sharing of feelings essential to open communication. In many cases, elderly persons' strong feelings about funerals, euthanasia, lying in state, and so on may reflect an effort at controlling events associated with something that is, in fact, not controllable. The writing of a will may also (Wass et al.,

1978–79) reflect a concern for the welfare of others. Kalish and Reynolds (1976) and Kastenbaum and Aisenberg (1976) discuss the fact that older persons "personalize" death more often than do the young. This personalization may take the form of wanting to be reunited with a departed loved one, or seeing God. This may reflect one's religious views, or simply represent a longing to be with those with whom one has shared life. It goes without saying that family, professionals, and others interested in helping the aged person should be sensitive and open to the elderly individual's feelings about such issues.

Wass (1979) and Kalish and Reynolds (1976) have provided us with some insight into the nature of death from the perspective of older persons. Wass (1979, p. 190) speaks of "the death taboo and the elderly." This avoidance of death specifically works against the older person's willingness to discuss very personal concerns; having lost a confidant often leaves the elderly person without anyone with whom to share his or her innermost feelings. Although depression in the aged in some cases is an outcome of the introspection accompanying reminiscence, more likely it stems from the lack of opportunity to share thoughts and relive previous conflicts with others who may be unwilling or unable to understand. Thus many factors may contribute to death-related depression in the aged, which may have a suicidal component. Ironically, depression, or an unwillingness to talk, could easily be interpreted as part of the older person's "preparations" for death (Kastenbaum, 1978).

Although an elderly person's feelings about death are sometimes seen as an outgrowth of specific environmental happenings (e.g., feeling helpless or being relocated or having failing health as a function of losing someone close through death), conclusions in this regard are difficult to reach due to the lack of information.

Of particular interest in this regard is a study by Keith (1979), who examined the relationship between life changes (marital status, health, church involvement, informal family/friendship contacts) and the elderly's response patterns toward life and death. Individuals were categorized as (1) positivists: those whose life goals are fulfilled and for whom death is not to be feared, (2) negativists: those who fear death and see it as something that cuts short their time on earth, (3) activists: who see death as a foreclosing of ambition, even though valued goals have been achieved, and (4) passivists: those who see death as a respite from life's disappointments, for whom death is actually a positive event. Keith (1979) found that the negativists or passivists experienced the most discontinuity. Women tended to be more accepting (positivists, passivists) of death than did men (negativists, activists); 40% of Keith's sample were described as negativists or passivists. Changes in marital status and in health tended to be associated with negativism in men; such events did not produce systematic changes in women, however. Religiosity did not seem to be as comforting for men as it did for women. Those with higher incomes tended to be positivists, whereas those with lower incomes tended to be passivists or negativists. Less formal/informal activity was associated with passivism in both men and women. Of particular interest was the finding that, among low-income groups where a spouse was ill, death was seen as a release (passivism). Given the frequency with which older persons favor euthanasia (see above), such feelings may reflect the value they place on ending their own lives.

SUICIDE IN THE ELDERLY

Perhaps one of the real tragedies of old age is that biases about the aged are often internalized by older persons who may or may not be potentially suicide prone (see Chap. 13). It is as if the aged person says to oneself, "If this is all that my life is worth, then could my death have more meaning?" It is no wonder that elderly suicides have been described by Stenback (1980) as "egoistic" (using Durkheim's terminology). Egoistic

suicides are those involving few commitments to interpersonal or cultural values, often resulting in (or stemming from) social isolation. Hence, for the elderly, the suicide act is highly individualistic. This characteristic quality of aloneness makes it particularly difficult to establish interpersonal resources upon which the older person can rely in dealing with stress and/or loss. The egoistic elderly suicide unfortunately also frequently encourages at best a wait and see attitude and at worst an attitude of we cannot do anything about the problem (willful ignorance) on the part of professionals and family. This, in turn, reinforces the older person's sense of isolation and hopelessness.

This situation results in an underestimation and ignorance of both the scope and seriousness of suicidal threats by older persons, leading to efforts to save the lives of only those who are perceived to have something worth saving.

One cannot help but be impressed with the diversity found among elderly persons (Botwinick, 1978; Maddox & Douglas, 1974). With regard to the treatment and prevention of elderly suicides, it seems best to acknowledge, not downplay, such individual differences. It is the recognition of this diversity that increases the effectiveness of what Shneidman (1980) has referred to as prevention, intervention, and postvention of suicide. In this light, although a number of factors do seem to correlate with the incidence of suicide among elderly persons, they are not necessarily causal, and their variety and potential for interaction would seem to argue against the construction of suicide-proneness scales for use with elderly clients (Miller, 1979a). Moreover, because the bulk of elderly suicides *are* seriously planned and carried out, each person must be dealt with on a case-by-case basis. Simply put, although generalizations about suicide-prone elderly remain attractive, it is the recognition of each aged person as a unique individual that facilitates the prevention of suicide. A belief in the appropriateness of death for the elderly, a valuing of youth and power, and excessive generalizations and myths about older persons are forces that reinforce suicide as the "final alternative" (Miller, 1979a).

Miller (1979a) has estimated that, while persons 60 years and older represent 18.5% of the United States population, they commit 23% of all suicides. Similar estimates have been made by the National Institute of Mental Health (1980) and by Pfeiffer (1977). These estimates all support the fact that older persons are taking their own lives at rates markedly above those of the general population. On the basis of this statistical evidence, there seems ample reason for professional helpers, service providers, and families to regard suicide among the elderly seriously.

Although data on attempted suicides are notoriously unreliable, the ratio of committed to attempted suicides seems to increase inversely with chronological age (Stenback, 1980). Perhaps the most intensive study of the older white male (who is at risk, relative to other elderly) (Manton, Blazer, & Woodbury, 1987) was undertaken by Miller (1978, 1979a, 1979b).

Miller (1978) conducted a systematic examination of 301 white elderly male suicides in Arizona during 1970–1975, supplemented by interviews with the widows of 30 of these men. His analyses suggested elderly in the following group do differ from those who died of natural causes during the same period. The "typical" older white male who takes his life:

1. Seldom attended religious services
2. Was not visited (or did not visit) friends or relatives at least once a week
3. Left a suicide note for someone
4. Left a will
5. Was experiencing chronic sleeping problems the year before his death
6. Was addicted to, or had a strong reliance on, drugs
7. Had a relative with an emotional or mental illness
8. Killed himself in the bedroom of his house

Other factors, although not statistically significant, nevertheless had clinical value and oc-

curred more often in the suicide group than in the control group:

1. Having had a domineering parent
2. Being described as a loner who had few close friends
3. Being bereaved by the death of a friend or relative (who served as a confidant) during the previous 2 years of his life
4. Owning a firearm (pistol) that was used to kill himself, purchased within 1 month prior to his death
5. Not being an active member of a civic, fraternal, or religious organization
6. Having been seen by a physician 1 month prior to his death
7. Suffering a serious, painful physical illness during the last year of life
8. Seeing himself as inadequate or useless
9. Being unhappy or depressed
10. Giving at least verbal/behavioral cues as to his impending suicide

Although this "profile" is purely descriptive, as Miller notes, it seems to present viable diagnostic possibilities for those working with elderly persons.

Dynamics of Elderly Suicide

Although much effort seems to have gone into the development of theory and into the compilation of suicide statistics, comparatively little research or intensive study has been conducted on elderly suicides. In most cases, discussions of the factors associated with suicide are reduced to speculation as to whether they are fundamental, contributing, or precipitative in nature. Such conclusions are based on interviews with survivors and/or frequently rest on research that lacks controls against which solid comparisons can be made (Miller, 1979a). Kastenbaum and Costa (1977) moreover point out that the withholding of treatment necessary to the construction of such controls would be considered unethical by most; client confidentiality (anonymity) makes evaluation difficult. In addition, those who attempt suicide (particularly if they are older) face professional bias in the kind of interventive/preventive care they receive. It is important to note that the motivations of those who only attempt suicide in fact differ from those who are successful. This distinction, however, does not seem to be as central to suicide among the elderly as it is to cases involving those who are younger.

Stenback (1980) suggested five major factors that seem to be related to elderly suicides: (1) general and age-specific losses and failures causing depression, hopelessness, and despair; (2) an "egoistic" personality—excessively individualistic, cold, and emotionally shallow; (3) a society unable to create social integration by means of family bonds, community interest groups, and supportive social services; (4) a personality trait of resolving problems by action and not by passive adaptation; and (5) a suicide-promoting environment that is personal or cultural in nature.

In his intensive study of white male suicides in Arizona, Miller (1979a) summarizes eight patterns of geriatric suicide: reactions associated with (1) severe physical illness, (2) mental illness, (3) the threat of extreme dependency and/or institutionalization, (4) the death of one's spouse, (5) retirement, (6) pathological personal relationships, (7) alcoholism and drug abuse, and (8) multiple factors. Similar conditions were found to be linked to elderly suicide by Shichor and Bergman (1979).

Although Miller notes that these factors rarely act independently of one another and that considerable variation can be found within patterns, suicides among the elderly are nevertheless associated with the *salient* motivational factors noted above. Miller (1979a, p. 7) states, "The crucial factor seems to be how well developed and efficacious are the person's coping abilities."

Regardless of whether suicide is conceptualized in terms of a loss of ego integrity (Erikson), biologically-based death wish (Freud), self-directed aggression (Menninger), lack of social integration (Durkheim), or loss of hope

(Farber), the fact remains that the factors must be interpreted by the elderly person in such a way as to suggest that taking one's own life is the only solution. Thus some elderly who have lived rather precarious lives become overwhelmed by loss; others, with a history of positive coping skills in dealing with change, seem to be resilient. This diversity in the emotional resources of elderly persons, with varying coping styles related to varying degrees of life satisfaction, is well documented in the gerontology literature (Filsinger & Sauer, 1978; Neugarten, 1977; Thomae, 1980). Thus, rather than focus on loss or change per se as a contributing/precipitating factor in elderly suicides, it seems more fruitful to examine the perceived degree of stress or loss by the individual, which is determined in part by the nature of the factor itself, its timing, the person's coping skills, and whether factors are experienced concurrently. Depending upon one's biases about human behavior in general, and upon one's perspective on aging in particular, suicide may be alternatively viewed as having an intentional component or, as Stenback (1980) advocates, as an act that does *not* involve free moral choice but instead is a behaviorial disorder with definite psychological, biological, and social determinants. Kastenbaum and Costa (1977), consistent with this view, treat suicide as an outgrowth of life-style. Peterson (1980), however, suggests that suicide has definite intentional elements, and that elderly persons are, to a large extent, conscious actors in their own demise. The premise adhered to will determine the focus of effort directed at suicide prevention/intervention: should one change the person or change the matrix of cultural factors that impel one to take one's own life?

Peterson (1980) has provided a theoretical framework that permits us to resolve this question. Included in this framework are the following considerations:

1. A social component, which includes forces over which the individual has no control, unrelated to personality dynamics
2. The interaction between the individual's cop-

ing strength and his or her subjective evaluation of low social cohesion (losses in social support associated with role loss (retirement, loss of spouse, physical mobility, sexuality)—in fact, individuals with high degrees of coping strength are frequently best able to deal with such loss in spite of little social support

3. Ideas associated with intrapersonal (Freud) and social organizational dynamics (Durkheim)

Thus, the taking of one's life (proneness to suicide) is a joint function of loss, social support, and coping strength. Peterson's analysis yields the following equation: Suicide proneness = social support (cohesion) × coping strength in dealing with loss. The greater the product of these factors, the lesser the mental health of elderly individuals in relation to death.

Miller (1979a) echoes a similar sentiment in his discussion of the balance between the "quality" and "quantity" of life. Each elderly person forms a personal equation whereby a "line of unbearability" is crossed and the aged person decides that the quality of his or her life is more important than its quantity. Thus, individual evaluations of what it takes to push one beyond this "line of bearability" are likely to differ. For some, this invisible line is derived from the mere prospect of growing old and dying in an institution; for others it may be living in pain, loss of a confidant, loss of a meaningful occupational "network," or simply feeling unloved, useless, unwanted, or alone.

Thus, lists of factors, more accurately interpreted as "correlates" of suicide, must be seen in this light; their significance and subjective impact will vary for different individuals in varying situations.

Such factors might include a history of mental illness, being socially isolated/lonely, being single, widowed, or divorced, and having retired. It must be noted that these factors are only correlated with the incidence of suicide among the aged; they are not necessarily causal. For example, the importance of living alone is paramount

among the widowed, particularly for elderly widowers. Widowed elderly are not only more prone to suicide within the first year of bereavement but, as Stenback (1980) notes, those who attempt suicide are more likely to have suffered the loss of a close relative in the past than otherwise; Miller's (1978, 1979a, 1979b) findings tend to support this point. Again, not widowhood per se, but the inability to replace confidant relationships is what makes the loss of a spouse pivotal with respect to elderly suicide (Schulz, 1978).

Retirement is typically considered to be a crisis for most elderly men. In spite of popular opinion, there is little direct evidence to support the notion that "retirement shock" is linked to suicide. Many elderly, in good health, with adequate retirement income, may in fact see retirement positively. For many elderly men, the psychological benefits of being freed from the responsibilities of work are positive aspects of retirement. For others who are unoccupied or are prevented from reorganizing their lives (e.g., developing a new circle of friends, avoiding role conflict with spouse, learning to live on a fixed income, developing new interests, avoiding age-discriminatory hiring practices or poor health and other changes associated with retirement), retirement can lead to lessened self-esteem, depression, and social isolation. In a comprehensive review of the literature, Rowland (1977) concluded that widowhood and death of a significant other, but *not* retirement, predicted death for elderly persons. In most cases, health status is confounded with retirement status, personality variables (i.e., financial, interpersonal), the ability to cope with and/or compensate for such losses, and health status. Consequently, it is inappropriate to state that for all elderly events such as retirement necessarily precipitate a suicidal crisis. Miller (1979a) suggests a link between retirement and suicide, but indicates that further research is necessary.

Death within institutions (nursing homes, mental hospitals, geriatric wards) is commonplace for many elderly, who perhaps resent being thus confined in the first place. Even when their families have consulted them and they concur in the placement, most elderly are, at best, reluctant to enter a nursing home. They are places from which people do not return; they are perceived (accurately or not) by many aged as depersonalizing, dehumanizing, lonely places (Kahana, 1973). The gerontological literature generally supports (Rowland, 1977; Schulz & Brenner, 1977) relocation as a precursor of death among the elderly. Poorly trained staff, limited resources, withdrawal of the family from the elderly person who dies a prolonged death (Kastenbaum, 1978), the indignity of not being able to care for oneself, and isolation from other comparatively well elderly within the nursing home are conditions defining a characteristic way of life seen as less bearable than a death that is self-chosen for many elderly. Miller (1979a) states that the mere prospect of being institutionalized was enough to precipitate suicide for some elderly men. When overt, quick means of taking one's life are not available, many elderly resort to other methods: self-starvation, refusal to follow physicians' orders, refusal to take medications, delaying treatment, voluntary seclusion, engaging in dangerous activities, excessive drinking, drug abuse, smoking, or dietary mismanagement. These persons are often regarded by staff and other residents as "problems," most probably increasing their sense of abandonment and isolation. They may be drugged, thus contributing to their depression.

Nelson and Farberow (1980) have explored the significance of indirect self-destructive behavior (ISDB) in elderly nursing home residents. ISDB differs from suicide in that its consequences are not immediately fatal, but it is thought to ultimately lead to an individual's premature death. It may be manifested in such diverse behavior as alcoholism, drug abuse, hyperobesity, self-starvation, passive–aggressive behavior, withdrawal, abuse of one's health, or excessive/compulsive risk taking. Although these behaviors may have a self-destructive component, they may also serve to alleviate feelings of powerlessness or low self-esteem. In an all-male sample of elderly, Nelson and Farberow

(1980) found relationships between ISDB and the following factors: experience of significant loss, confusion, dissatisfaction with the treatment program and with life in general, infrequent contact with family or friends, absence of religious commitment, and the limited possibility for release from the institution. Thus, ISDB tends to be associated with limited activity, chronic physical illness, and a loss of control/direction over one's life; it results in a great deal of depression, anger, and frustration. Farberow and Devries (1967) noted correlations between measures of ISDB and the MMPIS (Minnesota Multiphasic Personality Inventory Suicide Risk) scale and concluded that, in the face of cultural taboos on suicide, ISDB serves as a substitute for overt suicidal behavior. In spite of its psychological benefits in providing the individual with some means by which to cope with the environment, ISDB nevertheless tends to be associated with negative effects and isolation. As these authors note, further research is needed to clarify the distinction between the self-destructive and adaptive components of ISDB.

In a review of the limited literature on elderly suicide, Miller (1978, p. 294) concluded that ". . . research on geriatric suicide has tended to be fragmented, uncoordinated, noncomparable, and for the most part, lacking in control groups." More attention needs to be given to education about suicide per se directed toward elderly persons, their families, physicians, and the general public. In addition, a fruitful area to explore more fully might be the roles that family dynamics and elderly persons' feelings/cognitions about death play in understanding aged suicides. Balanced against these goals, of course, must be the ethical and practical questions involving confidentiality and the withholding of alternative forms of treatment. As Kastenbaum and Costa (1977) suggest with regard to suicide in general, it may be premature and/or impossible to develop general theories about suicide in the elderly, given the tremendous interindividual variability among elderly persons and the complexity of elderly suicides (involving loss, coping skills, and a social cohesion factor). Thus, it may be unwise to attempt to develop "suicide-prone" profiles or to attempt to rely too heavily on research findings in favor of clinical experience.

Suicide Prevention/
Intervention with the Elderly

Elderly suicides present a particularly difficult problem for the professional in that they are by and large egoistic/anomic in nature. Elderly persons seeking to take their own lives rarely use methods that are designed to attract attention; when they are unsuccessful it is often by accident. They are, in addition, unlikely to contact suicide prevention centers for help (Farberow & Moriwaki, 1975) and seem to be reluctant to take advantage of most of the social services available to them (Kramer, Taube, & Redick, 1973). Moreover, the negative attitudes of clinicians toward treating elderly persons are well documented (Birren & Renner, 1979; Ford & Sbordone, 1980; Lawton & Gottesman, 1974) and exacerbate the problem.

Given the above considerations, perhaps the most effective means for reducing the number of suicides among the elderly would involve (1) altering cultural attitudes toward aging in general; (2) educating the elderly, family members, health care professionals, and the public about suicide; and (3) bringing to the attention of potential suicides the existence of available psychological/supportive services.

Miller (1979a), in noting that aged males who committed suicide had visited their physicians 1 month prior to their deaths, suggests that the suicidal ideation might have been brought to the forefront if these physicians had been more skilled in asking probing questions. Given our society's prohibition against self-destructive behavior, simply being able to acknowledge suicidal thoughts is of vital importance to elderly persons, whose value systems stress self-reliance and independence. Miller (1979a) found that 60% of his sample had given a verbal or

behavioral clue as to their impending suicide; 37% of their survivors acknowledged such clues. Twenty-three percent did not recognize such clues; many did nothing when they were given advance information. "In one case the deceased told his wife and daughter every night for 2 weeks that he wanted to take his life, yet his family failed to secure the professional attention he so desperately needed. . . . In at least two of the cases . . . wives found suicide notes in advance of the men's deaths—one, one week in advance and the other the day before—but totally discounted the credibility of the notes" (Miller, 1979a, p. 78). It is also possible that the wives in these cases were implicitly cooperating with their husbands.

Admittedly, there are no easy solutions to the problem of suicide in the aged; a number of ethical and social–cultural questions must be squarely faced if older persons are to preserve their dignity and sense of belonging. Perhaps Miller (1979a) has identified the central issue with regard to the older person who takes one's life. In discussing suicide prevention research he states, "Although they (the research team) emphasized outreach services are imperative to reach depressed people who may have become withdrawn and isolated, they felt *the ultimate answer would be for old age itself* to offer the elderly something worthwhile for which to live" (Miller, 1979a, p. 19).

BEREAVEMENT—THE ELDERLY AS SURVIVORS OF LOSS

By the age of 65, half of elderly women have lost their husbands; by the age of 75, two thirds are widows (see Chap. 13). Kastenbaum (1978) feels that the aged are literally overwhelmed by grief; they suffer "bereavement overload" when a second death occurs before the impact of one death has been worked through.

Schulz (1978) concurs that the aged are at risk, both physically and psychologically, as a consequence of widowhood. Rowland (1977) concludes that widows have a greater chance of developing either a physical or psychological illness, or dying, within the first 6 months to 1 year after the deaths of their husbands than do nonwidows. This risk factor was even higher when the spouse's death was sudden. Schulz (1978), however, questions the assumption that such negative effects are a consequence of widow(er)hood per se. It may be that (1) those who are in better health tend to remarry, leaving those who are in poorer health behind; (2) those who are fit, tend to marry those who are also fit; (3) both widows and spouses live in a high-risk environment; (4) the loss of a spouse creates a sense of hopelessness, a surrender accompanied by a profound sense of depression/desolation, leading to lowered resistance to disease and/or stress; or (5) death of one's spouse robs one of the support and/or cues required in order to take one's medicine on time, eat balanced meals, keep doctor's appointments, and so on. Schulz (1978) rejects all of the above as explanations for the increased mortality/illness of widows, with the exception of the common unfavorable environment, hopelessness/depression, and the nongrief behavior change explanation (loss of support/cues). Obviously the termination, through death, of a relationship that has been nurtured by years of sharing, caring, and love is a terribly painful and disruptive event, one that is thought by many (Holmes & Rahe, 1967) to be the single most stressful experience that can befall one. In this light, the broken-heart syndrome probably accounts for a great deal of the illness/death experienced by widows. Contrary to folklore, Carey (1979–80) concluded that widowers were significantly better adjusted than were widows during the first year of bereavement. Although being "forewarned" (allowing one to rehearse, or grieve in an anticipatory sense) was important for widows, it was not for widowers. Younger widowed elderly (less than 57 years of age) were better adjusted than were those who were widowed at an older age. Widows who were more highly educated, had higher incomes, and lived alone (with no children to

care for/live with) made better adjustments. Such factors were not as important for widowers, however. Interestingly, those with uniformly happy marriages *and* those with constant, pervasive marital problems appeared to be better adjusted than widows. For both men and women, not facing the death and/or deterioration prior to death, and uncertainty about what life would be like after the death of their spouse (who would care for them, manage their personal lives and/or financial affairs, concerns over personal safety, worries over dependent children) were the major problems seen to be overcome. Physicians, nurses, chaplains, and, especially, neighbors, funeral directors, and family (Richter, 1987) were named by the widowed as sources of support, comfort, and help both before and after their spouses' deaths.

Sanders (1979–1980) notes that working through one's grief was especially difficult (reflected in denial, physical symptoms) when the death of a grown child was experienced. Grief reactions were often very intense and prolonged. This did not seem to vary with age, sex, or socioeconomic status. Older persons whose adult children die before them may experience a sense of impotence that is difficult to deal with; being a parent involves a sense of omnipotence relative to one's child that is most likely formed very early in life (Stevens-Long, 1979). Whereas Kalish and Reynolds (1976), Schulz (1978), and Jackson (1979) discuss "stages" (initial shock/disbelief, a working through of one's feelings and review of one's relationship with the deceased, and then a restructuring phase, where life moves on) that may last for varying periods of time, research by Barrett and Schneweis (1980–81) does not support the notion that one's reactions to or feelings about the degree of support needed vary with the length of time widowed (3 years or less to 20 years or more). On the other hand, Sanders (1980–1981) found, in a sample of younger (63 years or less) versus older (65 years or more) widows/widowers, that the young initially experienced intense grief reactions (denial, anger, guilt, feelings of loneliness, physical/sleep disturbances, loss of energy, rumination/preoccupation with the death) followed by a lessening approximately 18 months late, whereas the reverse was true for older widows/widowers. Thus, although being able to experience anticipatory grief and preparing oneself for the death may have beneficial effects upon later adjustment for a limited amount of time, the long-term effects of the loss of one's spouse are clearly important; loneliness is the chief problem. Moss and Moss (1980) have even discovered the tremendous impact that building one's identity around and investing oneself emotionally in a marital relationship has in the remarriage of those elderly who are widowed. Remarriage in old age usually occurs anywhere from 18 months to 4 years after the death of one's spouse, and many older women persist in relating to their new husbands in terms, both physically and psychosocially, reminiscent of their former relationships with the deceased husband. Thus, a triad of sorts is formed, and the new husband often serves as a "first husband surrogate." In many cases, this preoccupation with sanctification of the deceased spouse can interfere with the new relationship. In order for the second relationship to develop, ties with the first spouse must be acknowledged, understood, and respected by both parties, not ignored or denied.

Grief is a very complex and yet private experience; in many cases it may take years to be fully resolved; in some cases it is never resolved. To the extent that a widow/widower built a life on a primary relationship with the deceased spouse, caution must be exercised before judging extended grief reactions in the aged as "abnormal," especially when the surviving elder has no other source of emotional support, is in fact physically isolated from others, or has little access to eligible would-be partners. Grief is often composed of a multitude of responses at varying levels (affective, behavioral, physical) and seemingly contradictory emotions (e.g., an intense desire to maintain the image/memory of the dead spouse versus guilt/anger). It seems

wise to deal with grieving elders as individuals who are likely to be vulnerable, both psychosocially and physically.

OLDER PERSONS WHO ARE DYING

If we assume that older persons who are, in fact, terminally ill are "ready to die" or assume that their deaths are less socially important or tragic, we may deny them the opportunity to deal with what Kubler-Ross (1969) terms "unfinished business," as well as ourselves miss out on a rewarding experience by not getting to know someone who may have something very precious to teach us about *life*. Kastenbaum (1978) notes that it is, in fact, very difficult at times to determine if an older person is terminally ill. Sudden changes in personality *may* reflect an attempt to cope with feelings of imminent death that one cannot verbalize. Acknowledging any and all needs, both emotional and material, is the key to helping those elders who are dying face their imminent demise with a sense of "I am ready to go." Since the publication in 1969 of *On Death and Dying* by Elisabeth Kubler-Ross, a great deal of interest and enthusiasm has been generated in understanding/helping persons who are terminally ill. Unfortunately, Kubler-Ross's "stages," through which persons progress in reacting to their impending deaths, have been overinterpreted. The stages are composed of (1) denial (no, not me), (2) anger (directed at doctors, nurses, or those who will go on living), (3) bargaining (with others [God]) in order to prolong one's life, (4) depression (a reaction to one's worsening symptoms/deterioration and the knowledge that death will follow), and (5) acceptance (a sense of readiness about death, but without a loss of hope that life could be prolonged if a cure were found). Thus, staff/family may feel compelled to "push" the dying person to reach the final stage. Stopping at an earlier stage (denial, anger) is seen by the staff/family as a "failure" on their part. Similarly, Kubler-Ross's stages have been interpreted rigidly to the extent that *every* person *should* experience these stages in a given order. In contrast to this, a dying person–helper interaction model has been proposed as an alternative by Rodabough (1980). Moreover, Peterson (1980), Schulz (1978), and Kastenbaum (1978) all note that prolonged reactions such as denial or anger can have positive emotional consequences for many terminally ill, and that there is a great deal of movement back and forth between stages (including the simultaneous experience of two stages). Dismissing a person's behavior as ''simply anger'' may overlook important external reasons (e.g., poor quality of care) for that anger. Peterson (1980) notes that there may be degrees of denial and that a client's denial may simply reflect the aura of ''mutual pretense'' regarding discussing death that the patient and the medical staff/family have implicitly agreed upon during the course of care. Obviously, although it may save the staff and the person's family a great deal of trouble in discussing death and reinforce their own need to deny both their own and the older person's death, it robs the elderly person of the opportunity to draw the family closer, as well as finish unfinished business (make up for past sins and hurts, want to say the unsaid). Kubler-Ross (1974) herself states that these ''stages'' are not to be rigidly applied and reinforces the variability in their presence/absence and degree of intensity across persons. Likewise, apparently ''seeing'' acceptance increases the likelihood of interpreting this as an indication of older persons ''disengaging'' during their last days, in preparation for death. As Peterson (1980) notes, funerals often reinforce this denial of the person and/or apparent acceptance, by the use of comforting terms (passed on, slumber room), elaborate preparatory efforts to make the deceased look ''alive,'' or the use of eulogies and/or ceremonies that do not reflect the true nature of the deceased person. Likewise, anger, rather than being seen as a prelude to something more adaptive, is often a perfectly legitimate response to death and loss; if suppressed or internalized, it often becomes depression. Simply put, there is

some truth in the notion that we die as we have lived—angry, denying, depressed, constantly asking for another chance, or accepting of things that cannot be changed. The real message Kubler-Ross's work should give (regardless of its methodological deficiencies, see Kastenbaum [1978], Schulz [1978], and Peterson [1980] for discussions) is to deal with each dying person where one happens to be (emotionally speaking) at the moment. From a personal wish to deny, or from anger, often one would like to make death more predictable, to control it, when it is beyond control. To fail to recognize that every older person's feelings about impending death are unique is to deny that person the dignity of making decisions about his or her own life (as well as death), decisions that he or she may desperately want and need to make in order to die ''an appropriate death'' (in a desired manner). In so doing, one loses a bit of oneself in the effort to make these choices for others. Similarly, relating to those elderly who are bereaved and grieving demands the recognition that grief is very personal, that widows and widowers may grieve in various ways (see Lopata [1973] and Peterson & Briley [1977]) consistent with their feelings about the death (preventable or not, acute or anticipated), their relationship to the deceased spouse, available resources, sex, ethnic background, socioeconomic status, coping strength and weaknesses, and family dynamics.

Helping the Elderly Deal with Death

Perhaps one of the major themes implicit in our discussion of helping, and reflected in material pertaining to older persons and death, is a recognition of individual differences in views about death and dying and adjusting to loss. Imposing a number of ''shoulds'' on older persons can do nothing but suppress desires to share concerns regarding fears about death, the writing of a will, funeral planning, the wish to die at home, euthanasia, bodily disposal, the fate of survivors, and so on and communicate to the older person that the helper is not willing and/or able to accept the elder on his or her own terms as an *individual*. On the other hand, support can be offered simply by listening, remaining nonjudgmental, and indicating either verbally or nonverbally that it is permissible to talk about anything, or not talk at all. Available family/community resources (e.g., Compassionate Friends, Widow-to-Widow programs) can make the task easier. Although it has been argued that these programs may have the impact of stigmatizing the elder, they appear to be a valuable source of comfort and support at a time when such support is likely to be scarce. Such help, obviously, need not be professional; in fact, informal support may be more acceptable to aged persons who value family/neighborhood ties. Given the possibility of a younger counselor being more threatened by death-related issues when dealing with elderly clients who are dying and/or bereaved (Gilbert, 1977; Blum & Tallmer, 1977), peer help and support may actually be preferable. Although it may run counter to their own values, helpers should remember that death may be preferable to life for some older persons who are in pain, have no one, feel useless or unwanted, or who value their physical and/or mental capabilities. In some cases, these goals may be attained through hospice care, where dying persons are permitted to live out their final days free of pain, surrounded by friends, family, and valued possessions (if this is so desired), in full control of their own lives until death, knowledgeable of the impending demise. It should be made clear that, despite the popularity of hospice care as opposed to institutional (hospital, nursing home) care, a hospice is not for all persons. Some elderly persons need the security of the presence of medical staff, life-extending equipment, etc. Hospice care places tremendous psycho-emotional, financial, and interpersonal care-giving burdens on the family. As Hine (1979–1980) has discussed, these are responsibilities that all families do not wish to or cannot bear. Likewise, bearing the burden of emotional caring for an elderly person who is dying or bereaved is an immense responsibility, with the likelihood of the helper

becoming a key figure in the elderly person's life. Empathy, recognition of individuality, a commitment to life until death, whatever its quality, nonjudgmental support, and openness (to one's own feelings as well as those of the older) are the qualities needed by the helper to allow older persons to live until they die (Kubler-Ross, 1978). Although this chapter has dealt with death, its real value lies in the appreciation of the interconnectedness of life and death. As Wass and Corr (1981, p. 2) have noted, "We cannot grasp or evaluate the proportions and the significance of life if we do not bring death into the picture. Just as death must be construed through life, so also life must eventually be seen in the context of death. Certainly death is not the only perspective from which to understand life, but . . . it is indispensable as a constitutive element of human existence." Understanding and relating to older persons and death in this fashion will enrich both the helper's life and theirs.

SUMMARY

Myths about aging, as well as predominantly negative attitudes about older persons, have led to a devaluation of older persons' lives, with a consequent neglect of the importance of life versus death as a salient influence on their behavior.

Ideas about older persons' views about death are rooted in theories about aging, notably Erikson's psychosocial theory of ego development, Cumming and Henry's disengagement theory, and Butler's concept of the life review. Each tends to reinforce the view that the aged are preoccupied with fears of death. Objective data, however, suggest great variability among older persons in fear of death, which may or may not be manifest at a conscious level of awareness.

A recent concern is suicide among the aged, which occurs predominantly among older white males. Although younger suicides are often attention-getting cries for help, older suicides (both within and outside the institution) have an intentional focus to them that makes prevention difficult. Important, however, are the older person's resources and the efficacy of his or her coping skills in understanding why some aged are suicidal and others are not.

Older persons are more likely to be bereaved and are considered at risk for the negative effect of widow(er)hood, particularly when the spouse's death was sudden. However, a number of alternative factors can explain the enhanced death–bereavement association among older widows and widowers. In dealing with an elder who is grieving, compassion and an awareness of the importance of the primary relationship that has been lost through death are paramount. Likewise, dying older persons need to be treated as individuals who may respond to their own mortality in any number of ways.

In helping older persons deal with death, one must avoid value judgments and deal with each elder in a humane nonstigmatizing manner to preserve dignity, but yet facilitate an open expression of attitudes and feelings about death per se as well as issues surrounding the preparation for one's own death.

REFERENCES

Adams, E. B. (1979). *Reminiscence and life review in the aged: A guide for the elderly, their family, friends, and service providers.* Denton, TX: Center for Studies in Aging.

Barrett, C., & Schneweis, K. (1980–1981). An empirical search for stages of widowhood. *Omega, 11,* 97–104.

Bascue, L. O., & Lawrence, R. (1977). A study of subjective time and death anxiety in the elderly. *Omega, 8,* 81–89.

Bell, B., & Batterson, C. (1979). The death attitudes of older adults: A path analytical exploration. *Omega, 10,* 59–76.

Bengston, V., Cuellar, J., & Ragan, P. (1977). Stratum contrasts and similarities in attitudes toward death. *Journal of Gerontology, 32,* 76–88.

Birren, J., & Renner, V. J. (1977). Research on the psychology of aging: Principles and experimentation. In J. Birren & K. W. Schaie (Eds.), *Handbook of the psychology of aging.* New York: Van Nostrand Reinhold.

Birren, J., & Renner, V. J. (1979). A brief history of mental health and aging. *Issues in mental health and aging: Volume I: Research.* Rockville, MD: National Institute of Mental Health.

Blauner, R. (1966). Death and social structure. *Psychiatry, 28,* 378–394.

Blum, J., & Tallmer, M. (1977). The therapist vis-a-vis the older patient. *Psychotherapy: Theory, Research and Practice, 14,* 361–367.

Botwinick, J. (1978). *Aging and behavior.* New York: Springer.

Butler, R. (1963). The life review: An interpretation of reminiscence in the aged. *Psychiatry, 26,* 65–76.

Butler, R., & Lewis, M. (1981). *Aging and mental health: Positive psychosocial and biomedical approaches* (3rd ed.). St. Louis: Mosby.

Carey, R. (1979–1980). Weathering widowhood: Problems and adjustments of the widowed during the first year. *Omega, 10,* 163–175.

Chappell, N. (1975). Awareness of death in the disengagement theory: A conceptualization and an empirical investigation. *Omega, 6,* 325–343.

Christ, A. (1961). Attitudes toward death among a group of acute geriatric psychiatric patients. *Journal of Gerontology, 16,* 56–59.

Clayton, V. (1975). Erikson's theory of human development as it applies to the aged: Wisdom as contraindicative cognition. *Human Development, 18,* 119–128.

Cumming, E., & Henry, W. (1961). *Growing old.* New York: Basic Books.

Erikson, E. (1963). *Childhood and society* (2nd ed.). New York: Norton.

Farberow, N. L., & Devries, A. G. (1967). An item differentiation analysis of MMPIs of suicidal neuropsychiatric hospital patients. *Psychological Reports, 20,* 607–617.

Farberow, N., & Moriwaki, S. (1975). Self destructive crises in the older person. *Gerontologist, 15,* 333–337.

Fiefel, H., & Branscomb, A. (1973). Who's afraid of death? *Journal of Abnormal Psychology, 81,* 282–288.

Filsinger, E., & Sauer, W. (1978). An empirical typology of adjustment to aging. *Journal of Gerontology, 33,* 333–337.

Ford, C., & Sbordone, R. (1980). Attitudes of psychiatrists toward elderly patients. *American Journal of Psychiatry, 137,* 571–575.

Gilbert, J. (1977). Psychotherapy with the aged. *Psychotherapy: Theory, Research, and Practice, 14,* 394–402.

Glaser, B. G., & Strauss, A. I. (1965). *A time for dying.* Chicago: Aldine Press.

Hayslip, B., Pinder, M., & Lumsden, B. (1981). The measurement of death anxiety in adulthood: Implications for counseling. In R. Pacholski & C. Corr (Eds.), *Proceedings of the forum for death education and counseling.* Arlington, VA: Forum for Death Education and Counseling.

Hine, M. (1979–1980). Dying at home: Can families cope? *Omega, 10,* 175–187.

Holmes, T., & Rahe, R. (1967). The social readjustment scale. *The Journal of Psychosomatic Research, 11,* 213–218.

Jackson, E. (1979). Bereavement and grief. In H. Wass (Ed.), *Dying: Facing the facts.* Washington, DC: Hemisphere.

Jeffers, F., Nichols, C., & Eisdorfer, C. (1961). Attitudes of older persons toward death: A preliminary study. *Journal of Gerontology, 16,* 53–56.

Kahana, E. (1973). The humane treatment of old people in institutions. *Gerontologist, 13,* 31–35.

Kalish, R. (1985). The social context of death and dying. In R. Binstock & E. Shanas (Eds.), *Handbook of aging and the social sciences.* New York: Van Nostrand Reinhold.

Kalish, R., & Reynolds, D. (1976). *Death and ethnicity: A psychocultural study.* Los Angeles: University of Southern California Press.

Kastenbaum, R. (1978). Death and bereavement in old age: New developments and their possible implications for psychosocial care. *Aged Care and Services Review, 1,* 1–10.

Kastenbaum, R. (1985). Death and dying: A life span approach. In J. E. Birren & K. W. Schaie (Eds.), *Handbook of the psychology of aging.* New York: Van Nostrand Reinhold.

Kastenbaum, R., & Aisenberg, R. (1976). *The psychology of death.* New York: Springer.

Kastenbaum, R., & Candy, S. (1973). The 4 percent fallacy: A methodological and empirical critique of the use of population statistics in gerontology. *International Journal of Aging and Human Development, 4,* 15–22.

Kastenbaum, R., & Costa, P. (1977). Psychological perspectives on death. *Annual Review of Psychology, 28,* 225–249.

Keith, P. (1979). Life changes and perceptions of life and death among older men and women. *Journal of Gerontology, 34,* 870–878.

Kramer, M., Taube, R., & Redick, R. (1973). Patterns of use of psychiatric facilities by the aged: Past, present and future. In C. Eisdorfer & M. P. Lawton (Eds.), *The psychology of adult development and aging.* Washington, DC: American Psychological Association.

Kubler-Ross, E. (1969). *On death and dying.* New York: Macmillan.

Kubler-Ross, E. (1974). *Questions and answers on death and dying.* New York: Macmillan.

Kubler-Ross, E. (1978). *To live until we say goodbye.* Englewood Cliffs, N.J.: Prentice-Hall.

Lawton, M. P., & Gottesman, L. (1974). Psychological services to the elderly. *American Psychologist, 29,* 689–693.

Lopata, H. (1973). *Widowhood in an American city.* New York: Oxford.

Maddox, G., & Douglass, E. (1974). Aging and individual differences: A longitudinal analysis of social, psychological, and physiological indicators. *Journal of Gerontology, 29,* 555–563.

Manton, K. G., Blazer, D. G., & Woodbury, M. A. (1987). Suicide in middle age and later life: Sex and race specific life table and cohort analysis. *Journal of Gerontology, 42*(2), 219–227.

Marshall, V. (1975). Aging and awareness of finitude in developmental gerontology. *Omega, 6,* 113–127.

Marshall, V. (1979). Socialization for impending death in a retirement village. *American Journal of Science, 80,* 1124–1144.

Mathieu, J., & Peterson, J. (1970). Some social–psychological dimensions of aging. Paper presented at the Annual Convention of the Gerontological Society, Ontario, Canada.

Miller, M. (1978). Geriatric suicide: The Arizona study. *The Gerontologist, 18,* 488–495.

Miller, M. (1979a). *Suicide after sixty: The final alternative.* New York: Springer.

Miller, M. (1979b). A review of the research on geriatric suicide. *Death Education, 3,* 283–296.

Moss, M., & Moss, D. (1980). The image of the deceased spouse in remarriage of elderly widow(er)s. *Journal of Gerontological Social Work, 3,* 59–69.

Mullins, L., & Lopez, M. (1982). Death anxiety among nursing home residents: A comparison of the young-old and old-old. *Death Education, 6,* 75–86.

National Institute of Mental Health. (1980). NIMH seeks proposals on suicide and depression among the elderly. *Aging Research and Training News,* pp. 5–6.

Nelson, R., & Farberow, N. (1980). Indirect self-destructive behavior in the nursing home patient. *Journal of Gerontology, 35,* 949–957.

Neugarten, B. (1977). Personality and aging. In J. Birren & K. W. Schaie (Eds.), *Handbook of the psychology of aging.* New York: Van Nostrand Reinhold.

Peterson, J. A. (1980). Social–psychological aspects of death and dying and mental health. In J. E. Birren & R. B. Sloane (Eds.), *Handbook of aging and mental health.* Englewood Cliffs, NJ: Prentice-Hall.

Peterson, J., & Briley, M. (1977). *Widows and widowhood: A creative approach to being alone.* New York: Association Press.

Pfeiffer, E. (1977). Psychopathology and social pathology. In J. Birren & K. W. Schaie (Eds.), *Handbook of the psychology of aging.* New York: Van Nostrand Reinhold.

Pinder, M., & Hayslip, B. (1981). Cognitive, attitudinal, and affective aspects of death and dying in adulthood: Implications for care providers. *Educational Gerontology, 6,* 107–124.

Preston, C., & Williams, R. (1971). Views of the aged on the timing of death. *Gerontologist, 11,* 300–304.

Reynolds, D., & Kalish, R. (1974). Anticipation of futurity as a function of ethnicity and age. *Journal of Gerontology, 29,* 224–231.

Rhudick, P., & Dibner, A. (1961). Age, personality, and health correlates of death concerns in normal aged individuals. *Journal of Gerontology, 16,* 44–49.

Richter, J. M. (1987). Support: A resource during crisis of mate loss. *Journal of Gerontological Nursing, 13*(11), 8–22.

Riegel, K., & Riegel, R. (1972). Development, drop and death. *Developmental Psychology, 6,* 306–319.

Roberts, J., Kimsey, L., Logan, D., & Shaw, G.

(1970). How aged in nursing homes view dying and death. *Geriatrics, 25,* 115–119.

Rodabough, T. (1980). Alternatives to the stages models of the dying process. *Death Education, 4,* 1–19.

Romaniuk, M. (1981). Reminiscence and the second half of life. *Experimental Aging Research, 7,* 315–336.

Romaniuk, M., & Romaniuk, J. (1981). Looking back: An analysis of reminiscence functions and triggers. *Experimental Aging Research, 7,* 477–490.

Rosenmayr, L. (1985). Changing values and positions of aging in Western culture. In J. E. Birren & K. W. Schaie (Eds.), *Handbook of the psychology of aging.* New York: Van Nostrand Reinhold.

Rowland, K. (1977). Environmental events predicting death for the elderly. *Psychological Bulletin, 84,* 349–372.

Sanders, K. (1979–1980). A comparison of adult bereavement in the death of a spouse, child, and parent. *Omega, 10,* 303–322.

Sanders, C. (1980–1981). A comparison of older and younger spouses in bereavement outcome. *Omega, 11,* 217–232.

Schulz, R. (1978). *The psychology of death, dying and bereavement.* Reading, MA: Addison-Wesley.

Schulz, R., & Brenner, G. (1977). Relocation of the aged: A review and theoretical analysis. *Journal of Gerontology, 32,* 323–333.

Shichor, D., & Bergman, S. (1979). Elderly suicides in Israel. *Gerontologist, 19,* 169–174.

Shneidman, E. (1980). *Death: Current perspectives* (2nd ed). Palo Alto, CA: Mayfield.

Simpson, M. (1979). Social and psychological aspects of dying. In H. Wass (Ed.), *Dying: Facing the facts.* Washington, DC: Hemisphere.

Stenback, A. (1980). Depression and suicidal behavior in old age. In J. E. Birren & R. Sloane (Eds.), *Handbook of mental health and aging.* Englewood Cliffs, NJ: Prentice-Hall.

Stevens-Long, J. (1979). *Adult life: Developmental processes.* Palo Alto, CA: Mayfield.

Sundow, D. (1967). *Passing on: The social organization of dying.* Englewood Cliffs, NJ: Prentice-Hall.

Swenson, W. (1961). Attitudes toward death in an aged population. *Journal of Gerontology, 16,* 49–52.

Templer, D., Ruff, C., & Franks, C. (1971). Death anxiety, age, sex, and parental resemblance in diverse populations. *Developmental Psychology, 4,* 108.

Thomae, H. (1980). Personality and adjustment to aging. In J. E. Birren & R. Sloane (Eds.), *Handbook of mental health and aging.* Englewood Cliffs, NJ: Prentice-Hall.

Veatch, R. (1979). Defining death anew. In H. Wass (Ed.), *Dying: Facing the facts.* Washington, DC: Hemisphere.

Wass, H. (1977). Views and opinions of elderly persons concerning death. *Educational Gerontology, 2,* 15–26.

Wass, H. (1979). Death and the elderly. In H. Wass (Ed.), *Dying: Facing the facts.* Washington, DC: Hemisphere.

Wass, H., Christian, M., Myers, J., & Murphy, M. (1978–79). Similarities and dissimilarities in attitudes toward death in a population of older persons. *Omega, 9,* 337–354.

Wass, H., & Corr, C. (1981). *Helping children cope with death: Guidelines and resources.* Washington, DC: Hemisphere.

Wass, H., & Sisler, H. (1978). Death concern and views on various aspects of dying among elderly persons. Paper presented at the International Symposium on Dying, Tel Aviv, Israel.

Watson, W., & Maxwell, R. (1977). *Human aging and dying.* New York: St. Martin's Press.

Appendix

NORMAL NUTRITIONAL NEEDS

Normal nutritional needs of the aged may be determined so that each person may consume the desirable amount of calories.

Basal calories are first determined. This number equals the desirable or ideal body weight (IBW) multiplied by ten. Then calories are added for activity levels. Calories for a sedentary person equal the IBW (stated in pounds) multiplied by three. For a person of moderate activity, the IBW (pounds) is multiplied by five; for someone engaged in strenuous activity, the IBW (pounds) is multiplied by ten. Then 10% of the total is added to it to cover specific dynamic action of food. Calories may be added for indicated weight gain at a rate of 500 calories per day to gain 1 pound per week. Likewise, 500 calories per day may be subtracted to yield a weight loss of 1 pound per week.

The IBW may be quickly estimated in this manner. For females, begin with 100 pounds and add 5 pounds for every inch of height over 5 feet. For males, begin with 110 pounds and add 5 pounds for each inch of height over 5 feet.

NEEDS FOR SPECIFIC NUTRIENTS

Most nutrients are needed in amounts equal to those required in younger years, but the total calories consumed need to be decreased 2–8%

for each decade of life past the age of 20 years. Thus, "empty calorie" foods should be avoided so that each food eaten contributes to a well-balanced diet. Unfortunately, nutritious foods are often not chosen because of mastication and digestive problems.

Protein

Because of lessened ability to digest and absorb protein, an aged person needs to consume as much protein as was consumed in younger years. A combination of animal and plant sources of protein is preferable in order that all of the amino acids are obtained.

Fiber

Increasing the intake of dietary fiber or roughage found in unprocessed grains, fruits, and vegetables helps correct the problem of constipation common among the aged. A supplement of bran is also helpful. Because fiber is filling, it contributes to a sensation of satisfaction and helps reduce total caloric intake. Because laxatives interfere with the normal muscular action of the intestines, they should be avoided. Also, they cause decreased absorption of nutrients due to speeding the passage of food through the intestines. Mineral oil is especially dangerous since it limits the absorption of fat-soluble vitamins.

Sugar

Reduced glucose tolerance necessitates a restriction on the intake of sugar and sweets.
Starchy foods may be substituted because they
are burned more slowly than sugar. Excess sugar
may also contribute to atherosclerosis by raising
the level of fats in the blood.

Fat

The proportion of fat in the diet should be reduced, especially the saturated fats. The American Heart Association has recommended that
only 30–35% of one's total caloric intake be
derived from fats. Fats may lead to indigestion
due to reduced liver and pancreatic function;
therefore, fat intake should be distributed among
all meals.

Vitamins

Vitamin requirements remain the same with
aging, and proper vitamin intake may resolve
many general health problems commonly associated with aging. A balanced diet is preferable
to the administration of vitamin medications. Vitamin deficiencies are common among the aged.
They may be due to an inadequate diet, to incomplete digestion and absorption, or to less desirable methods of preserving foods. Many vitamins are lost by cooking vegetables and fruits
at high temperatures with lots of water. Preser-
vatives may also cause loss of vitamin content.

Minerals

Only a small percentage of dietary calcium is
absorbed so that the aged need a daily intake
of two 8-ounce glasses of milk or milk
substitutes.

Anemia is another frequent problem of the
aged due to insufficient iron intake. Iron is more
efficiently absorbed from meats than from vegetables and eggs, which makes sufficient iron intake even more difficult for the aged, who eat
less meat due to chewing difficulties and cost.

Fluids

An intake of five to eight glasses (8 oz) of water
each day is desirable to aid diminished kidney
function of the aged, to aid digestion, and to
prevent constipation.

RECOMMENDED DAILY INTAKE

The "basic four" is applicable as a daily food
guide for the aged. Two or more servings—each
equal to an 8-ounce cup of milk—of the milk
group should be included. The meat group
should be represented by two or more servings,
each equivalent to 2 ounces of cooked lean meat,
poultry, or fish. Four or more servings of the
vegetable/fruit group and of the bread/cereal
group are necessary. One serving of vegetable or
fruit equals one half cup or one portion, e.g., one
banana or one potato. At least one citrus fruit to
supply vitamin C and one dark green or dark
yellow vegetable/fruit to supply vitamin A
should be included. Other wholesome foods may
be chosen to round out meals and meet energy
requirements. Condiments, margarine, and jam
may be used sparingly.

PHYSICAL INDICATORS OF POOR NUTRITION

Many clinical symptoms may be traced to deficiencies in one or more nutrients. A summary of
these problems may be found in Table A–1.

Deficiencies of vitamins A and C, protein,
calcium, and iron are common among the aged.
Disease processes necessitating diet modification merely further limit already restricted dietary intake of aged persons.

INTERACTIONS

Absorption of all nutrients is affected by interactions with other nutrients and with various medications. For example, folic acid enhances the

TABLE A–1. PHYSICAL SIGNS INDICATIVE OR SUGGESTIVE OF MALNUTRITION

	Normal Appearance	Signs Associated with Malnutrition	Possible Disorder or Nutrient Deficiency	Possible Non-nutritional Problem
Hair	Shiny; firm; not easily plucked	Lack of natural shine; dull and dry Thin and sparse Silky and straight; fine Dyspigmented Flag sign Easily plucked (no pain)	Kwashiorkor and, less commonly, marasmus	Excessive bleaching of hair Alopecia
Face	Skin color uniform; smooth, pink, healthy appearance; not swollen	Nasolabial seborrhea (scaling of skin around nostrils) Swollen face (moon face) Paleness	Riboflavin Iron Kwashiorkor	Acne vulgaris
Eyes	Bright, clear, shiny; no sores at corners of eyelids; membranes a healthy pink and moist; no prominent blood vessels or mound of tissue or sclera	Pale conjunctiva Red membranes Bilot's spots Conjunctival xerosis (dryness) Corneal xerosis (dullness) Keratomalacia (softening of cornea) Redness and fissuring of eyelid corners Corneal arcus (white ring around eye) Xanthelasma (small yellowish lumps around eyes)	Anemia (e.g., iron) Vitamin A Riboflavin, pyridoxine Hyperlipidemia	Bloodshot eyes from exposure to weather, lack of sleep, smoke or alcohol
Lips	Smooth, not chapped or swollen	Angular stomatitis (white or pink lesions at corners of mouth) Angular scars Cheilosis (redness or swelling of lips and mouth)	Riboflavin	Excessive salivation from improper fitting dentures
Tongue	Deep red in appearance; not swollen or smooth	Scarlet and raw tongue Magenta tongue (purplish) Swollen tongue Filiform papillae atrophy or hypertrophy	Nicotinic acid Riboflavin Niacin Folic acid Vitamin B_{12}	Leukoplakia

(continued)

343

TABLE A–1. (*Continued*)

	Normal Appearance	Signs Associated with Malnutrition	Possible Disorder or Nutrient Deficiency	Possible Non-nutritional Problem
Teeth	No cavities; no pain; bright	Mottled enamel Caries (cavities) Missing teeth	Fluorosis Excessive sugar	Malocclusion Periodontal disease Health habits
Gums	Healthy; red; do not bleed; not swollen	Spongy, bleeding Receding gums	Vitamin C	Periodontal disease
Glands	Face not swollen	Thyroid enlargement (front of neck swollen) Parotid enlargement (cheeks become swollen)	Iodine Starvation	Allergic or inflammatory enlargement of thyroid
Skin	No signs of rashes, swellings, dark or light spots	Xerosis (dryness) Follicular hyperkeratosis (sandpaper feel to skin)	Vitamin A	Environmental exposure
		Petechiae (small skin hemorrhages)	Vitamin C	
		Pellagrous dermatosis (red swollen pigmentation of areas exposed to sunlight)	Nicotinic acid	
		Excessive bruising Flaky paint dermatosis Scrotal and vulval dermatosis Xanthomas (fat deposits under the skin around joints)	Vitamin K Kwashiorkor Riboflavin Hyperlipidemia	Physical abuse
Nails	Firm; pink	Koilonychia (spoon-shaped) Brittle; ridged	Iron	
Subcutaneous tissue	Normal amount of fat	Edema Fat below standard Fat above standard	Kwashiorkor Starvation; Obesity	
Muscular and skeletal systems	Good muscle tone; some fat under skin; can walk or run without pain	Muscle wasting	Starvation; Kwashiorkor	
		Frontal and parietal bossing (round swelling of front and side of head) Epiphyseal enlargement (swelling of ends of bones) Knock knees or bow legs	Vitamin D	

Body system	Physical signs	Nutrient deficiency
	Musculoskeletal hemorrhages	Vitamin C
	Calf muscle tenderness	Thiamin
	Thoracic rosary	Vitamin D; vitamin C
	Fractures in elderly	Osteoporosis
Cardiovascular system	Normal heart rate and rhythm; no murmurs or abnormal rhythms; normal blood pressure for age	
	Cardiac enlargement	Thiamin
	Tachycardia	
	Elevated blood pressure	Sodium?
Gastrointestinal system	No palpable organs or masses (in children, however, liver edge may be palpable)	
	Hepato-splenomegaly	Kwashiorkor
Nervous system	Psychological stability; normal reflexes	
	Psychomotor changes	Kwashiorkor
	Mental confusion	Nicotinic acid; thiamin
	Depression	Pyridoxine; vitamin B_{12}
	Sensory loss	
	Motor weakness	
	Loss of position sense	Thiamin
	Loss of vibration	
	Loss of ankle and knee jerks	
	Burning and tingling of hands and feet (paresthesia)	

Adapted with permission from Krause, M. & Mahan, L. (1979). Food, nutrition, and diet therapy. Philadelphia: Saunders.

absorption of iron. Calcium absorption is improved by vitamin D, ascorbic acid, an equal calcium/phosphorus ratio, lactose, and certain amino acids.

Malabsorption of vitamin A may be caused by decreased bile secretions, laxatives, and antibiotics. L-dopa and INH contribute to the malabsorption of vitamin B_6, whereas aspirin causes loss of folic acid and vitamin C. Folic acid is also lost because of anticonvulsants that cause the loss of vitamin D as well. Vitamin K is malabsorbed in the presence of coumarin and cholestyramine.

Absorption of phosphate is inhibited by aluminum hydroxide. Calcium absorption is especially vulnerable because it is lessened by many substances—prednisone, phenobarbital, glutethamide, fat, oxalic acid (found, e.g., in spinach and cranberries), and phytic acid (found, e.g., in whole grain cereals).

INDEX